'This is a timely and important book for anyone working or living with someone with atypical communication. I am delighted that the editors have gathered together chapters from such well-respected experts in this field. The result is a really well-researched, up-to-date, practical guide. This is sure to be an essential "go to" reference.'

Nikki Kiyimba, *PhD, Consultant Clinical Psychologist and Senior Academic, Bethlehem Tertiary Institute, New Zealand*

A Guide to Managing Atypical Communication in Healthcare

This book presents a supportive and practical guide for healthcare professionals and trainees in a way that considers a wide spectrum of atypical communication conditions, their impact on everyday healthcare interactions, and the social and cultural contexts in which interactions with atypical communicators take place.

A growing number of patients have been reporting atypical capacity for communication, creating unique challenges for healthcare professionals and patients in forming meaningful clinical interactions. In this book, leading international scholars from a range of healthcare professions provide insight into optimal management for those with atypical communication conditions. This includes speech, language, and hearing impairments. Chapters provide optimal management strategies, case examples, clinical recommendations, and recommended resources relevant for a range of healthcare professionals. The first collection of its kind, this book supports inter-professional practices and serves as a useful guide for those with an interest in clinical communication, and communication and diversity.

This book will be a valuable resource for health and mental healthcare professionals, as well as undergraduate and postgraduate students in healthcare and allied healthcare courses. It can be included as recommended reading material in clinical communication curricula.

Riya Elizabeth George, BSc (Hons), MSc, PhD, PGCAP, SFHEA, is an associate professor/reader in clinical communication & diversity education at Queen Mary University, London. Riya is a creative and committed medical educationalist, academic, and health psychologist working at Barts and The London School of Medicine and Dentistry, London, and has extensive and varied experience in leading innovations in how healthcare students and professionals can be taught diversity to ensure they deliver high quality care to a range of patients and understand how their own perspectives may influence the care they provide.

Michelle O'Reilly, BSc (Hons), MSc, MA, PhD, PGCAPHE, SFHEA, is an associate professor of communication in mental health at the University of Leicester, Leicester. She is a research consultant and quality improvement advisor for Leicestershire Partnership NHS Trust. Michelle is also a chartered health psychologist with an interest in child and adolescent mental health research.

A Guide to Managing Atypical Communication in Healthcare

Meaningful Conversations in Challenging Consultations

Edited by
Riya Elizabeth George and
Michelle O'Reilly

Routledge
Taylor & Francis Group
LONDON AND NEW YORK

Designed cover image: © Getty Images

First published 2023
by Informa Law from Routledge
4 Park Square, Milton Park, Abingdon, Oxon OX14 4RN

and by Informa Law from Routledge
605 Third Avenue, New York, NY 10158

Informa Law from Routledge is an imprint of the Taylor & Francis Group, an informa business

British Library Cataloguing-in-Publication Data
A catalogue record for this book is available from the British Library

Library of Congress Cataloging-in-Publication Data
Names: George, Riya, editor. | O'Reilly, Michelle, editor.
Title: A guide to managing atypical communication in healthcare : meaningful conversations in challenging consultations / edited by Riya George & Michelle O'Reilly.
Description: Abingdon, Oxon ; New York, NY : Informa Law from Routledge, 2023. | Includes bibliographical references and index. | Identifiers: LCCN 2022041154 (print) | LCCN 2022041155 (ebook) | ISBN 9780367696122 (hardback) | ISBN 9780367696139 (paperback) | ISBN 9781003142522 (ebook)
Subjects: MESH: Communication | Professional-Patient Relations | Communication Disorders—psychology | Communication Barriers | Communication Aids for Disabled | Culturally Competent Care
Classification: LCC R118 (print) | LCC R118 (ebook) | NLM W 62 | DDC 610.1/4—dc23/eng/20230120
LC record available at https://lccn.loc.gov/2022041154
LC ebook record available at https://lccn.loc.gov/2022041155

ISBN: 9780367696122 (hbk)
ISBN: 9780367696139 (pbk)
ISBN: 9781003142522 (ebk)

DOI: 10.4324/9781003142522

Typeset in Times New Roman
by codeMantra

Contents

Figures

Acknowledgements

The editors have many to thank for making this edited collection possible. We take this opportunity to pass on our gratitude to all those who have helped in the development of this book. First, we thank the team at Routledge who have assisted in the planning, development, and publishing of this book. We appreciate their guidance, time, and effort. Second, we are grateful to the authors of the chapters. Without them there would not be a collection and their expertise and time are very much valued. Third, the reviewers of the chapters played an instrumental role in assuring the quality of the book and we thank them for their comments and advice. Finally, as editors we have supportive families and colleagues that have helped this book come to fruition.

Riya also acknowledges the role of her faith:

> *'For I know the plans I have for you,' declares the LORD, 'plans to prosper you and not to harm you, plans to give you hope and a future.'*
>
> (Jeremiah 29:11)

Thank you to God, who has graced my life with unimaginable opportunities.

Editor biographies

Riya Elizabeth George

Riya Elizabeth George is an Associate Professor/Reader in Clinical Communication Skills and Diversity Education at Barts and The London School of Medicine & Dentistry, Queen Mary's University of London (QMUL). Riya has extensive and varied experience in teaching communication skills to healthcare students and in providing strategic direction in the development and implementation of diversity initiatives in a range of health educational settings. Riya has several senior, active roles within health educational bodies such as General Medical Councils, Medical Schools Council, and Health Education England Equality and Diversity Committees. Riya continues to be inspired by diversity and clinical communication issues in healthcare, and this book represents an amalgamation of these two interests in a practical resource.

Michelle O'Reilly

Michelle O'Reilly is an Associate Professor of Communication in Mental Health at the University of Leicester and a Research Consultant and Quality Improvement Advisor for Leicestershire Partnership NHS Trust. Michelle is also a Chartered Psychologist in Health. Michelle has research interests in mental health and social media, self-harm and suicidal behaviour, neurodevelopmental conditions, and child mental health services, such as mental health assessments and family therapy. Michelle recently won the Anselm Strauss Award for Qualitative Family Research for her co-authored contribution on discursive psychology in this area (with Nikki Kiyimba and Jessica Lester). Michelle has expertise in qualitative methodologies and specialises in discursive psychology and conversation analysis. Michelle has written considerably in the field of research methods and has written practical guidance for clinical practitioners.

Contributors

Jonathan Beebee, Registered Nurse in Learning Disabilities with over 20 years of experience. He is the Royal College of Nursing's Professional Lead for Learning Disabilities and Nurse Consultant for PBS4, a social care provider that specialises in supporting people with learning disabilities and complex needs. Jonathan has a Master's in Positive Behaviour Support and supporting people with learning disabilities who have behaviours that are described as challenging is his area of expertise. Prior to his current appointments, Jonathan has worked in a variety of roles across the NHS, social care, the Care Quality Commission, and the Department of Health.

Kaddour Bouazza-Marouf, PhD, Associate Professor/Reader in Mechatronics at Loughborough University. Kaddour Bouazza-Marouf completed his BSc and PhD from Newcastle University, UK. He teaches robotics and control engineering. He is a Chartered Engineer (CEng), Fellow of the Institution of Mechanical Engineers (FIMechE), and Associate Editor of the IFAC *Journal of Mechatronics.* His area of specialisation is in mechatronics in medicine applications, including augmentative and alternative communication research and development.

Anne Carney, MS, CCC-SLP is a Lecturer in the Department of Speech, Language and Hearing Sciences at Boston University's Sargent College. She teaches in the MS-SLP program and supervises graduate students completing their clinical practicums in the Boston University Aphasia Resource Center. Anne's clinical and research interests include group treatment for aphasia, intensive comprehensive aphasia programs, and interprofessional education and practice. She is a certified member of the American Speech-Language-Hearing Association. Since 2020, Anne has served as the Chair of the Aphasia Access Resource Exchange working group.

Alison Drewett, PhD, Senior Lecturer in Speech and Language Therapy at De Montfort University and leads the teaching portfolio on Learning

Disabilities and Mental Health. She is in her fourth year of a part-time PhD studentship funded by ARC-EM (NIHR) based at the University of Leicester and supervised by Dr Michelle O'Reilly and Professor Terry Brugha. Her PhD research uses a video-reflexive ethnographic design to investigate staff and autistic patient interactions in a mental health hospital in order to facilitate quality improvements in care and communication practices. Alison also works as an independent speech and language therapist with adults with mental health conditions and autism. She is an Honorary Fellow at the University of Leicester and has an honorary contract with Leicestershire Partnership (NHS) Trust.

Graham Easton, MBBS, MSc, MEd, FRCGP, Professor of Clinical Communication Skills at Barts and The London School of Medicine & Dentistry, Queen Mary's University of London. Graham is a general practitioner (GP) and medical educationalist. Graham is also an experienced medical journalist. He has presented a wide range of radio programmes including *Case Notes* on BBC Radio 4 and *Health Check* for BBC World Service, and was an editor at the *British Medical Journal* for four years. His passion is communication – whether broadcasting about health for the general public or training doctors and students in the art and science of communicating with patients. As well as co-editing the prize-winning textbook *General Practice at a Glance* and *How to Pass the CSA Exam for Trainee GPs*, he has published a book about general practice for a general audience called *The Appointment* – the story of a fictional morning surgery. As a GP trainee in the 1990s he had several poems published. He trained in medicine at the Royal London Hospital and then on the Oxford Region GP Training scheme.

Louise Edwards, BSc (Hons), speech and language therapist, Leeds Metropolitan University graduate, 1998. She has worked clinically across the healthcare journey, including community, paediatric acute, rehabilitation, medico-legal, and education settings. Louise has extensive knowledge and skills in working with infants, children, and young people with congenital and acquired communication and eating, drinking, and swallowing issues. In 2021, Louise commenced a professional doctorate in health exploring compassionate care with a focus on children and young people with technology needs (tracheostomy, non-invasive ventilation) at the University of Central Lancashire.

Yasmin Elsahar, PhD, researcher in biomedical engineering systems and augmentative and alternative communication (AAC) technologies at the Wolfson School of Mechanical, Electrical and Manufacturing Engineering, Loughborough University, UK. Yasmin completed her PhD in Electronic, Electrical, and Systems Engineering at Loughborough University in July 2021. Her area of specialisation is in smart sensing technologies in healthcare. Yasmin's research interests are centred on the development of intelligent healthcare engineering systems through the utilisation of machine learning and deep learning technologies. She authored several publications on the subjects of smart sensors and AAC.

Sarah Griffiths, PhD, MRCSLT, Senior Research Fellow at the University College. Her background is in speech and language therapy (SLT), specialising in adults with neurogenic communication disorders. She was Senior Lecturer in SLT for 14 years; with areas of expertise including motor speech disorders, psychology, and evidence-based practice. She has employed qualitative methods in applied healthcare research, for example using conversation analysis to examine how adults with atypical communication and their interlocuters collaborate to manage everyday conversations. As a dementia researcher in recent years her work has encompassed complex interventions development, realist methodology, and implementation. Her most recent work, on large-scale dementia research programmes, has focused on developing primary care led post-diagnostic support for people with dementia and their informal carers.

Elizabeth Hoover, PhD, CCC-SLP, BC-ANCDS is a Clinical Professor in Sargent College of Health and Rehabilitation Sciences at Boston University. She is a licensed speech-language pathologist and holds board certification in adult neurogenic communication disorders from the Academy of Neurogenic Communication Disorders and Sciences. Her research and clinical practice are focused on socially oriented intervention approaches for people with aphasia with a specialty in conversational treatment. Liz directs the Sargent College Aphasia Resource Center and is a board member of the Aphasia Access organization. Her current research investigates mechanisms of recovery in conversation group treatment for aphasia.

Sijung Hu, PhD, Associate Professor/Reader in Biomedical Engineering. Sijung is a Leader of Photonics Engineering and Health Technology Research Group, Loughborough University, UK since 2002. After being awarded a PhD at Loughborough University in 2000, Sijung was invited to join Kalibrant Ltd as a Senior Scientist for R&D *in vitro* diagnostics in 1998. Sijung has successfully supervised 29 completed PhDs (2002–21) with very satisfactory outcomes of original research reflecting a broad range of biomedical engineering with over 100 leading journal publications, and over five granted patents. Recently, Sijung with his led team has created an avenue for dynamic airflow pressure detection for augmentative and alternative communication based upon the principles of breath characterisation.

Anne Hurren, PhD, MRCSLT, Senior Lecturer in Speech and Language Sciences at Leeds Beckett University. Prior to this she held a clinical post as Chief Speech and Language Therapist (SLT), specialising in laryngectomy and voice disorders for 25 years with research, undergraduate and post-graduate teaching integrated into her role. Her research publications are within her specialist clinical field and include the development of a validated scale to assess voice quality in individuals who have undergone surgical voice restoration after laryngectomy. A key area of research interest concerns how people perceive their own voice post-surgery and how this may differ from the perspectives of their family, SLTs, ENT surgeons, and members of their community.

Linda Jose, BSc (Hons), MRCSLT, speech and language therapist and Lecturer in Speech & Language Sciences at Newcastle University. Prior to joining the Speech and Language Sciences team in 2013, Linda worked as a generalist and specialist therapist in the NHS. Her area of specialism was in primary and secondary school-age pupils with autism spectrum disorder (ASD). Her work involved working as part of a multidisciplinary team accessing children with possible ASD or complex communication disorders. It also involved collaboration with parents, carers, and other members of the multidisciplinary team in developing appropriate packages of care for individuals with speech, language, and communication needs. This sparked an interest in teaching which motivates her within her current position.

David Kerr, PhD, Senior Lecturer in Mechatronics and Optical Engineering. David joined the Wolfson School of Mechanical, Electronic and Manufacturing Engineering, Loughborough University in 1985, obtaining his PhD in Laser Metrology in 1992. His research areas include computer vision, digital image processing and optical metrology. He has 13 publications in the fields of image processing, machine vision, and augmentative and alternative communication (AAC) in the last five years. David with his colleagues created an AAC prototype system in 2015 to use breathing patterns as 'breath signals' then converted into words.

James Law OBE, Professor of Speech and Language Sciences at the University of Newcastle. James originally qualified in linguistics (1978) and in speech and language therapy (1981), becoming a professor in 1999 at City University, London. He was the Director of the Centre for Integrated Healthcare Research, Queen Margaret University, Edinburgh between 2004 and 2009. Since 2010, he has been a Professor of Speech and Language Sciences at Newcastle University and a member of the Royal College of Speech and Language Therapists since 1989 and received the fellowship of the College in 2000. In 2018 he was made an Officer of the Order of the British Empire for his dedicated services to speech and language therapy. He also received a lifetime contribution award from the International Association of Logopedics and Phoniatrics.

Penny Levickis, PhD, Senior Research Fellow at the Research in Effective Education in Early Childhood (REEaCh) Hub, in the Melbourne Graduate School of Education, University of Melbourne, Australia. In 2013,

Penny was awarded her PhD, which examined the contribution of parent responsive behaviours to child language development. In 2016, she was awarded a Marie Sklodowska-Curie Fellowship which she carried out at Newcastle University, UK, with Prof. James Law and Prof. Cristina McKean. This work included developing and testing the implementation of the Parental Responsiveness Rating Scale (PaRRiS) as a measure to assist health professionals with identifying children at risk of language difficulties. Her current research focuses on enhancing adult–child interactions in early childhood education settings and the home environment to promote child language development and reduce social inequalities.

Kirsty Mclachlan, MPhil, BSc, MRCSLT, qualified speech and language therapist (SLT) from Strathclyde University (1999). This was followed by a master's degree at Newcastle University (2004). She has held the post of Lead SLT in head and neck cancer for NHS Lothian since 2006. This role involved establishing a fibreoptic endoscopic evaluation of swallowing service for head and neck cancer patients and setting up a modified voice prosthesis (VP) service for laryngectomy patients with complex surgical voice restoration needs. She established a laryngectomy VP database to record VP changes prospectively and has published the results of this work (currently in press). She considers herself lucky to lead a group of excellent SLT clinicians and one SLT assistant, who all contribute and support these innovative service developments.

Nick Miller PhD, FRCSLT, Emeritus Professor of Motor Speech Disorders at the University of Newcastle. Throughout his career he combined clinical management of people with acquired progressive and non-progressive neurological communication disorders in community and hospital settings with lecturing and research on these and related topics. His internationally acclaimed research has been based on single case and small group studies through to large scale investigatory and experimental approaches, qualitative as well as quantitative methods. A thread throughout his clinical and research work has been to understand the impact on the individual and their family of receiving a diagnosis of communication disorder and the experience of living with such challenges, and from this to learn lessons for the optimization of support and intervention for people affected.

Jean Neils-Strunjas, PhD, Professor and Chair in Communication Sciences and Disorders at USC, Columbia, USA. Within her specialties as a certified speech-language pathologist, she is trained in geriatric assessment and intervention. She is guided by the goals to provide maximum support and humane treatment for older adults with cognitive impairment. To that end, she focuses her research on the development of behavioural interventions for speech, language, communication, and memory impairment for persons with dementia. As Principal Investigator of an

NIH-funded grant, she investigated the writing ability of persons with mild dementia and Alzheimer's disease symptoms. Her interdisciplinary approach creates interprofessional and interdisciplinary teams that combine strategies from linguistics, exercise science, and speech-language pathology that increase the physical, communicative, and social activities for the geriatric community.

Rosalind Pawar, BSc (Hons), MSC, Qualified Speech and Language Sciences at Newcastle University. She has worked in community and acute speech and language therapy roles. She specialised in stroke and neurology with interests in social communication disorders and dysphagia rehabilitation. She is currently seconded to the role of Clinical Lead Speech and Language Therapist at Barnet Hospital, Royal Free London NHS Foundation Trust. Rosalind has undertaken postgraduate studies including advanced clinical decision making and cognitive communication disorders.

Philip Robinson, BA MMedSci, speech and language therapist in independent practice who works exclusively with stammering in adults and children age 11+. He holds a bachelor's degree in linguistics and a Master's in Clinical Communication Studies from the University of Sheffield, and has been a practising speech and language therapist since 2014. He has worked in both the NHS and for a large independent clinic where he was Clinical Lead for Dysfluency, and now sees patients from his own private practice on Harley Street in Central London. Stammering runs in his family, and personal experiences with a childhood stammer brought Philip into the speech and language therapy profession.

Crystal Rolfe, Associate Director for RNID Health Strategy and involved in roles such as being the Audiology Specialist and England Director. Crystal has worked as an audiologist in the NHS, training in the private sector and guest lecturer at UCL. Crystal also has an MSc in Health Psychology and is a trustee for a small health charity.

Gavriella Simson, BSc (Hons), MSc, Qualified Speech and Language Sciences. Gavriella completed a Bachelor of Health Sciences and Master of Speech Pathology (Honours) at Latrobe University, Melbourne, Australia. She has worked in the acute, rehabilitation, and community settings in Australia and England. Her current role is in the voice and head and neck cancer services at Barnet Hospital, Royal Free London NHS Foundation Trust.

Gareth Smith, Consultant Clinical Scientist in Audiology at Mid and South Essex Hospitals Group, Essex. Dr Smith has over 20 years' experience in the field of clinical audiology; over this time he has served as President of the British Academy of Audiology and Secretary to the British Society of

Audiology. He is currently audiology editor for *ENT & Audiology News*, an international professional magazine.

Trini Stickle, PhD, Associate Professor of English at Western Kentucky University, United States of America. As an applied linguist, her research interests are broadly focused on factors that negatively affect persons' access to meaningful interaction within their communities. She focuses on individuals with dementia, individuals with autism, and individuals learning English as a second language to better understand the interaction barriers unique to each group and specific participant strategies to overcome these difficulties. Dr Stickle is currently investigating the aging and healthcare experiences of immigrant and refugee populations living in the southern regions of the United States. She is also developing trainings for K-12 teachers on embracing dialect diversity. She is the current section editor on old age for *The Palgrave Encyclopedia of Critical Perspectives on Mental Health.*

Samuel Tromans, PhD, Associate Professor in the Department of Health Sciences at the University of Leicester, and an Honorary Consultant in the Psychiatry of Intellectual Disability at Leicestershire Partnership NHS Trust. He completed his PhD in psychiatric epidemiology at the University of Leicester under the supervision of Professor Traolach Brugha, where he investigated adult autism prevalence within acute psychiatric inpatient settings. He has published over 30 book chapters and journal articles, predominantly relating to autism and intellectual disability. He has a postgraduate certificate in medical education from the University of Dundee and is a Fellow of the Higher Education Academy. He has been a Member of the Royal College of Psychiatrists since 2015 and graduated from University of Leicester Medical School in 2011.

Mari Viviers, MCommPath, PhD, Mari is a highly specialist speech and language therapist at St Mary's Hospital, Imperial College Healthcare NHS Trust. She obtained her PhD at the University of Pretoria (South Africa) in 2017 with specialism in neonatal dysphagia. Her career has spanned public and private healthcare in South Africa and the United Kingdom with a focus on infant feeding disorders and early communication intervention. She previously served as Associate Professor at a university in South Africa. Mari serves as a committee member on two Royal College of Speech and Language Therapists Clinical Excellence Networks. Currently she holds a joint role as Education Lead for Allied Health, Psychology, and Healthcare Scientists and highly specialist speech and language therapist at Guy's and St Thomas' NHS Foundation Trust. She has presented nationally and internationally at various conferences and has published numerous peer-reviewed papers.

Abbreviations

AAC	augmentative and alternative communication
AD	Alzheimer's dementia
ADHD	attention deficit hyperactivity disorder
AHA	American Heart Association
AI	artificial intelligence
APA	American Psychiatric Association
ASD	autism spectrum disorder
AT	assistive technology
BCI	brain computer interface
BSL	British Sign Language
CA	conversation analysis
CCC	Carolina Conversation Collections
CCN	complex communication needs
CSA	Clinical Skills Assessment
DA	discourse analysis
DLD	developmental language disorder
DSM-5	*Diagnostic and Statistical Manual of Mental Disorders*, 5th Edition
DVD	digital video disc
EOL	end of life
GBD	Global Burden of Disease Study
GMC	General Medical Council
GP	general practitioner
HCP	healthcare professional
HNC	head and neck cancer
HoH	hard of hearing
ICD-10-DCR	International Classification of Diseases
ICU	intensive care unit
IWA	individual with aphasia
LD	language disorder
MND	motor neuron disease
MS	multiple sclerosis

NAA	National Aphasia Association
NHS	National Health Service
NIA	National Institute of Aging
NICE	National Institute for Health and Care Excellence
OME	otitis media with effusion
PD	Parkinson's disease
PND	progressive neurological disorder
PPE	personal protective equipment
PTSD	post-traumatic stress disorder
PTSS	post-traumatic stress symptoms
PWS	person who stammers/people who stammer
RCN	Royal College of Nursing
RCSLT	Royal College of Speech and Language Therapists
SBAR	situation, background, assessment and recommendation
SCA™	Supported Communicaton for Adults with Aphasia
SCD	social (pragmatic) communication disorder
SLCN	speech, language, and communication needs
SLT	speech and language therapy/therapist
SVR	surgical voice restoration
UK	United Kingdom
UN	United Nations
VRE	video-reflexive ethnography
WHO	World Health Organization

Preface

About the book

Dr Riya Elizabeth George

Meeting Jonathan

My usual Thursday shift as a healthcare assistant typically began with serving tea and breakfast to the patients on the hospice ward. As I peered round the corridor to see a new patient, named Jonathan, I remember the eerie silence that filled the room as I opened the door. My initial thought was 'perhaps he's not in?' But as I turned round, I saw a man sitting in a wheelchair. His body was so contorted and convoluted, his back permanently arched forward causing his face to be looking downwards and his legs and arms were twisted amongst each other, grappling to find a comfortable position.

I remember pausing, not knowing how to begin to converse with someone I could not even have eye contact with and whose body language and facial expressions appeared unwelcomely immobilised. Jonathan has multiple sclerosis, which increasingly over time had taken control of his body. Cautiously, I kneeled, to try and catch sight of Jonathan's face, but even that proved challenging, with only glimpses of his eye lashes flickering, being seen. I introduced myself and informed Jonathan that I had tea and some slices of toast and jam for him to eat. As I spoke, I thought to myself, 'how can he possibly eat like this?', 'Shall I make breakfast for him?', 'Is he even listening?' Filled with uncertainty, I asked 'can I … help you with breakfast?' To which he did not reply. I asked the question again, this time speaking slower and somewhat louder, and anxiously waited for a response. Silence.

I just assumed perhaps he could not communicate or maybe that he could not hear me. Unsure and trying to appear helpful, I began making a cup of tea for him, leaving a few sachets of sugar next to it and then started to open a small pot of butter and strawberry jam to spread over his toast.

'No. I can do that myself, thank you.'

From the awkward silence that continued to fill the room, Jonathan suddenly spoke in a clear and authoritative manner. Startled, I quickly apologised, not quite sure what to say or how to act. My assumptions suddenly challenged. Jonathan can speak. Jonathan can hear. Jonathan can communicate. With compassion for my incorrect assumptions, he explained to me that spreading butter and jam was something he could still do despite his condition. A small but treasured act of independence. He conveyed his struggles with communication as well as his ingenious ways around them. Jonathan was all too familiar with the communication errors I had made, the sound of hesitation in my voice and my uncertain proactiveness to try and do something rather than to wait and listen.

These challenges may sound familiar to you. This story was one of my earliest encounters of a communication issue I dealt with as a healthcare professional. Since then, I have experienced a repertoire of communication challenges ranging from ascertaining an accurate clinical history to negotiating treatment plans, practising shared decision making, and trying to understand the patient's experience as well as their healthcare needs. Practising in a variety of culturally diverse clinical settings meant conversing with patients and healthcare professionals with differing abilities to communicate with one another. Communication is a ubiquitous concept in the field of healthcare and one that to some extent has been taken for granted. The ability to articulate, express, recount, listen, and understand one another in a fast paced, ever-changing healthcare system is often unquestioned. However, communicating in this context requires skill and training to ensure all parties are fully engaged in the process. The myriad of complex healthcare environments present, with unfamiliar people, locations, and terminology makes having everyday meaningful conversations challenging in itself and these challenges are even more insurmountable for those with atypical communication conditions. Even with the best of intentions, often healthcare professionals can help too little, too much and in some cases not help at all.

Atypical communication can arise from a multitude of health conditions (such as aphasia due to stroke or aphonia from a total laryngectomy) and results in patients having difficulty expressing and /or comprehending language. Recent research highlights that 20 percent of the UK population is likely to experience having a communication difficulty at some point in their lives (Royal College of Speech and Language Therapists, 2022), thereby increasing the likelihood that healthcare professionals will interact with atypical communicators. Communication is not just simply about the ability to speak but also the ability to hear and understand what is being said. The impact of atypical communication is varied, with some individuals finding it hard to ask a question or keep the same pace as normative communication; whilst others may have speech difficulties that make it difficult for them to be understood or have communication devices that require time to create a message. Atypical communication can often leave patients without a voice or a voice that presents as a variation from the norm. Communication is the primary vehicle for establishing meaning in clinical narratives and both patients and healthcare professionals have reported experiencing major challenges and frustrations during healthcare encounters because of communication barriers (Morris et al., 2013; Burns et al., 2018). Adults and children with atypical communication conditions experience higher risk for adverse events in healthcare (Barlett et al., 2008) and report lower satisfaction with the healthcare services they receive (Hoffman et al., 2005). Over- (helping too much) or under-accommodation (helping too little) can frequently occur among healthcare professionals in their interactions with atypical communicators for a variety of reasons; these can include a lack of knowledge about particular communication conditions and patients' preferences, a lack of awareness as to when accommodations are needed, and erroneous assumptions on the part of healthcare professionals regarding the patient's communicative abilities (Fox et al., 2005; Parr et al., 2006).

Clinical communication is a mandatory requirement in many healthcare curricula and a plethora of healthcare bodies advocate the inclusion of teaching on the management of atypical communication conditions among patients (General Medical Council, 2019; Nursing Midwifery Council, 2009). However, current resources are often piecemeal in nature, focusing on particular communication condition, rather than considering the wide spectrum of atypical communication conditions that healthcare professionals are likely to experience. Furthermore, many of the existing resources are targeted at healthcare professionals specialised in speech and language and are either not accessible or sufficiently appealing to a broader healthcare audience.

Meaningful conversations in challenging consultations presents a supportive and practical guide for healthcare professionals that considers the spectrum of atypical communication conditions and its impact on everyday healthcare interactions. A growing number of patients have an atypical capacity for communication (both acquired and developmental), creating unique challenges for healthcare professionals and patients in forming meaningful clinical interactions. In this book, leading scholars from a range of healthcare professions provide supportive, practical guidance, and insight into optimal management for those with atypical communication conditions. Drawing on a range of evidence-based recommendations and clinical experiences, the spectrum of atypical communication conditions is explored, which includes speech, language, and hearing impairments. The assumption that understanding typical communication development will inform our understanding of atypical communication, and vice versa, is not without controversy. This collection of chapters not only highlights communication challenges experienced by healthcare professionals and atypical communicators, but also the competencies and often novel forms of communication displayed.

References

Bartlett, G., Blais, R., Tamblyn, R., Clermount, R., & MacGibbon, B. (2008). Impact of patient communication problems on the risk of preventable adverse events in acute care settings. *Canadian Medical Association Journal, 178*(12), 1555–1562.

Burns, I. M., Baylore, C., Dudgeon, B. J., Starks, H., & Yorkston, K. (2018). Healthcare provider accommodations for patients with communication disorders. *Topics in Language Disorders, 37*(4), 311–333.

Fox, A., & Pring, T. (2005). The cognitive competence of speakers with acquired dysarthria: judgements by doctors and speech and language therapists. *Disability & Rehabilitation, 27*(23), 1399–1403.

General Medical Council (GMC). (2009). *Medical students: professional values and fitness to practice.* London: General Medical Council.

Hoffman, J., Yorkston, K., Shumway-Cook, A., Ciol, M., Dudgeon, B., & Chan, L. (2005). Effects of communication disability on satisfaction with health care: a survey of Medicare beneficiaries. *American Journal of Speech Language Pathology, 14*(3), 221–228.

Morris, M., Dudgeon, B., & Yorkston, K. (2013). A qualitative study of adult AAC users' experiences communicating with medical providers: disability and rehabilitation. *Assistive Technology, 8*(6), 472–481.

Nursing Midwifery Council (2009). *The Code. The professional standards of practice and behaviour for nurses, midwives and nursing associates.* Retrieved from www.nmc.org.uk/globalassets/sitedocuments/nmc-publications/nmc-code.pdf

Parr, S., Pound, C., & Hewitt, A. (2006). Communication access to health and social services. *Topics in Language Disorders Communication Access: Models and Methods for Promoting Social Inclusion, 26*(3), 189–198.

Royal College of Speech and Language Therapists (2022). *The Royal College of Speech and Language Therapists (RCSLT) strategic vision: 2022–2027.* Retrieved from www.rcslt.org/wp-content/uploads/2022/03/RCSLT-Strategic-Vision-2022-2027.pdf

Introduction

Atypical communication in healthcare

Riya Elizabeth George and Michelle O'Reilly

Chapter contents:

Introducing atypical communication

Communication skills begin in infancy with the development of language. In typical development an infant will have basic language skills by the age of one year, and during those early years will grasp a greater fluency and vocabulary (Fletcher & O'Toole, 2016). During infancy the child learns to associate the sounds they hear in the environment with people and objects (Pinker, 1994) and over time learns the art of communication and social interaction, which transcends merely the spoken word. Indeed, the child refines pronunciation, extends their vocabulary, attains a command of syntax, learns politeness strategies, and understands what gets them into trouble (Pinker, 1994). By the age of 5 years, a typically developing child may have a vocabulary of over 5000 words and understand the basic art of communication (Keenan et al., 2016). Notably, not all children learn language at the same rate, and not all children master communication in what is considered a 'typically developing' way. For some children they can experience language difficulties, of which there are two main types, receptive and expressive. Receptive language refers to the child's ability to understand the spoken word, sentences, and meanings of what is said by others, whereas expressive language refers to the child's ability to be able to express their thoughts

DOI: 10.4324/9781003142522-1

through sentences in a way that is grammatically correct (Fletcher & O'Toole, 2016).

In this context, it is important to recognise that while there are many attempts to define communication, there has not been a universal or perfect definition, with communication being more than language (Littlejohn et al., 2017). Some work and practices will emphasise some aspects of communication over others, which has consequences for how we understand impairment (Andersen, 1991). While defining atypical communication does have some tensions, in general terms it tends to refer to social interactions where one or more of the interlocutors has an impairment that is evident in consequential ways within that interaction (Wilkinson, 2019). Atypical communication then, is generally understood as when any part of communication is not developing in the usual way and when this impacts pre-verbal communication, development of speech, vocabulary, social communication skills, verbal and written literacy, fluency, and/or language (Fletcher & O'Toole, 2019).

Atypicality and health

Difficulties in communication are often attributable to a present disability, developmental disorder, or health condition (Goldbart & Caton, 2010), and in this book it is these forms of atypical communication that is our primary focus. Goldbart and Caton reported that those individuals experiencing complex communication needs tend to require significant support from their communication partners; and this is something that has important implications for healthcare settings. It is also important to recognise that those groups of individuals cannot and arguably should not be treated as a homogenous group, and their communication impairments are also likely heterogeneous, even within groups. Nonetheless, these do tend to be individuals who have poorly developed communicative and social skills, which are often present with sensory, intellectual, and/or behaviour challenges (Nind & Hewett, 2001).

It is arguably helpful then, to differentiate the types of conditions that may impact on communication. Wilkinson (2019) differentiated between those that are congenital/developmental and thus occur before birth or during early childhood development, and those that are acquired, in that they occur after the person has developed communication. Wilkinson also differentiated between disorders that have an organic basis, that is anatomical, physiological, or neurological, and those that are functional, where there is no such known basis. Wilkinson further differentiated communication disorders by different areas of competency in terms of the production of coherent and intelligible talk and other social conduct, whereby he offered the following categories:

- *Disorders in which speech is impaired*: this included motor speech disorders.

- *Disorders in which hearing is impaired*: this includes congenital hearing loss and hearing loss associated with ageing.
- *Disorders in which fluency is impaired*: the most common impairment example here is stammering or stuttering.
- *Disorders in which language is impaired*: these can include language disorders like aphasia, and those where cognitive abilities are impaired such as memory or attention or the motor speech subsystems are impacted (e.g., through a stroke or Parkinson's).
- *Disorders in which cognition is impaired*: there are many disorders where cognitive functioning is regularly impaired in some manner. These individuals are described as having a pragmatic impairment.

Benefits and challenges of atypical communication in healthcare settings

Many individuals with these atypical communication types will engage with various physical and/or mental health care practitioners either directly because of their disability/disorder/condition, or like the typically developing population, with unrelated health problems. It is important that healthcare professionals can communicate with these individuals in effective ways, and while they may have training in the specific condition if that is the purpose of the appointment, it may not necessarily be the case (for example, someone with aphasia or dementia may visit a dentist with toothache, a GP with an ear infection). Thus, while a psychiatrist may have specialist communication training to converse with an autistic person, a nurse in the emergency department may have less experience. It is therefore incumbent on professionals to try to make reasonable adjustments for diversity, including disability (The Equality Act, 2010).

Healthcare settings are imbued with asymmetry, as the skilled professional is often in a more powerful position than the lay patient or client. In cases where there are additional diversity factors the asymmetry can be widened and this can create situations of challenge for those individuals. In healthcare, the language of consultation places the patient at a disadvantage, a gap that is widened for those with a communication disability (Law, this volume). Law notes that this therefore puts an emphasis of responsibility on the practitioner to elicit the appropriate responses from the patient, and to ensure they have been understood.

In healthcare settings, communication barriers are already a challenge and so is the input of the healthcare system (Mason et al., 2019). Mason et al. argued that there needs to be a flexibility of healthcare providers to be open to alternative communication styles and use of accessible language. This is compounded further by other factors like limited services, accessibility of facilities, socio-economic factors, and referral pathways (Bradshaw et al., 2019). A recent review has also illustrated barriers in relation to healthcare for those with atypical communication. In the context of autism, specifically, Malik-Soni et al. (2021) argued that there are six broad domains of barriers encountered, which are: (1) shortage of services, (2) lack of clinician knowledge, (3) cost, (4) family and individual knowledge, (5) language, and (6) stigma.

In practice, therefore, it is necessary for practitioners to recognise the individuality of the person they are working with, but also have a commitment to inclusion and subscribing to the social competence paradigm by accounting for the active agency of those individuals in communicative exchanges (Biklen & Burke, 2006). Indeed, by using the concept of atypical communication to help reposition the communication as a *difference* rather than as a pathology, it helps us think more carefully about the way in which we adapt and flex to the needs of those individuals (Drewett, 2021).

Structure of the book

There are 16 chapters in this book, beginning with four introductory chapters which explore the spectrum of typical to atypical communication conditions, illustrate the impact of the cultural and social context of communication development, highlight the importance of storytelling in facilitating meaning in healthcare interactions and consider the application of technology. These four chapters form the necessary theoretical background to which the subsequent chapters are built. The latter chapters, authored by a range of different healthcare professions, provide practical based recommendations, with clinical examples grounded in both research evidence generated by healthcare professionals and clinical practices. We list here the abstracts from the chapters to provide an overview.

Part I Theoretical and social debates in the field of atypical communication

Chapter 1 Considering the spectrum of typical to atypical communication: deficit or difference?

Riya Elizabeth George

Healthcare interactions are increasingly restrained by limitations in time, capacity, and resources, making communication between parties challenging. Much of the literature for healthcare practitioners on consultation skills, clinical reasoning, and developing therapeutic healthcare relationships assumes typical communication from both the healthcare practitioner and the patient. The comparison between typical and atypical communicators, two categorically different groups has been an endemic, classic approach in the field of communication development. Much of our knowledge on atypical communication has been built on variants of this dichotomised approach.

By comparing discrete groups, it tends to narrow one's focus on differences rather than similarities between groups. This comparative approach is generally founded on the assumption that typically developing individuals are the benchmark for normative functioning and the measuring stick for optimal development. This creates the potential to overlook the ways in which atypical individuals may be advantaged in communication development and the processing of information. By exploring the characteristics that fall along the spectrum from typical to atypical communication it can help highlight the fundamental similarities in communication development and may also aid in the social de-stigmatisation of individuals with particular conditions.

In this chapter, the author introduces the focus of the book by illuminating for the reader a body of literature that explores how to take a dimensional approach in considering the full spectrum of variation, ranging from typical to atypical communication development in a culturally and socially diverse healthcare context; with the understanding that insight gained from both typical and atypical communication is mutually informative. The impact of comparative approaches to how atypical communication is understood in healthcare and the challenges it presents in everyday healthcare interactions is also considered.

Chapter 2 The social and cultural context of meaningful conversations

James Law

Communication is essentially a social phenomenon and although it is driven by cognition, sometimes associated with intelligence and thus perceived to be 'determined', it is socially loaded and context dependent. This chapter begins by exploring what we mean by communication; disentangling traditional distinctions between language (what is language per se) and parole (the use of language, and the behaviour that we experience and share with others). Culture is transferred through communication often at the individual level. However, it is clear that different cultures communicate differently with one another, and this can present challenges when interacting in a culturally diverse healthcare setting. While linguistic differences make a change, they are not the whole story. For example, differences in the use of tones in person-to-person communication can affect the perception of the speaker.

Superficially, we all have equal access to our language, yet it is clear that some have a greater opportunity than others and we see this transpire in the types of vocabulary used, the language structures adopted, accent and the 'way' that people communicate with one another, especially if there is a perceived power differential, as there commonly is between health practitioner and patient. While this is true in all consultations to some degree, it is exacerbated when the relationship is especially asymmetric, as it can be when one of the parties has a communication difficulty. With time-constrained healthcare appointments, invalid assumptions can be made regarding the communicative and intellectual abilities of patients. These assumptions can be aggravated by healthcare conditions that further skew a patient's communicative abilities.

This chapter aims to reflect the reality of clinical interactions with atypical communicators, considering the implications of a culturally and socially diverse healthcare context in how we communicate. It provides examples and clinical case scenarios and includes a series of exercises to draw the attention of the reader to the experiences of those with atypical communication conditions in a diverse healthcare setting.

Chapter 3 Finding meaning through storytelling in healthcare

Riya Elizabeth George and Graham Easton

Traditional forms of storytelling can often be thought of as merely a childhood experience. However, stories (sometimes referred to as narratives) are part of our everyday lives. Storytelling is an important and undervalued communication tool, particularly with atypical communicators. A patient generally describes their symptoms using a narrative and introduces key people (or characters) that are part of their experience. Storytelling necessitates both listening and sharing and is a two-way process. Evidence shows that storytelling can help healthcare professionals develop deeper relationships with patients and form a greater understanding of their individual needs. Narrative medicine is a relatively new concept that is gaining traction in different spheres of healthcare. It describes the importance of going beyond merely the collection of symptoms in an acute encounter to understanding the patient's experience and journey.

This chapter explores the notion of storytelling in healthcare and its use in facilitating meaning and depth when communicating with patients. By describing and providing examples of the use of storyboarding, illustrations, journaling, graphics, and pictorial charts, these tools can be used to establish meaningful conversations with atypical (and typical) communicators in a range of healthcare settings.

Chapter 4 Technology and atypical communication: a healthcare context

Yasmin Elsahar, Sijung Hu, David Kerr, and Kaddour Bouazza-Marouf

Efficient patient-provider communication is an integral aspect of the healthcare setting. Within this context, difficulties arise when medical conditions are compounded by a condition of speech disability, restricting the patients' abilities to communicate their needs and concerns. Augmentative and alternative communication (AAC) methods have been utilised across the medical setting to help address this problem. Nonetheless, challenges regarding efficient patient–provider communication are still existent, given the variety of AAC tools and the range of conditions related to the disabilities encountered by healthcare practitioners. In this chapter, the benefits and challenges associated with the utilisation of current AAC technologies are presented and discussed in the healthcare context. Ways in which available and forthcoming AAC technologies can enable healthcare providers to optimise communication are illustrated.

Part II Practical guidance for working with children and families

The chapters in the second part of the book, focus primarily on working with children and families. This part of the book reflects the expertise of different practitioners exploring the challenges of triadic consultations, where different expectations and levels of communication are simultaneously present. Issues around participation, consent, and engagement frequently arise when working with children and families, and the presence of atypical communication can create further complexity. Part II, therefore, provides an entire tool kit for those who practice with this population, providing case examples, practical tips, and guidance for how to establish meaningful conversations.

Chapter 5 Children and young people with atypical communication in healthcare

Mari Vivers and Louise Edwards

Children and young people with atypical communication are increasingly seen in a variety of healthcare settings. This chapter presents information around possible atypical communication and strategies to support communication exchanges, including practical tips and signposting to resources. This offers an opportunity for the healthcare practitioner to further develop their skills in supporting diverse communication needs. This chapter is of clinical relevance to ensure children and young people are not restricted in their participation in educational, vocational, family, and community environments, including healthcare.

Chapter 6 Communicating with children and young people with speech, language, and communication needs

James Law, Penny Levickis, and Linda Jose

The prevalence rates for children and young people with speech, language, or communication needs are high (three in every school class) and it is likely that healthcare practitioners will come across them in their own right (i.e., because they have a difficulty) or because their difficulties are associated with some health conditions. Child development drives both what a child can understand and how their parents respond to them, and it is critical that all practitioners are aware of how this might affect the interaction between the healthcare professional and the young person, whether they are two or 15. This chapter looks at the communication skills of children and young people where the primary concern is their speech and language difficulties. In the United Kingdom, these children and young people are commonly referred to as having speech, language, and communication needs (SLCN). This group of children is of particular concern because their difficulties are not always obvious and health practitioners may find it challenging to recognise them. This chapter begins with a brief introduction to the diagnostic categories used for these children alongside the functional difficulties that they can experience. We explore the association between children's environments and their language abilities. We then look at the locations where practitioners are most likely to encounter children with SLCN and the role that the context plays in how best to communicate with them. Finally, we provide five clinical practice recommendations that are critical to understanding the needs of children with communication difficulties.

Chapter 7 Conversing with families of atypical communicators

Rosalind Pawar and Gavriella Simson

Families of atypical communicators play a key role in facilitating communication with healthcare professions. However, atypical communicators and their families frequently experience communication barriers when accessing the healthcare system. This can have an impact on the quality of the care provided and treatment outcomes. Through two case studies and research, this chapter presents an insight into how a communication disorder impacts the life of the individual affected and their family. It explores the communication barriers within the healthcare system. Practical communication recommendations for healthcare practitioners are provided and key guidance and legislation are presented. Recommendations for supporting individuals from culturally diverse backgrounds and those where English is not the first language are discussed. This chapter explores how families can act as a facilitator and barrier when communicating with healthcare professions. Recommendations for assisting families in maximising communication opportunities for the atypical communicator are presented. This chapter also highlights the evidence on the impact of the COVID-19 pandemic on communication with families.

Chapter 8 Communicating with people with tracheostomies and head and neck cancers

Anne Hurren, Kirsty McLachlan, and Nick Miller

This chapter explains why and how people with a tracheostomy and/or head and neck cancer experience altered communication. Some, but not all, patients with head and neck cancer will require a tracheostomy but most tracheostomy procedures are performed for reasons unrelated to local carcinoma. Tracheostomy and laryngectomy are frequently confused as both have a visible neck stoma; the critical distinctions are outlined and related to their communication needs and the rehabilitation options. Cultural and psychosocial issues are discussed, and two case examples illustrate how this population may present in both an emergency and a community setting. We conclude with guidelines for optimising communication and minimising any negative impacts and list key resources for those who would like to learn more about issues concerning this population.

Part III Atypical communication in progressive neurological disorders

Progressive neurological disorders (PNDs), such as multiple sclerosis and Parkinson's disease significantly interfere with patients' lives, and those of their families. There is a growing recognition that language impairments and pragmatic deficits occur in different neurodegenerative disorders. Changes in communication, brought about by neurological disorders, are most often defined and described in terms of the individual's impairments of speech and voice or language. Communication is per definition an interaction, a joint effort that makes the conversational partner a key player. This is true in all types of everyday conversations, but especially so when one of the interacting persons has a communicative impairment. Part III of this book pays special attention to the communication challenges that can arise from PNDs. It considers its implications in relation to the patient, but also their families and the wider healthcare team, providing illustrative examples, guidance, and practical recommendations.

Chapter 9 Atypical communication in Parkinson's disease, multiple sclerosis, and motor neuron disease

Sarah Griffiths and Nick Miller

PNDs such as Parkinson's, motor neuron disease, and multiple sclerosis can cause significant communication difficulties. Listeners may hear distorted speech or quiet voice, but challenges for the person can extend way beyond speech itself, to encompass cognition, language, and non-verbal communication. These changes can impact greatly on a person's sense of self and well-being. This chapter summarises PND-associated communication changes, and explains how to recognise communication hurdles, highlighting the collaborative nature of effective communication, whereby listeners play as important a role as speakers. The chapter examines how health and social care workers can ensure the voices of people affected are heard and understood. Evidence-based strategies are presented, to equip professionals to take a tailored approach to encounters with people with PNDs, thereby assuring maximum support for communication, and person-centred care.

Chapter 10 Dementia and conversation patterns helpful to practitioners

Trini Stickle and Jean Neils-Strunjas

Stickle and Neils-Strunjas explore the challenges that common dementia symptoms often create for doctor–patient communication. Clinical visits, like everyday interactions, are affected by word- or concept-finding difficulties, the loss of memory, perseveration, and severe syntactic disfluency. As such, these difficulties may erode rapport and impede efficacy of care and treatment. In this chapter, we present strategies that work toward productive and positive experiences for medical staff and patients with dementia. We also highlight conversational practices to avoid: ones that yield little progression and are evidenced by patient stress and/or withdrawal from the conversation. Finally, we demonstrate ways to move unproductive conversations toward more productive outcomes and enjoyable experiences. Each conversational strategy or difficulty is illustrated through actual conversation excerpts and aided by practical guideline summaries.

Part VI Practical guidance on specific conditions resulting in atypical communication

Chapter 11 Supporting meaningful conversations in stroke-induced aphasia

Elizabeth Hoover and Anne Carney

Stroke is a leading cause of chronic disability in adults and approximately one third of stroke survivors develop aphasia. Aphasia is the loss or reduction of language affecting the production or comprehension of spoken and written language. Many individuals with aphasia (IWAs) recover some language function; however, the communication difficulties associated with aphasia are often chronic and may limit the ability to return to work and hobbies, engage in social relationships, and may lead to stigma and isolation. Thus, the consequences of aphasia can be wide reaching and severe for IWAs, their community, and the healthcare system.

This chapter briefly describes different types and causes of aphasia, along with the incidence and prevalence of the condition. Case studies are included to illustrate the psychosocial and health consequences associated with aphasia across the continuum of care and to highlight the potential for communication breakdown in healthcare environments. IWAs and their families report feeling excluded from healthcare discussions, receiving inadequate information to make decisions, and reduced involvement in decision making particularly surrounding hospital discharge. Further, observations of clinical interactions between clinicians and IWAs reveal unbalanced conversations, with the clinician directing the topic, timing, and flow of the conversation. The chapter provides strategies and illustrated examples to address the issues described above and support successful communication in healthcare environments, such as conducting a clinical interview and understanding health information, establishing patient-centred goals, and gaining informed consent. Finally, the chapter reviews patient-centred research relating to living successfully with aphasia.

Chapter 12 Communication and people with learning disabilities

Jonathan Beebee

People with learning disabilities should have the same rights to accessing healthcare as everyone else. They should be as involved in decisions about their care as much as possible. However, cognitive and communication disabilities can appear to create a barrier to this. For some people, their learning disabilities will be an invisible disability and may go unnoticed. For others, they may have physical characteristics or unusual behaviours that make their needs more visible. For practitioners who are not experienced in supporting people with learning disabilities it can be an intimidating experience. This chapter aims to explore some of the communication needs for people with learning disabilities and provides advice on strategies to help overcome these challenges.

Chapter 13 Communication with autistic adults

Alison Drewett and Samuel Tromans

This chapter will discuss principles to facilitate effective communication with autistic adults, with reference to two research studies involving this patient group, both conducted within adult mental health settings. The purpose of presenting the two research studies, each from a different research paradigm, one qualitative and one quantitative, is to offer principles grounded in research findings and researcher reflections. Each study takes a distinct methodological approach, reflecting the diversity of autism research, but both nonetheless present recommendations relevant to clinical practice. Following a general introduction to autism and communication, the studies are discussed in turn with subsequent presentation of communication guidelines.

Chapter 14 Improving engagement with people who stammer

Philip Robinson

Stammering is a disorder of fluency that can have profound and lifelong effects on the well-being and life experiences of the speaker. While observable levels of dysfluency sit within a spectrum, the underlying thoughts and feelings about one's own stammer can have a dramatic impact on self-esteem and affect the ways in which one interacts with the world. This chapter proposes, through reference to the author's experiences with a stammering caseload, a set of tangible guidelines to help healthcare professionals interact successfully and productively with this population, and to help treat them with the dignity and parity they can often find to be lacking in interactions with other service providers.

Chapter 15 Communication, hearing loss, and deafness

Gareth Smith and Crystal Rolfe

With 1 in 6 people in the United Kingdom having hearing loss and 87,000 British Sign Language (BSL) users, healthcare professionals in all disciplines are likely to encounter hard of hearing (HoH) and deaf people. Many countries have in-place legal frameworks to support the needs of deaf and HoH individuals, however the published literature and lived-experiences of individuals demonstrates that often they face major challenges in accessing services and, once they have accessed the service, barriers to communication continue. This chapter highlights the extent of hearing loss in the population, introduces the concept of the deaf community, highlights the challenges faced by those with hearing loss, and offers practical solutions and considerations to improve the experience of both the service users and the healthcare professionals they interact with.

Chapter 16 Conclusion and reflections

Michelle O'Reilly and Riya Elizabeth George

This chapter provides an overview of key learning messages mentioned across the collection of chapters and outlines a list of further recommended readings and resources for healthcare professionals. In this chapter we bring together some of the core recommendations from across the book to provide a simple communication 'toolkit' for all areas of healthcare. This will be a practical conclusion to a book that is diverse in its approach and its focus.

Intended audience

The first collection of its kind, this book aims to appeal to a broad international audience and includes international contributors to recognise the different healthcare systems and organisations globally. This book will examine a wide range of atypical communication conditions as well as the social and cultural context in which interactions with atypical communicators takes place. It will consider and provide optimal management strategies, case examples, clinical recommendations, and recommended resources relevant for a range of healthcare professionals. This book will be a valuable resource for undergraduate and postgraduate students on healthcare and allied healthcare courses as well included as recommended reading material in clinical communication curricula. The contribution of authors from varied fields of healthcare will support inter-professional practices and will be a valuable resource for those with an interest in clinical communication and communication and diversity.

References

Andersen, P. (1991). When one cannot not communicate: a challenge to motley's traditional communication postulates. *Communication Studies*, *42*(4), 309–325.

Biklen, D., & Burke, J. (2006). Presuming competence. *Equity and Excellence in Education*, *39*(2), 166–175.

Bradshaw, P., Pellicano, E., van Driel, M., & Urbanowicz, A. (2019). How can we support the healthcare needs of autistic adults without intellectual disability? *Current Developmental Disorders Reports*, *6*, 45–56.

Drewett, A. (2021). A PhD learning journey: The value of conversation analysis and discourse approaches for speech and language clinical practice. In M. O'Reilly, and J.N Lester (Eds.). *Improving communication in mental health settings: Evidence-based recommendations from practitioner-led research*. London: Routledge.

Fletcher, P., & O'Toole, C. (2016). *Language development and language impairment*. Oxford: Wiley Blackwell.

Goldbart, J., & Caton, S. (2010). *Communication and people with the most complex needs: what works and why this is essential*. Manchester: MENCAP.

Keenan, T., Evans, S., & Crowley, K. (2016). *An introduction to child development* (3rd ed.). New York: Sage.

Littlejohn, S., Foss, K., & Oetzel, J. (2017). *Theories of human communication* (11th ed.). Longrove, IL: Waveland Press.

Malik-Soni, N., Shaker, A., Luck, H., Mullin, A. E., Wiley, R. E., Lewis, M. E. S., & Frazier, T. W. (2021). Tackling healthcare access barriers for individuals with autism from diagnosis to adulthood. *Pediatric Research, 91*(5), 1028–1035.

Mason, D., Ingham, B., Cos, M., Birtles, H., Brown, T., James, I., Scarlett, C., Nicolaidis, C., & Parr, J. R. (2019). A systematic review of what barriers and facilitators prevent and enable physical healthcare services access for autistic adults. *Journal of Autism and Development Disorders, 49*, 3387–3400.

Nind, M., & Hewett, D. (2001). *A practical guide to intensive interaction*. BILD.

Pinker, S. (1994). *The Language Instinct*. New York: Penguin Press.

The Equality Act (2010). Retrieved from www.legislation.gov.uk/ukpga/2010/15/contents

Wilkinson, R. (2019) Atypical interaction: conversation analysis and communicative impairments. *Research on Language and Social Interaction 52*(3), 281–299.

Part I

Theoretical and social Debates in the field of atypical communication

1

Considering the spectrum of typical to atypical communication

Deficit or difference?

Riya Elizabeth George

Chapter contents:

- The endemic practice of comparison
- Considering models of cultural diversity
- Moving forward: exploring dimensional approaches
- References

Healthcare interactions are increasingly restrained by limitations in time, capacity, and resources, making communication between parties challenging in itself. Much of the literature for healthcare professionals on consultation skills, clinical reasoning, and developing therapeutic healthcare relationships assumes typical communication from both the healthcare professional and the patient. Patients with a capacity for atypical communication are more likely to struggle when communicating their needs to healthcare professionals, and this is further compounded by the fast paced and unfamiliar healthcare environment.

Atypical development of communication is defined as a deviant or difference in any part of communication that is not developing as expected for the age of the individual. The different areas of communication that are impacted (i.e. speech, language, or fluency) give rise to a multitude of labels that are used to describe the developmental or acquired delays or deficits. Whilst these labels are sometimes used interchangeably with different terms, they generally refer to a set of symptoms and this information is used to determine what therapy/intervention and or treatment is most suitable. The comparison between typical and atypical communicators, two categorically different groups, has been an endemic, classic approach in the field of communication development.

In this chapter, we introduce the focus of this book by considering the impact of comparative approaches on how atypical communication is understood in healthcare and the challenges it presents in everyday healthcare

DOI: 10.4324/9781003142522-3

interactions. We intend to begin to illuminate for the reader how to take a dimensional approach in considering the full spectrum of variation, ranging from typical to atypical communication development in a culturally and socially diverse healthcare context; with the understanding that insight gained from both typical and atypical communication is mutually informative.

The endemic practice of comparison

How should differences between 'typically developing' individuals and other populations be interpreted? To what extent should the emphasis be on advocating remediation for individuals who are on a developmental trajectory that differs from the norm versus embracing different developmental trajectories as equally valid contributions to the diversity of human experiences? Akhtar and Jaswal (2013) pose these very questions when trying to interpret diverse developmental paths. Many studies in communication development involve group comparisons, whether clinical groups or cultural groups. Comparisons inadvertently predicate on or lead to valuing one group over the other; meaning one group or its performance is often taken as the 'standard' and is considered desirable and the norm and the other is unfavourably compared to it (Medin, Bennis, & Chandler, 2010). Implicit in this approach is the assumption that individuals who possess condition X or disorder Y represent a distinct, non-overlapping population or category from individuals who do not have this condition or disorder.

Generally, the performance of privileged groups in society, those in the majority and/or holding the most power, are considered to be the norm and that of others is considered to have 'deficits' relative to this norm. For example, autism is often always defined by the challenges experienced by autistic individuals. However, there are things that people with autism excel at, which are not commonly considered in the profile of the autism spectrum disorder. For example, some individuals with autism sometimes do better than those without autism on perceptual tasks like visual searches (Joseph et al., 2009). Based on this evidence, would it be appropriate to claim that individuals without autism suffer from perceptual impairments? Or is it possible to go beyond a simplistic deficit model and recognise some of the differences associated with autism may be advantageous in some contexts (Robinson, 2011)?

The use of groups comparison approach has deep roots in developmental psychology – we can see this categorical approach mirrored in classic theoretical discussions from debates around the distinct roles of nature and nurture in explaining phenomena to deliberations on the characterisation of development as continuous or discontinuous. Although contemporary psychology has largely moved beyond such dichotomised approaches to the questions posed by Akhtar and Jaswal (2013), the group comparison approach is endemic in our methodological approaches to questions on cognitive and communication development.

A contributing factor as to why this approach is so frequently used may reflect the fact that thinking about distinct groups reflects fundamental aspects of how we, as humans, organise our world. Categorisation offers a way to make sense of the messiness and complexity of the world we live in. We label individuals based on personality characteristic, we classify life forms according to a taxonomic system and we group artefacts into categories. Akhtar and Menjivar (2011) explain that we seek to impose order on our social world by classifying individuals into discrete social groups. Research shows our human tendency to organise diverse entities into unifying categories and to then use these categories to guide reasoning about shared characteristics and properties of category members emerges early in development (e.g., Baldwin, Markman, & Melartin, 1993). This early-emerging tendency to categorise, combined with evidence that categorical information is easier to remember and reason about, suggests that categorical representations may be privileged in our cognitive systems (see Cimpian, 2016). Put simply, humans find it easier to think about and process information in a categorical fashion. Another contributing factor for the comparison approach reflects the dominant classification approach that has been applied to mental and development disorders. The most used systems are the *Diagnostic and Statistical Manual of Mental Disorders*, 5th Edition (APA, 2013) and the World Health Organization's (2016) *International Classification of Diseases and Related Health Problems*, which treat disorders as categories based on a set of defining features. This categorical approach to the assessment of psychological disorders has continued to dominate the fields of psychology and psychiatry, despite considerable research demonstrating that most presenting symptoms exists on a continuum (Esterburg & Compton, 2009; Lahey et al., 2008). Furthermore, the on-going use of a comparison approach is likely sustained by practical advantages; for example, comparing the speech and language development of a group of 2-year-olds with a group of 4-years-olds on a particular task will allow one to collect insights into the unfolding communication development more rapidly. Conversely, longitudinal research is time-consuming, costly as well as labour intensive. However, many authors such as Paterson, Parish-Morris, Hirsh-Pasek, and Golinkoff emphasise that despite practical challenges of longitudinal research, a longitudinal approach does give a more nuanced perspective on the development of an individuals over time that simply cannot be attained using a cross-sectional comparative approach.

Although the comparison approach has many disadvantages, the use of this approach has led to seminal insights into multiple aspects of cognitive development. For example, comparisons of deaf and hearing individuals have yielded insights into how early language experiences, or lack thereof, shape the language system and enhance our understanding of the neural bases for language (e.g., Ferjan Ramirez et al., 2014; Goldin-Meadow & Mylander, 1998). Studies comparing children who are blind to those who are sighted have helped us understand the role of sensory experience in the development of spatial and conceptual knowledge (e.g., Bedny & Saxe, 2012; Bigelow, 1996). Furthermore, our understanding of the developmental course of language development in typically developing children has led to the identification of specific difficulties in children not following this path, including children with specific language impairment (e.g., Bavin et al., 2005; Collisson et al., 2015; Norbury & Bishop, 2002).

Comparing discrete groups tends to focus one's lens on differences rather than on similarities between groups. Yet, as illustrated by Ferjan et al. (2014), the elucidation of similarities (i.e., an intact multiple object tracking system) between individuals from atypical groups and typical groups highlights fundamental similarities in the human cognitive system, can describe strengths that can be built upon in the context of interventions, and may also aid in de-stigmatisation of individuals with particular conditions. 'Othering' can be a by-product of comparison, influencing our understanding and treatment of others whose behaviours, values, or capacities appear to differ from what we perceive to be the norm. Another potential disadvantage of the comparison approach as applied to atypical and typical groups surrounds the reliance on typically developing individuals as the benchmark of normative or typical functioning. As illustrated by Bialystok's (2011)'s discussion of attention in individuals, this comparative focus, with typically developing individuals as the standard, can lead researchers to overlook ways in which atypical individuals may be advantaged in processing information. As we identify differences, it is essential that we consider the impact – both positive and negative of these labels (Pearson, Conner & Jackson, 2013).

Considering models of cultural diversity

Culture shapes behaviour, and standards of what is and is not acceptable behaviour are culturally determined (Bruner, 1990). In addition, the measures used to sample behaviours of interest and the evidence base on which diagnostic decisions are made are also subject to cultural biases. What are the implications of these challenges for understanding developmental disorders? There is growing recognition in mainstream developmental psychology and communication literature that much of what is published about human perception, cognition, and communication development is derived from research studies conducted in Western societies and that these cohorts reflect a tiny minority of the world's population that is often not representative of the majority (Henrich, Heine, & Norenzayan, 2010). Thus, the conclusions that researchers draw about typical human development may be limited to a rather narrow subsample of privileged individuals (i.e., those who are educated, live in democratic societies, and have high socio-economic status).

Medin et al. (2010) highlighted the powerful but subtle 'home field disadvantage' that so malevolently seeps into our interpretations of cultural groups other than our own. Two of their cautionary points are particularly important. First, there is an imbalance in the way that we view heterogeneity (in behaviours, motivations, values, capacities, etc.) in our own cultural groups as compared with others. We tend to assume strong heterogeneity within our own cultural group, but all too often tacitly assume that there is considerable homogeneity along these same dimensions in other cultural groups. Second, we tend to consider our own cultural group as the 'unmarked', or normative case, leaving other groups as the 'marked' case. Consider, for example, the wide-spread assumption that assessments that were developed by and for members of White middle-class majority Western cultural groups can be handily applied to members of different groups. Similarly, Gutierrez and Rogoff (2003) focused on potential pitfalls of characterising diversity in educational settings. They argued against viewing culture itself as a 'trait' or entity harboured within all members of a given group. Instead, they take a cultural-historical perspective on culture as a dynamic analysis of repertoires of practices. Like Medin et al. (2010), Gutierrez and Rogoff caution against the assumption of homogeneity (e.g., that particular learning styles are true of all children from a given culture) and propose instead that educators consider particular children's school performance within the context of the cultural practices that they actually engage in with their families. Finally, Claude Steele's work (e.g., Steele, 1997) on stereotype threat paints a vivid depiction of how detrimental the expectations we hold of others can be. Through a rich series of studies, Steele has clarified how deficit interpretations of students' performance cause more problems than they solve. All three models argue against settling for simple models in which culture is considered a cause, particularly because multifaceted clusters of factors tend to correlate with one another in determining complex outcomes such as academic performance or language development. Taken together, these three cultural models raise four warning signals; these are:

1) *Avoiding assumptions of homogeneity*: It is important to consider the broad within-group variation among individuals. With so much within-group diversity, it is unclear whether it makes sense to include all individuals under a single label.
2) *Designing assessments from within the culture being studied rather than transplanting assessments from other groups*: Medin et al.'s (2010) observation that in research and in practice we tend to 'mark' other cultures, leaving our own culture as 'unmarked'. This leads to assumptions that the mainstream culture is the standard and the other non-majority cultures are the ones that are different or deficient.
3) *Avoid overly simple causal models, given the complex clusters of factors involved*: The examples included in these models remind us that our understanding of aetiology or cause can be only as good as our current understanding (or misunderstanding) of a phenomenon, that our

understanding is coloured not only by the breadth (or restrictedness) of the individuals or groups we have considered but also by the assumption of the majority culture community.

4) *Carefully consider the impact of labels, expectations, and stereotype threat*: The authors ask us to consider how we can appropriately factor in the impact of perceptions (both by self and others) of a deficit label or deficit interpretation?

Moving forward: exploring dimensional approaches

Whereas comparative approaches tend to classify individuals into categorically distinct groups, dimensional approaches aim to study the full spectrum of variation, ranging from typical to atypical, on a given construct or in a diverse population of individuals with the understanding that knowledge gleaned on both typical and atypical development is mutually informative (Cicchetti & Toth, 2006). In dimensional approaches, an index is provided marking an individual's relative position compared to others. For example, a dimensional approach to understanding child attention involves ascertaining one child's relative standing compared to other children in a given population (Fox & Henderson, 1999). Of course, identifying the relevant population for comparison for a given child is a nontrivial task. Nonetheless, this approach lends itself well to the study of typical and atypical development, as it more closely reflects the reality of individual variation within a population.

The traditional approach to studying clinical conditions has been deeply rooted in the medical model. From a medical perspective, disease conditions are often considered categorical in nature (e.g., presence or absence of diabetes, cancer, or Parkinson's disease, etc.). In the formulation of some diagnosable mental disorders, a similar classification approach to the medical literature is applied, in that a symptom, such as psychosis, is either present or not. This categorisation of mental disorders is based on an individual meeting a minimum threshold on a set of diagnostic criteria. Traditionally, the classification of mental disorders has been a helpful practical approach to diagnosis, as it can determine the need for treatment and the type of treatment that should be received. Of course, one problem with this categorical approach is the use of artificial boundaries in carving symptoms into categories. For example, two children, one just meeting and one just failing to meet diagnostic criteria, will be treated as categorically distinct when these two children may, in fact, be more similar than they are different. Moreover, the need for children to meet a certain symptomatic threshold to receive a diagnosis may limit the availability of resources and services accessible to children who are struggling but who fall below this clinically significant threshold.

To paraphrase a familiar saying, one approach will not fit all research questions. However, when examining typical and atypical development, we would encourage readers to consider a dimensional approach when possible. This book aims to showcase the spectrum of differences that can arise from typical to atypical communication. The practice of categorising and comparing variables or populations as 'typical' or 'atypical' can lead to a loss of information and/or inappropriate classification of individuals. For example, if a sample of participants is split at the mean (or median) of the distribution, with those above the distribution considered typical and those below considered atypical, misclassification is most likely to occur among the participants clustered around the mean. As a result, participants who are statistically similar are treated as categorically different based on a small cut-point difference. This practice of dichotomisation has the potential to lead to misunderstanding of the relation between variables in developmental science, which in turn has considerable implications for the translation of knowledge to practice and policy (Dawson & Weiss, 2012). For example, if results from analyses that divided typical and atypical at a designated cut point (e.g., mean) revealed differences between the two groups in terms of degree of deficits (i.e., language delay, intelligence) or level of symptomatology (e.g., inattention), the clinical recommendations may be to treat these 'typical' and 'atypical' groups as qualitatively different. Thus, children falling on the atypical side of the cut point may have access to specialised services to attenuate deficits or symptomatology, while those falling on the typical side may not have the same privileged access to such services as they failed to meet the designated threshold, but as noted previously, the degree of deficit and level of symptomatology of those clustering around the mean may be more similar than they are different.

When using the comparative approach to studying typical and atypical development, a consideration should be made as to when this method is best employed. This approach may be best utilised when the presence or absence of a condition is more easily characterised, like a condition (deafness, brain lesion, chromosomal abnormality), as opposed to creating cut points of typical or atypical on constructs (e.g., attention, working memory) that are best captured as dimensional in nature. A viable avenue for attaining a greater understanding of whether a construct is best captured as categorical or dimensional is a data-analytic tool called taxometric analysis. Taxometric research seeks to determine whether a set of indicators correlate in a manner more consistent with a distinction as dimensional or categorical (Waller & Meehl, 1998). To date, taxometric research has largely been conducted in the clinical literatures, such as the research described by Lahey et al. (2008) on the underlying dimensions of psychopathology. Another example from this field of research, which has relevancy for the examination of attention in cognitive development, stems from research by Marcus and Barry (2011) who sought to examine the widespread notion that attention deficit hyperactivity disorder (ADHD) is a discrete condition. They applied a taxometric analysis to data from the National Institute of Child Health and Human Development Study of Early Child Care and Youth Development and found that ADHD symptoms have a dimensional rather than categorical structure. The taxometric approach has also been applied to developmental and cognitive-related constructs as well.

Drawing on this literature, we suggest that any consideration of differences between typical and atypical individuals needs to entail attention towards a construct like clinical significance. That is, does this difference reflect a meaningful impact on everyday functioning for an individual? Is this difference meaningfully related to the critical mechanisms that underpin a condition or disorder? If considering a clinical group, does this difference between the typical and atypical groups inform treatment options and selection? Much of our knowledge on atypical communication has been built on variants of this dichotomised approach. By comparing discrete groups, it tends to narrow one's focus on differences rather than similarities between groups. This comparative approach is generally founded on the assumption that typically developing individuals are the benchmark for normative functioning and the measuring stick for optimal development. This creates the potential to overlook the ways in which atypical individuals may be advantaged in communication development and the processing of information. By exploring the characteristics that fall along the spectrum from typical to atypical communication, it can help highlight the fundamental similarities in communication development and may also aid in the social de-stigmatisation of individuals with particular conditions.

References

Akhtar, N., & Jaswal, V. K. (2013). Deficit or difference? Interpreting diverse developmental paths: An introduction to the special section. *Developmental Psychology*, *49*, 1–3.

Akhtar, N., & Menjivar, J. A. (2011). Cognitive and linguistic correlates of early exposure to more than one language. *Advances in Child Development and Behaviour*, *42*, 41–78.

American Psychiatric Association (APA). (2013). *Diagnostic and statistical manual of mental disorders* (5th ed.). Washington, DC: Author.

Baldwin, D. A., Markman, E. M., & Melartin, R. L. (1993). Infants' ability to draw inferences about nonobvious object properties: evidence from exploratory play. *Child Development*, *64*, 711–728.

Bavin, E. L., Wilson, P. H., Maruff, P., & Sleeman, F. (2005). Spatio-visual memory of children with specific language impairment: evidence for generalized processing problems. *International Journal of Language & Communication Disorders*, *40*, 319–332.

Bedny, M., & Saxe, R. (2012). Insights into the origins of knowledge from the cognitive neuroscience of blindness. *Cognitive Neuropsychology*, *29*, 56–84.

Bialystok, E. (2011). Reshaping the mind: The benefits of bilingualism. *Canadian Journal of Experimental Psychology/Revue canadienne depsychologie expérimentale, 65*, 229–235.
Bigelow, A. E. (1996). Blind and sighted children's spatial knowledge of their home environments. *International Journal of Behavioral Development, 19*, 797–816.
Bruner, J. (1990). Culture and human development: a new look. *Human Development, 33*, 344–355.
Cicchetti, D., & Toth, S. L. (2006). Building bridges and crossing them: translational research in developmental psychopathology. *Development and Psychopathology, 18*, 619–622.
Cimpian, A. (2016). The privileged status of category representations in early development. *Child Development Perspectives, 10*, 99–104.
Collisson, B. A., Grela, B., Spaulding, T., Rueckl, J. G., & Magnuson, J. S. (2015). Individual differences in the shape bias in preschool children with specific language impairment and typical language development: theoretical and clinical implications. *Developmental Science, 18*, 373–388.
Dawson, N. V., & Weiss, R. (2012). Dichotomizing continuous variables in statistical analysis: a practice to avoid. *Medical Decision Making, 32*, 225–226.
Esterberg, M. L., & Compton, M. T. (2009). The psychosis continuum and categorical versus dimensional diagnostic approaches. *Current Psychiatry Reports, 11*, 179–184.
Ferjan Ramirez, N., Leonard, M. K., Davenport, T., Torres, C., Halgren, E., & Mayberry, R. I. (2014). Neural language processing in adolescent first-language learners: longitudinal case studies in American Sign Language. *Cerebral Cortex, 26*, 1015–1026.
Fox, N. A., & Henderson, H. A. (1999). Does infancy matter? Predicting social behavior from infant temperament. *Infant Behavior and Development, 22*, 445–455.
Goldin-Meadow, S., & Mylander, C. (1998). Spontaneous sign systems created by deaf children in two cultures. *Nature, 391*, 279–281.
Graham, S. A., & Madigan, S. (2016). Bridging the gaps in the study of typical and atypical cognitive development: a commentary. *Journal of Cognition and Development, 17*(4), 671–681.
Gutiérrez, K. D., & Rogoff, B. (2003). Cultural ways of learning: individual traits or repertoires of practice. *Educational Researcher, 32*(5), 19–25.
Henrich, J., Heine, S. J., & Norenzayan, A. (2010). The weirdest people in the world? *Behavioral and Brain Sciences, 33*, 61– 83.
Joseph, R. M., Keehn, B., Connolly, C., Wolfe, J. M., & Horowitz, T. S. (2009). Why is visual search superior in autism spectrum disorder? *Developmental Science, 12*, 1083–1096.
Lahey, B. B., Rathouz, P. J., Van Hulle, C., Urbano, R. C., Krueger, R. F., Applegate, B., & Waldman, I. D. (2008). Testing structural models of DSM-IV symptoms of common forms of child and adolescent psychopathology. *Journal of Abnormal Child Psychology, 36*, 187–206.
Marcus, D. K., & Barry, T. D. (2011). Does attention-deficit/hyperactivity disorder have a dimensional latent structure? A taxometric analysis. *Journal of Abnormal Psychology, 120*, 427–442.
Medin, D., Bennis, W., & Chandler, M. (2010). Culture and the home-field disadvantage. *Perspectives on Psychological Science, 5*, 708–713.

Norbury, C. F., & Bishop, D. V. (2002). Inferential processing and story recall in children with communication problems: a comparison of specific language impairment, pragmatic language impairment and high-functioning autism. *International Journal of Language & Communication Disorders*, *37*, 227–251.

Pearson, B. Z., Conner, T., & Jackson, J. E. (2013). Removing obstacles for African American English-speaking children through greater under-standing of language difference. *Developmental Psychology*, *49*, 31–44.

Robinson, J. E. (2011). *Be different: Adventures of a free-range Aspergian with practical advice for Aspergians, misfits, families, and teachers*. New York, NY: Random House.

Steele, C. (1997). Claude Steele's stereotype threat experiment. *Study.com*, 15 May 2016, retrieved from study.com/academy/lesson/claude-steeles-stereotype-threat-experiment.html

Waller, N. G., & Meehl, P. E. (1998). *Multivariate taxometric procedures: distinguishing types from continua*. Thousand Oaks, CA: Sage.

World Health Organization (WHO). (2016). *ICD-10: International statistical classification of diseases and related health problems* (Volume 2, Instruction Manual, 5th ed.). Geneva, Switzerland: World Health Organization.

2

The social and cultural context of meaningful conversations

James Law

Chapter contents:

- Communication in healthcare
- Values in healthcare communication
- Values and language competence
- The healthcare consultation
- Communication skills assessments
- Considering epistemic in justice
- Intercultural communication
- New and old media
- Considering the effect of improved communication on outcomes
- Promoting meaningful conversations
- References

Communication in healthcare

Everyone understands what it means to talk to people because we do it all the time and probably spend relatively little time reflecting on the process. However, meaningful conversations require many different skills and attributes from both parties, which must fit together to work effectively. In the extreme situation where one person can talk and the other either is not able to or chooses not to, conversation cannot occur at all. Of course, speech can be supplemented by gesture, manual signing systems, or alternative and augmentative communication (AAC), but their use is challenging unless both parties understand them well. Clearly, if your conversation partner is deaf and is using British Sign Language or has athetoid cerebral palsy and needs to use a communication device, this is obvious. However, if they have a speech disorder such as dysarthria or dyspraxia, they do speak but they may be unintelligible. This is often true for a child with a developmental language disorder, but it is also true for someone whose speech intelligibility declines

DOI: 10.4324/9781003142522-4

following a stroke or with advanced Parkinson's. While it is tempting to focus on the person with a communication disability, perhaps because their communication difficulties are so obvious, it is also important to consider that the need for effective communication applies to everyone in a health consultation whether the patient has a disability, a different first language, mental health difficulties, or may simply be because they are anxious. A better understanding of how we communicate will help us to respond appropriately whenever we encounter such difficulties.

This chapter examines some of the key issues underpinning professional communication, specifically in the context where communication between healthcare professional and patient can be challenging because of the asymmetry in power relations between the two, an asymmetry based on professional knowledge, of course, but also on other characteristics that mark the interaction. These challenges can be exacerbated when the patient has a communication disability and finds it difficult to understand what is being said or to express themselves. It is relatively straightforward to identify poor interactions and specific behaviours on the part of the practitioner that may offer some redress, but effective communication also depends on the values of both practitioner and patient and the desire to find common ground. All these issues, while central to face-to-face communication, are equally important in the context of telehealth and the world of online interaction between patient and practitioner. In short there is much that the professional can do in modifying their behaviour to facilitate effective communication but, without a thorough understanding of the issues concerned, such changes may have limited impact on patient outcomes. Finally, we consider the evidence for whether improved communication makes a difference to patient outcomes.

Values in healthcare communication

There is more to effective communication than just the behaviour of the professional. Healthcare professionals in the United Kingdom do receive training and assessment in communication skills, and there are lists of things to do and to avoid (we shall see examples later), but effective communication also depends on values, which may be unaffected by training.

To begin engaging with values it is necessary to consider how communication works in society, especially between partners when there is an imbalance of power. The language of healthcare consultations commonly puts the patient at a disadvantage; this is amplified when that patient has a communication disability and needs to have adaptations in place to make the interaction work. This puts the responsibility on the practitioner both to ensure that the patient understands what is said to them, and to elicit the responses from the patient that will ensure that the practitioner has all the necessary information. These points are illustrated in the following case study.

Case study 2.1 Keith

Keith is 48 and married, living with his wife Catherine and with his two children. He has aphasia following a stroke ten months ago. He finds it difficult to understand what others are saying in conversation and to construct his own sentences. He also has dysarthria and sometimes struggles to make himself understood, especially with unfamiliar listeners. He received speech and language therapy while in hospital but has had difficulties accessing services in the community. He also has been having headaches and wants to discuss both issues with his general practitioner (GP). Catherine, his wife, has offered to come with him and helps arrange the appointment but he is insistent that he goes on his own when she is at work. The GP is a locum, not familiar with his case and has been too busy to read the notes. She is looking at them on her computer screen when he arrives. She asks him how he is and what he wants and he replies 'speech therapy over' with a sweep of his hand. Continuing to look at her screen she asks him whether he has had any and he says 'in hospital'. It is clearly difficult for him to speak and the interaction is effortful and frustrating. She wants to help and ask him if he wants to see a speech and language therapist and says that she will refer him. He nods. She has to get on to her next patient and he leaves having been unable to discuss his headaches. She makes the referral but the interaction is clearly frustrating for both parties.

Keith's story highlights the first common imbalance occurring in health consultations, that based on the professional's knowledge and patient's lack of it. This disparity is further amplified when there is a second imbalance caused by a patient's communication problem. But there is often also a third level of asymmetry where there is *epistemic injustice*. When this occurs, like the first imbalance, it is caused by the patient's lack of knowledge, not just the lack of professional knowledge but a more general lack because of a difference in background, culture or education. When the communication is about illness, there may also be different cultural narratives, and the practitioner needs to be able to hear what the patient is trying to convey about what his situation means to him. All these asymmetries may be exacerbated by the technologies increasingly adopted in attempts to improve access to services, including social media and other forms of digital communication.

The importance of effective communication should be at the centre of any debate about access to healthcare. The construction of meaning is a complex process that moves beyond the simple roles of sender and receiver and encoding and decoding information. There is the 'continuous interplay of perception and action in a co-regulated social context' (Fogel, 1993, p. 15).

In health consultations, both practitioner and patient are active contributors, involved in interpreting the message and in drawing inferences based on the context and knowledge of the other person (Sperber & Wilson, 1995). Kagan (1998, p. 817) refers to the 'equation' of communication, which is balanced by the skills, experiences, and resources that those involved in the interaction can draw on. Imbalances will occur whenever one person has difficulties in understanding the other or in formulating their questions or answers. The difficulties can be because of communication disabilities, cultural, or language differences. Barriers arise from the mismatch between an individual's capacity for communication and the unmodified demands of the communication environment, leading to an increased risk of communication breakdown where patients' questions remain unanswered, and diagnoses are tentative.

Communication of healthcare professionals with patients is one dimension of their workplace communication, covering everything from a power point presentation to delivering information and to relationships among colleagues, management, staff. Failures of workplace communication are commonly the subject of discussions and concerns in every walk of life (Schnurr, 2013). However, in the context of healthcare such failures can be particularly damaging, and every effort should be made to minimise them.

Values and language competence

The practical competence of speakers is of course not uniformly distributed through a society in which the same language is spoken. Different speakers possess different amounts of *linguistic capital* – that is, the capacity to produce expressions for a particular type of recipient. Moreover, the distribution of linguistic capital is related to the distribution of other forms of capital (such as economic and cultural capital) that define the position of an individual within the society. Hence differences in terms of accent, vocabulary, and narrative are indices of the social positions of speakers and reflections of the quantities of linguistic and other capital that they possess. The more linguistic capital that speakers possess, the more they are able to exploit the system of differences to their advantage and thereby obtain some advantage from their interactions. The forms of expression that are accorded the greatest value and secure the greatest profit are those that are most unequally distributed. They are unequal both in the sense that the conditions for the acquisition of the capacity to produce them are restricted and in the sense that the expressions themselves are relatively rarely used in the situations where they appear. The healthcare professional often has considerably more language capital than the patient. While this is clearly true in the specific detail of the technical language of the health professional, it is often also true of language associated with their social background, commonly middle class and invariably highly educated. It may be possible to mitigate the effects with awareness raising for the professionals, but it may not be possible to remove this power imbalance altogether. Indeed, it could be argued that professionals have little interest in removing it because that power may give them an advantage in terms of fostering the patient's belief and compliance with the intervention process.

This sense of power is highlighted in the Roberts et al. 2014 report.

> Power is an important topic of concern in linguistics and the means by which speakers exert power in interaction have been variously argued (such as interruptions, questioning strategies, highlighting mistakes). The GP consultation is typically characterised by asymmetric power, with the GP holding the ability to provide treatment. Power differentials by their nature mean speakers don't quite align, although a sense of alignment can be talked into being (Drew 1991: 21).
>
> (Taken from Roberts et al., 2014, p. 37)

Good communication requires the practitioner to reflect closely on their own communication skills and how they may be perceived by others.

The healthcare consultation

Here the term *consultation* refers to any interaction between a healthcare practitioner and patient. This may be formal meetings between a patient and a GP, the interactions occurring on ward rounds, or the less formal communications between patients and nurses or allied health professionals giving advice or ongoing therapy. More formal procedures, where roles are clear cut and specific goals must be met in a limited time, present the greatest challenge for the person with communication difficulties. The efficiency needed in such interactions may militate against effective communication precisely because questions are asked and decisions are made at speed and the views of the patient with communication difficulties may be sacrificed. This has long been recognised and various trainings have been put in place, to improve practitioner communication skills.

For patients, another problematical feature of many consultations is that the professionals assume that they are interchangeable and that it is possible for someone to just pick up the notes and continue where the previous practitioner left off. While such lack of continuity may be necessary for operational reasons, the patient and especially the person with a communication disability may find this especially challenging. It is often distressing to a patient to have to repeat answers to questions previously asked by someone else, especially if the patient has difficulty speaking or understanding.

There are plenty of guides on how to communicate with patients and this is routinely taught in the courses designed to train healthcare professionals in medical schools and elsewhere in higher education. Much of the training focuses on things to avoid and things to do. Here is an example adapted from Travaline, Ruchinskas, and D'Alonzo (2005).

Things to avoid

- Using highly technical language or jargon when communicating with the patient.
- Not showing appropriate concern for problems voiced by the patient.
- Not pausing to listen to the patient.
- Not verifying that the patient has understood the information presented.
- Using an impersonal approach or displaying apathy in communications.
- Not being sufficiently available to the patient.

Things to do

- Find out what the patient already knows.
- Find out what the patient wants to know.
- Be empathic.
- Slow down.
- Keep it simple.
- Tell the truth.
- Be hopeful.
- Watch the patient's body and face .
- Be prepared for a reaction.

These desirable features of interactions are easy to list, but in reality, we find that knowledge does not translate into action in an obvious way. We need to look closely at who does and does not interact effectively with patients, both in terms of outcomes and how the client experiences the interaction.

Communication skills assessments

The Royal College of General Practitioners (Roberts, Atkins, & Hawthorne, 2014) considered performance on the Clinical Skills Assessment (CSA) carried out with GPs in the United Kingdom. Those performing poorly had difficulties giving explanations to patients, misunderstood the consultation process, had more difficulty repairing misunderstandings, experienced more moments of misalignment with the patient that would impact on the unfolding consultation and sounded formulaic to examiners.

The interpersonal skills domain is characterised by requirements for 'empathy', 'rapport', 'connection', and 'alignment'. Stokes and Hewitt (1976) suggest that assessment of such qualities is difficult. 'Rapport', 'empathy', and 'warmth' are tricky if not impossible to judge. Although we all may have an intuitive understanding, ultimately these are inner emotional experiences of the interactants that are hard to observe from the outside. It is doubly subjective as observers can only guess at the individual, inner reactions of listeners. Empathy, as an emotional response to another person, becomes complicated in the artificial setting of an assessment where there are other intense emotions at play.

CSA assessments of interpersonal skills are based only on the candidate's side of the interaction. However, the interaction is a complex joint production, and this joint work is part of the evidence. 'Alignment' is a social/behavioural way of assessing consulting skills rather than a psychological way – looking at evidence of professional performance rather than inner feelings. This functional evaluation is useful in assessing simulated encounters.

Alignment also describes aspects of the consultation that deal with its overall management (managing the interaction, its speed and rhythm, and making appropriate inferences from the other's talk), as well as explicit strategies to show understanding and, where appropriate, agreement.

The institutional and professional constraints of the GP's role mean that not every ethical stance expressed by the patient can be supported with empathy. However, the doctor is expected to maintain the flow of the interaction and demonstrate a level of mutual understanding. The term 'alignment' allows for the tension between sustaining social relations but not necessarily fully supporting/endorsing the patient's stance. All verbal interactions carry 'metacommunication', a level of meaning through which the message implicitly defines the relationship between the communicators. In healthcare consultations this unspoken layer of meaning can also include 'signposting' – letting the patient know where the consultation is going and what's coming next. When a CSA candidate adds 'but it's nothing for us to worry about at the moment', she is signalling how a piece of medical information she has just given should be interpreted, as well as being attentive to the relationship with the patient and their concerns.

Metacommunication is important in any setting with an overhearing party, and in the CSA it shows the examiner the structure the candidate is working to, why they are doing something, and how attentive they are to patient-centredness. Effective metacommunication and signposting are features of many successful CSA candidates' interactions. No one is perfect, and all those involved in professional interactions experience moments of misunderstanding and/or misalignment, but poorer performing CSA candidates have been shown to demonstrate slightly more. Misunderstandings were caused by mishearing, forgetting, and missing clinical information. Other misalignments were caused by dysfluencies in speech and causing patient confusion. These could compound each other in multifactorial misunderstandings. Dysfluencies occur in all talk but are more likely in the exam context, raising the question of whether a position of communicative tolerance could be adopted. Much of this misalignment results from poor metacommunication and signposting, and failure to repair the resultant misunderstandings. Patients normally need to know why a physical exam is being undertaken, what is routine and what is a possible cause for concern. CSA candidates and examiners need to pay special attention to this. Once misunderstandings occur, they are difficult to repair, but if repaired swiftly a tense moment could be rapidly diffused. Misunderstandings and misalignments are common, and the identification and repair of misunderstanding in the professional communication is a litmus test of how well an interaction is working.

Considering epistemic justice

In recent years considerable interest has been shown in the concept of 'epistemic injustice'. This term was first introduced by British philosopher Miranda Fricker to describe the injustice associated with knowledge, specifically not taking into account the understanding of others or the testimonies of those from marginalised groups (Fricker, 2007). The concept highlights the power imbalance inherent in knowledge, which can lead to exclusion, silencing, systematic distortion, or misrepresentation of a person's meanings or contributions. Fricker split this into *testimonial* injustice and *hermeneutic* injustice. Testimonial injustice is unfairness related to trusting someone's word, when someone is ignored or not believed because of their sex, sexuality, gender, race, or disability. Hermeneutic injustice relates to how a person's experience is interpreted in relation to societal norms. This influences how they make sense of their lives when experiences are not well understood by themselves or by others. Both testimonial and hermeneutic injustice relate directly to the experience and self-awareness of the practitioner, although Fricker does not restrict her analysis to health contexts.

In their paper on epistemic injustice in healthcare, Carel and Kidd (3024) suggest 'that health professionals are considered to be epistemically privileged, in both warranted and unwarranted ways, by virtue of their training, expertise and third-person psychology' (p. 2). They decide which patient testimonies and interpretations to act upon. They are able to contrast cases in which patients are unconsciously (or consciously) assigned undeservedly low credibility with cases in which patients' credibility is undeservedly high. These are two ways in which health professionals' clinical judgement can be skewed as a result of assigning too little or too much credibility to patients. In cases where a doctor is especially paternalistic, patients may not be regarded as epistemic contributors to their case in anything except the most basic information – confirming their name or 'where it hurts'.

This is well recognised in psychiatry where people with mental health difficulties are much more likely to be a victim of this type of injustice than those with somatic problems (Crichton, Carel, & Kidd, 2017) and with those, for example, with chronic fatigue syndrome or myalgic encephalomyelitis, where there may be marked differences of perspective from patient and practitioner (Blease, Carel and Geraghty 2017). Case study 2.2 is an illustration from psychiatry (Crichton, Carel, & Kidd, 2017).

Case study 2.2 Chris

Chris was admitted to a psychiatric hospital on Section 2 of the Mental Health Act, even though he had agreed to be admitted and remained in hospital as a voluntary patient. He had been standing near the edge of a high cliff for an hour before he was noticed, and the police were called. The staff involved in his care on admission did not believe that he could be trusted to remain in hospital voluntarily and argued in the tribunal for the maintenance of the Section. His community psychiatric nurse attended the tribunal, arguing that it was not necessary for him to be sectioned as he had suicidal thoughts for many years, had gone to the same cliff many times in the past, had been admitted to hospital on several occasions as a voluntary patient, and had misgivings about the stigma attached to being sectioned. All this had been documented in the hospital notes. She conceded that there would always be a risk of self-harm, but that it was a matter of managing the risk without compulsory detention and with the help of his friends and family. After hearing this evidence, the tribunal members decided to rescind the Section.

Recently the voices of those with disabilities and the challenges they experienced have been highlighted more visibility for the public (Scully, 2020). For those with specific communication difficulties, the issue is only now beginning to be recognised, but the right to freedom of expression can be tested (UN, 1948).

> Looking closer, there are other – often unnoticed – reasons why citizens cannot make themselves heard. There are citizens who are not fighting to have a place on any particular platform, rather, many citizens are without a mode of communication, full stop. Those with communication disabilities are unable to express their views at all. And so the question of interfering with their expression of their views, or unjustly preventing them from accessing media and platforms to make themselves heard, cannot even arise.
>
> (Klausen, 2019)

Klausen takes a rather binary view. Experience would suggest that communication disability is more likely to lead to partial communication rather than a complete lack of it, although for many this may be more difficult to negotiate than immediately defaulting to managing a case through a proxy – a carer, parent, or spouse. Case study 2.3 gives an example.

Case study 2.3 Erin

Erin is 35, lives in a care home, and has a learning disability. She finds it difficult to understand what others have said to her, unless they control the amount of information, and struggles to explain more than her basic needs. She has a job in the kitchen of the care home but has not found it possible to get a job outside. She finds it difficult to express herself and when asked to talk about the pain she experiences she only points to where it hurts and winces. The doctor tries to understand but in the end she decides that the only way to find out what Erin is experiencing is through palpation alone. She finds nothing and invites Erin's key worker, Sara, in from the waiting room to see if she can help. The doctor asks Sara what she thinks is the problem and she replies that Erin quite often indicates that she feels uncomfortable, but they think that she is a bit of a hypochondriac and often do not pay much attention to her complaints, as things usually tend to go away. The doctor is unsure what to do but sends them back to the care centre with guidance on what to look out for in terms of symptoms. A month later Erin returns. She continues to complain of pains in her side. The doctor decides to explore this in more detail and contacts the speech and language therapist who is working with Erin. She attends the clinic and takes out a 'Talking Mat' which allows her to carry out a detailed analysis of the options presented by the doctor. This allows the doctor to focus on what is wrong and to question her about other symptoms such as fatigue, cramps, thirst, irregular periods etc. She concludes that Erin most probably has Addison's disease. Without this careful questioning this would have remained unnoticed.

In the end, the extent to which a practitioner considers these issues will be driven by the importance they attach to them. While we take for granted the right to self-expression, the reality for those with communication disabilities is that their right to be effectively listened too is often ignored. This must change if we are to reduce the chance of epistemic injustice (McCormack, Baker, & Crowe, 2018).

Intercultural communication

Whatever the means of communication – oral, written, e-mail, or social media – one of the key issues is how well they translate across different groups of patients, especially those who have different cultural and linguistic backgrounds. This issue is less about the understanding of messages, although this will be an issue if the practitioner and the patient are monolingual in different languages, but rather it is about how the interaction is affected by three critical intercultural variables:

- The relationship of the individual to the other person.
- The application of norms.
- The role of context in communication (Thatcher 2001).

As Thatcher (2001) eloquently stated, existing research methods 'seem derived from and designed for predominantly U.S. cultural and rhetorical values', which need to be 'critically adapted for intercultural studies' (p. 459). To directly transfer methods 'designed by U.S. scholars in the United States and for use in monocultural inquiry' to intercultural research is dangerous because it would create 'significant risks for neo-colonialism, orientalism, or ethnocentrism' (p. 5) (cited in Ding & Savage, 2013). This intercultural communication clearly has the potential to function at the individual level of the consultation, causing problems associated with the assumptions about the communication context, which are not shared by both parties in the interaction. Just as power imbalances are there in all professional interactions and are exaggerated when the patient has a communication disability, they are especially prominent when intercultural communication is an issue, not just concerning the language itself but for the cultural interpretation of those interactions.

New and old media

Most of the discussion so far has been about oral communication, especially in the context of healthcare consultations. The practitioner and patient are often discussing a matter of common interest – the illness, the disability, or the environment, which may or may not be modifiable. This is what most of us mean by a consultation, but while it may remain the most desirable process, it can no longer be taken for granted. Practitioners and their patients will increasingly be using a variety of media to communicate about their needs and options. This was already the case before the Covid-19 pandemic, but it has been amplified by it. Of course, this approach offers tremendous potential for allowing access to services for people who live remotely from centres of practice or who have problems with mobility.

Prior to Covid-19, practitioners would routinely see patients in their clinic, office, or on community home visits; the first stage in the process is the negotiation of the medium to be used. Superficially this may appear easy but in practice there are many constraints on what people are able to choose to use. Access to and ability to use digital media is less common in older age groups and among those whose work experience has not included the use of computers. The extent to which health services do or do not accept specific platforms may also be an issue. This is an aspect of the digital divide, where experience and resources may affect what is possible in many areas of life. The key issue is that structural societal problems of power associated with communication can be amplified by this process. Of course, there may be situations where the patient knows much more about the technology than the practitioner, which reverses the power balance to some extent, but the pattern remains essentially the same. The constantly changing technology and software also put additional demands on the practitioner. The following case study aims to illustrate these points.

Case study 2.4 Samara

Samara is 68 and lives at home with her family. She has a slight tremor, is worried that it might be something serious, and feels she needs to go to the doctor. She drops into the surgery and asks for an appointment, only to be told that everything is now online, and she needs to make an appointment from her home if possible, describing her symptoms for the doctor to consider before they have an online consultation. Samara does not use a mobile phone and is not at all familiar with computers although her son has one. He helps her get online but cannot be there for the consultation. She finds the keys difficult to manipulate – she has a slight tremor – and struggles to coordinate the camera. The signal comes and goes because they only have a limited broadband contract, and the consultation proves to be a frustrating experience. She does not manage to explain her concerns to the doctor and he finds it difficult to make an assessment. In the end the consultation breaks down and the GP tells Samara to come down to the clinic, where she can be seen in person. She does this, and the doctor suspects that she is in the early stages of Parkinson's disease. He sends her for further assessments, and this is confirmed. As the condition progresses, she does manage to order medicines online, but her tremor makes computer use prohibitively difficult. She finds it a challenge to make herself understood online and she must ensure that future consultations are in person.

In their efforts to improve access, practitioners should not assume that all their patients can make effective use of digital media, nor should they assume that all difficulties can be overcome by working through a family member or carer. The patient's autonomy should always be respected. In attempting to improve communication in healthcare settings, it is tempting to focus on oral communication because it is so salient in our everyday lives, but as increasing use of telehealth continues and the role played by social media expands into professional consultations, every aspect of communication needs to be taken into consideration.

Considering the effect of improved communication on outcomes

There is little evidence of the effect on outcomes of improving communication in healthcare settings: it will be a fruitful area of future research. Some quality improvement initiatives are aimed at improving communication. One of these is the Safe Surgery Checklist, now in routine use in most countries and credited with reducing adverse outcomes due to poor communication by at least a third. Another is the SBAR (situation, background, assessment, and recommendation) tool for facilitating and strengthening communication between nurses and prescribers. Mackintosh and Sandall (2010) believe that using it has the potential to reduce the chance of 'failure to rescue' in cardiac management. The SBAR handover tool is expected to improve patient safety and the patient experience, but more research is needed into its effects. Efforts to improve communication in all healthcare settings should benefit everyone, but those with communication disabilities will always need special consideration.

Central to work on improving communication in healthcare is the issue of values. It is the responsibility of every practitioner to recognise and understand the implication of the power imbalance and take responsibility for their own communication skills to maximise the effectiveness of the interaction with the patient whilst at the same time reducing the potential for errors with the associated costs to all those concerned.

Promoting meaningful conversations

This chapter and in particular the case studies hope to demonstrate the complexity of cultural and societal factors at play in patient experiences and the challenges this adds to the communication between patients and practitioners. It aims to highlight the importance of practitioners in considering their personal values as this dictates the nature and quality of the communication process in terms of how questions are asked and how the patient is facilitated in expressing their story.

Here are some key points and suggestions for improving communication in any conversation, but especially those in healthcare settings.

- Values make a difference. Remember what Elvis said '*Values are like fingerprints. Nobody's are the same, but you leave 'em all over everything you do*'. Our values affect our behaviour and also our metacommunications. Raising our awareness of our own assumptions and values improves our communication skills.
- Adapting our own behaviours to make us better communicators can be difficult. If it were easy, we would surely have already done it! We can often only see the need for change through discussion with others.

- We need to be alert to the fact that any conversation, clinical or otherwise, may not be equally meaningful to all parties.
- It is always good to check that the person we are talking to understands what we are saying. If, in doubt, ask.
- Intercultural communication is not just about language. There are a host of cultural expectations and norms that are brought to the forefront of a healthcare consultation. Discussing these openly can be helpful, but we are often not aware of the assumptions we are making and both practitioner and patient may not be comfortable exploring assumptions in this way.
- Exploring our assumptions takes time, something that practitioners rarely possess in abundance. In the end mutual consideration and tolerance is central to promoting optimal communications.
- Consider the medium for the interaction. If face to face meetings are impractical and digital interaction is necessity, make sure that the same standards of communication are applied.
- Consider whether you are giving enough time for the consultation. Where communication is a challenge for a patient for any reason, always consider giving double appointments. Time pressured appointments may be inefficient if there is not enough time to explore the patient's needs. If a patient with a communication difficulty becomes stressed by time pressure, they may become less fluent in being able to express themselves.

Returning to the central issue of values, here are some questions to ask of yourself and your colleagues. They are taken from the National Centre for Family Philanthropy (NCFP) list of ten 'to help start the values conversation'.

- What does the word 'values' mean to me personally and in the context of my family and friends?
- What are some of the values that have guided and sustained me through life?
- Where did these values come from?
- What family stories or role models have instilled my values and worldview?
- How do these values show up in my actions? In decision making and the way we relate to one another?

Here are a further five questions specifically related to language and communication skills in practice.

- What are my own experiences of not being able to communicate a message effectively? How did others respond and how did I feel about the response?
- To what extent do I believe that communication is a 'right'?

- Have I been made aware of any examples where I have not listened effectively to others and what were my feelings about this?
- How much is it my responsibility to adjust to others when I am communicating with them?
- How much do people's views about their communication come through what they say and do during my healthcare consultations and what difference does that make?

References

Blease, C., Carel, H., & Geraghty, K. (2017). Epistemic injustice in healthcare encounters: evidence from chronic fatigue syndrome. *Journal of Medical Ethics*, *43*, 549–557.

Carel, H., Kidd, I. J. (2014). Epistemic injustice in healthcare: a philosophical analysis. *Medicine, Health Care and Philosophy*, *17*, 529–540.

Crichton, P., Carel, H., & Kidd, I. J. (2017). Epistemic injustice in psychiatry. *British Journal of Psychiatry*, *41*(2): 65–70.

Ding, H., & Savage, G. (2013). *Guest editors' introduction: new directions in intercultural professional communication*. Technical Communication Quarterly, *22*(1), 1–9.

Fogel, A. (1993). Two principles of communication: co-regulation and framing, in: J. Nadel & L. Camaioni (Eds.), *New perspectives in communication development*. London: Routledge, 9–22.

Fricker, M. (2007). *Epistemic injustice: power and the ethics of knowing*. Oxford, Oxford University Press.

Kagan, A. (1998). Supported conversation for adults with aphasia: methods and resources for training conversation partners. *Aphasiogy*, *12*, 817–830.

Klausen, C. (2019). Knowledge, justice, and subjects with cognitive or developmental disability. PhD thesis. University of Waterloo, Ontario, Canada. Retrieved from https://uwspace.uwaterloo.ca/bitstream/handle/10012/15099/Klausen_Catherine.pdf?isAllowed=y&sequence=3

Mackintosh, N., & Sandall, J. (2010). Overcoming gendered and professional hierarchies in order to facilitate escalation of care in emergency situations: the role of standardised communication protocols *Social Science and Medicine*, *71*, 1683–1686.

McCormack, J., Baker, E., & Crowe, K. (2018). The human right to communicate and our need to listen: Learning from people with a history of childhood communication disorder. *International Journal of Speech-Language Pathology*, *20*, 142–151.

Roberts, C., Atkins, S., & Hawthorne, K. (2014). Performance features in clinical skills assessment: linguistic and cultural factors in the Membership of the Royal College of General Practitioners examination by London: Centre for Language, Discourse & Communication, King's College.

Schnurr, S. (2013). *Exploring professional practice: language in action*. London: Routledge.

Scully, J.L. (2020). Epistemic exclusion, injustice, and disability. In: Adam Cureton and David T. Wasserman (Eds.), *The Oxford handbook of philosophy and disability*. Oxford: Oxford University Press.

Sperber, D., & Wilson, D. (1995). *Relevance, communication and cognition* (2nd ed.). Oxford: Blackwell.
Stokes, R. and Hewitt, J. (1976). Aligning actions. *American Sociological Review, 41*(5), 838–849.
Travaline, J. M., Ruchinskas, R., & D'Alonzo, G. E. (2005). Patient–physician communication: why and how. *Journal of the American Osteopathic Association, 105*, 13–17.
Thatcher, B. (2001). Issues of Validity in intercultural professional communication research. *Journal of Business and Technical Communication, 15*(4), 458–489.
United Nations. (1948). *Universal declaration of human rights (UDHR).* Retrieved from www.un.org/en/universal-declaration-human-rights/

3

Finding meaning through storytelling in healthcare

Riya Elizabeth George and Graham Easton

Chapter contents:

- Storytelling and narrative-based practice in healthcare
- Stories in clinical consultations
- Identifying what makes a story: story elements and classic story structures
- Narrative consultation skills
- Storytelling and the challenges of Covid-19
- References

In the field of healthcare, it is often all too easy to forget a central concept: behind every patient is a story. So much of healthcare is about stories; the ones we hear, the ones we tell, and the ones we participate in. Stories can be used to untangle complicated clinical histories, patient experiences, explain healthcare information, and for healthcare advocacy (Zaharias, 2018). Traditional consultation frameworks largely address generic communicative skills and tend to analyse a consultation from a transactional point of view. In doing so, the nuances and subtleties of the clinical encounter are often missed. Additionally, the extent to which a healthcare practitioner can establish a human connection and understand what an illness *means* to a patient is less well defined. Patient narratives (a term interchangeably used with 'stories') repeatedly attest to the significance of these aspects, as do the narratives of healthcare practitioners who have experienced illness (Myers, 2008; Kiltzman, 2007). Yet, finding meaning in a clinical encounter remains a challenge – a challenge, that is further amplified for those with atypical communication.

This chapter explores the importance of storytelling and narrative-based practice and its use in facilitating meaning when communicating with patients. It discusses the different stories that are told in healthcare and how

DOI: 10.4324/9781003142522-5

this affects both the narrator and the listener. It identifies key components of what makes a story, describing how a patient typically tells a story and how a practitioner may interpret this. It discusses how we define what we really mean by 'story', outlining the key elements and structures of a story, and then goes on to think about a novel story model, which can be a useful way to identify and engage with stories in consultations. Narrative consultation skills are discussed with specific examples (such as storyboarding) included to support meaningful conversations with atypical communicators. Furthermore, how Covid has influenced how we tell and listen to stories in healthcare is also discussed.

Storytelling and narrative-based practice in healthcare

Despite advances in communication skills training, patients still frequently report complaints about healthcare practitioners not listening, appearing disinterested, interrupting, making assumptions, and not addressing patient concerns (Sincott et al., 2013). The changing landscape of healthcare, with unfamiliar people, locations, and terminology makes having everyday meaningful conversations challenging and patients have frequently reported that healthcare practitioners have lost sight of what really matters to patients. Narrative-based practice seeks to address this. According to Charon (2009), four factors may be contributing to these issues; firstly the 'context of illness', which describes the tendency for practitioners to view illness as a biological phenomenon, which may contrast to patients, who view their illness within the framework of their entire lives. Secondly, 'beliefs about disease causality'; patients generally have a different level of medical knowledge compared to practitioners, causing their notions of illness and its causes to differ widely. The third factor, 'the relation to mortality' denotes the many emotions that illness can elicit due to it being an unexpected event. These emotions colour one's attitude which is shaped by previous experiences, and this has the potential to conflict with the practitioner's perspective. Lastly, 'shame, blame, and fear', which describes the vulnerability that is implicitly inherent in clinical encounters. Patients may feel reluctant to share intimate aspects of themselves and practitioners may feel unsure or embarrassed to ask personal questions. Feelings of shame, blame, and fear can be inherent by-products of the experience of illness. Charon (2009) argues that acknowledging these four factors is essential to understanding the illness experience and what it means to the patient. This represents a fundamental shift from the practitioner's traditional stance of 'needing to solve the problem' to 'needing to understand'.

A fundamental tenet of narrative-based practice is that meaning is derived from stories (Claudini et al., 2011). Various definitions of narrative-based practice exist, many of which are found within medicine, Table 3.1 summarises key defining elements. Charon et al. (2016) defines narrative competence as the ability 'to recognise, absorb, interpret and be moved by the stories of illness' (p. 2). Healthcare practitioners spend much of the lives immersed in stories and narrative. From the beginning of when symptoms first started to appear to the completion of treatment, the experience of illness is told through a story. In every of episode of care, these stories are further proliferated into multiple accounts (either through interpretations, written reports, or comments passed between healthcare professionals) as different healthcare professionals attend to the patient's care. Despite great textual variation, these stories represent, what Ofri (2015) defines as a 'multi-voiced narrative of illness that is fundamental to and determining of a patient's care'. Launer (2013) argues that it is through conversation(s) between a patient and a practitioner that a shared understanding or a 'new story' is created. This understanding for the practitioner represents a closer approximation to the patient reality. Launer (2018) suggests we must see 'reality more like a tapestry of language that is continually being woven … we construct our view of reality by telling stories'. The benefits of narrative-based practice are summarised in Table 3.2.

Table 3.1 Definitions of narrative-based practice

What is narrative-based practice?
• Fundamentally about storytelling, the patient's story primarily, but also the doctor's (or healthcare practitioners) story and how these stories interweave in the clinical encounter to create a new story with new meaning and understanding and the possibility for change. • Acknowledging the uniqueness of each patient, validating their story and emphasising through genuine interest and concern. • Recognising the divide that can exist between the doctor (healthcare practitioner) and the patient and taking steps to bridge that divide by developing and strengthening connections. For the doctor (or healthcare professional) this entails listening closely, exploring fears, feelings and emotions; and developing a deeper understanding, not only of the illness experience but also of the patient and of the self.

Table 3.2 Advantages of narrative-based practice

Benefits of narrative-based practice
• Intrinsically therapeutic for the patient (in the telling and in being listened to). • Prevents the disconnect that might otherwise occur between the doctor (healthcare professional) and patient. • Promotes a deeper understanding of the patient and empathy. • Improves rapport and strengthens the doctor–patient relationship. • Enhances the doctor's (healthcare professional) powers of reflection (with respect to both patient and doctor). • Increases awareness. • Facilitates management as well as having the potential for considerable change.

Stories in clinical consultations

As a patient meets a healthcare practitioner, a conversation begins. The clinical consultation is brimming with stories. McWhinney's (1995) patient-centred interviewing model, shown in Figure 3.1 helpfully summarises three key stories present in the clinical encounter: the doctor's (or the healthcare practitioner's), the patient's, and the shared story they create. The model exemplifies the need to bridge the healthcare practitioner agenda, which emphasises the need to determine 'what is the matter with the patient' with the patient's agenda, which involves establishing 'what *matters* to the patient'. Patients may present several stories or just one – these may be complete or unfinished. They may change over time or vary according to who is listening. However they present themselves, these stories or narratives represent how the patient wishes to recount their experience of illness. These stories are often personal and add important context and meaning; failing to account for this in the diagnosis and treatment may likely compromise the care the patient receives (Easton, 2017). McWhinney (1995) claimed the

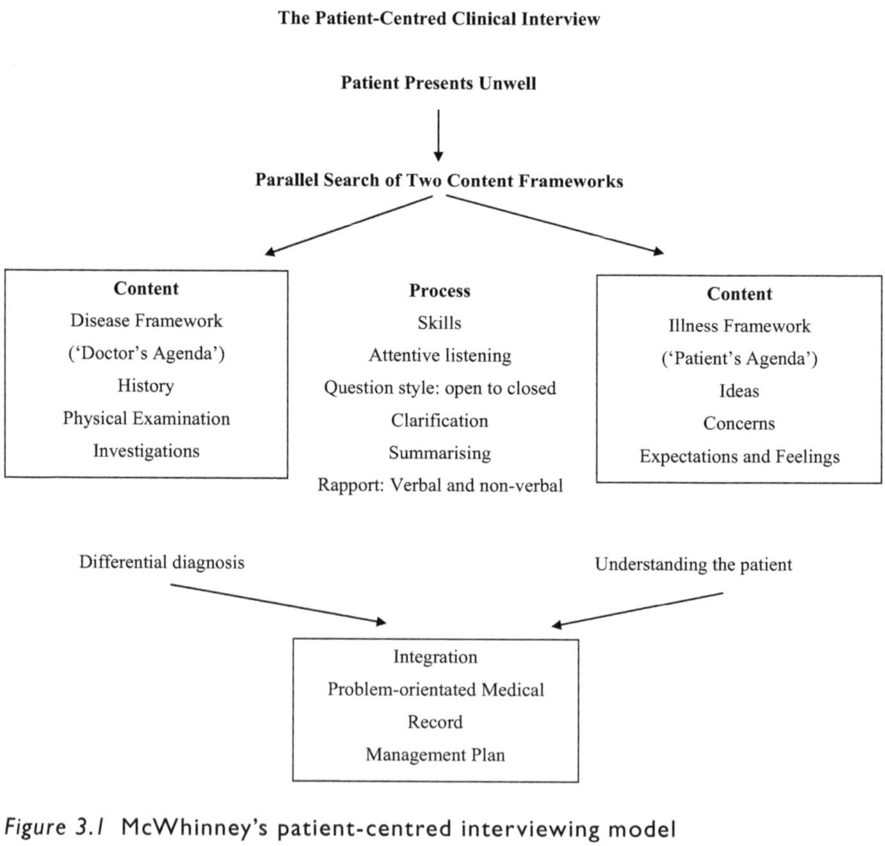

Figure 3.1 McWhinney's patient-centred interviewing model

greatest single problem in clinical interviewing is the failure to let the patient tell their story.

The practitioner also has their own story to 'tell'; these accounts are often driven by healthcare training and traditional notions of consultation interviewing skills. Medical narrative structures such as traditional clinical history taking tools (e.g. such as gathering the presenting complaint (PC), history of presenting complaint (HPC), past medical history (PMH), family history (FH), social history (SH), drug history (DH) etc.) and models for how to structure a consultation (e.g. the Cambridge Calgary Model) enable a stratification of the patient's story, filtering clinical and scientific details of disease from the patient's experience. Whilst these tools and models are hugely efficient at gathering relevant clinical information to guide diagnoses and treatments, they risk dehumanising patients by stripping the objective, factual details of disease from an individual's narration of suffering (Sobel, 2000). Clinical interviewing requires a careful balance of attending to both the practitioner's and patient's agenda and communicating in a way that puts the patient at the centre. Some patients may be not interested or reluctant to share their story and not every topic raised calls for detailed narrative exploration. This difficult juggling act can sometimes feel like rubbing your head whilst patting your stomach at the same time. Narrative-based practice goes beyond disease-framed, chronically ordered history taking, to seeing the patient as a person, and considers the entirety of their illness within their lived experience.

Storytelling is also an interactive social activity, a co-creation between the narrator and the listener. Mishler (1984) defines interplay between the two voices in a discourse as the voice of medicine and the voice of the patient's 'life-world'. In practical terms, this co-creation means involving the patient in decision making, negotiating a shared management plan, and often re-balancing the power dynamics in the consultation towards a patient-centred approach, thereby featuring the patient's story at the heart of the consultation (Easton, 2017). Multiple pieces of research strongly suggest that the patient-centred consultation correlates with clinical measures such as prescribing the right treatments, taking a reliable history and giving appropriate information (Roter & Hall, 2006). Furthermore, patient-centred interviewing facilitates a greater opportunity to empathise with patients and thereby enhance the practitioner–patient relationship. Growing evidence exists showcasing the benefits of shared decision making such as improved patient satisfaction, greater patient involvement, more confidence in decision making, and a greater likelihood of patients adhering to treatment and medical advice (De Silva, 2012).

Identifying what makes a story

Storytelling seems to be an almost in-built human instinct to bring order from the chaos of life. Yet how many of us could really describe what a story is? What are its key elements and recognisable patterns? What makes one account a story, and another not? If as health professionals we want to use stories as a useful consulting (or even therapeutic) tool, surely, we need to know what a story is, how to spot one, and how to construct useful ones?

Dictionaries tend to define a story along these lines:

> *a* description, *either* true *or* imagined, *of a* connected series *of* events.
> (Cambridge Dictionary online)

They are often very 'plot-driven' definitions; in other words, they focus on *events* unfolding over time. In most dictionaries, *story* is virtually synonymous with *narrative*, but they are different. It may seem pedantic to dwell on this, but the difference is important in order to grasp the elements that turn a basic narrative sequence of events into a potentially powerful and engaging story; the sort that our patients might tell in a consultation. The definition below is derived from an understanding of narrative from a wider pool of literature, including the fields of narratology, literary criticism, and linguistics:

> A sequence of events connected together in a way that gives them meaning.

Even though this definition of narrative introduces the importance of 'meaning' attached to a sequence of events (so distinguishing a narrative from a simple list, for example), it is still focused on the sequence of *events*. But within this very plot-driven definition of narrative there are many different genres of narrative (Riessman , 2002, p. 231); and story is just one, albeit a special type of narrative. All stories are narratives, but not all narratives are effective stories.

Story elements

Stories tend to be character-driven, and often have recognisable elements such as a protagonist or hero, some sort of struggle or conflict, and a climax and resolution. This is Scholes's widely used interpretation of story. He starts with a basic description of narrative, but then develops it to include those crucial 'story' elements:

> a telling or recounting of a string of events with at least three basic elements: 1) a situation involving some predicament, conflict or struggle, 2) an animate protagonist who engages with this situation for a purpose, 3) a plot during which the predicament is somehow resolved.
> (Scholes, 1982, p. 59)

Haven's definition of story pulls together the key elements into a succinct description:

> A detailed, character-based narration of a character's struggles to overcome obstacles and reach an important goal.
>
> (Haven, 2007, p. 79)

It is these key elements that seem to make stories so naturally appealing to humans and may explain why we make sense of life and our own identities through story (Bruner, 1986, 2002; Polkinghorne, 1988, 1996). We can identify with authentic characters and their struggles, we develop emotional connections with them, and we are invited to fill in any gaps in the stories using our imagination (Haven, 2007). As mentioned above, storytelling is a social activity too, so can be the glue that holds together cultural identity and meaning. It is no coincidence that we live in a 'story-shaped' world.

Classic story structures

In the classic story, these story elements are arranged into a story structure which has been used in Western cultures for thousands of years, from Greek myths and Bible stories to childhood fairy tales and Hollywood blockbusters. The simplest structure is the three-act structure which divides a story into three parts (acts), often called the Set Up, the Confrontation, and the Resolution. Act 1 (the Set Up) depicts the scene and the characters and ends by confronting the main character with a major challenge; Act 2 (the Confrontation) tells how the character struggles to overcome this challenge, usually failing; and Act 3 (the Resolution) resolves the story and its subplots, including the climax, the most intense point of the story.

In the 19th century, novelist Gustav Freytag further developed this basic 3-act structure into a narrative pyramid, describing the five key stages of a story, from start to finish. These stages are:

1. *Exposition* [setting the scene, the characters, and the world in which the story takes place].
2. *Rising action* [from the inciting incident, from which there is no turning back, the character's motivations, goals, and struggles, become clear].
3. *Climax* [when the story's conflict reaches a peak, and we learn the fate of the main characters].
4. *Falling action* [the aftermath of the climax, returning to a new normal].
5. *Resolution* [tying up loose ends].

Freytag's pyramid offers a visual representation of the classic story arc:

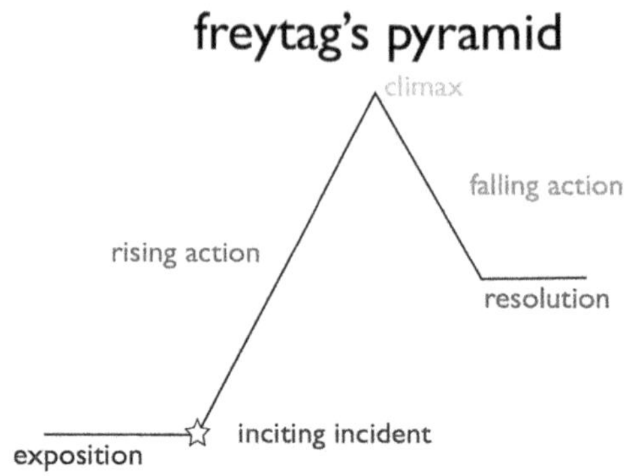

Figure 3.2 Freytag's pyramid – symbolising his theory of dramatic structure (Glatch, 2020)

Interestingly, story structures can vary across the globe and between cultures. Eastern cultures' stories often don't end with a clear resolution and tend to deal with multiple characters and sub plots, in contrast to the more individualistic journey of classic Western stories. In some native American Indian cultures story structures are not always linear with a beginning, middle, end. Rather, they are more circular and return to the starting point.

A structure for personal narratives

The classic 3- or 5-act story structure is a tool of the trade for film directors, TV producers, and writers. It is a tried and tested formula to engage an audience and hold the attention. But for most of us in daily life – including our patients – we don't tend to tell stories that way. We might include some of the key elements, or snippets of the classic structure. But most patient stories in consultations tend to be far less structured, and the elements not as carefully thought through. So what sorts of story structures do people tend to use when they are telling stories about themselves in everyday conversations?

William Labov is an American sociolinguist who studied hundreds of natural conversations in New York in the 1960s and 1970s (Labov & Waletsky, 1967) and concluded that *fully formed* natural personal narratives have six key ingredients:

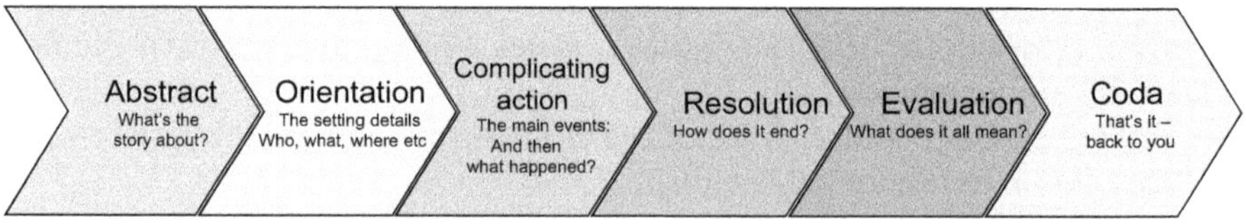

Figure 3.3 Adapted from Labov's sociolinguistic model of personal narratives (Labov & Waletsky, 1967)

Whilst there is debate over the merits and limitations of this model, particularly its focus on events rather than experience (Patterson, 2008), Labov's structural approach has been used widely in the field of personal narrative research – and most investigators either refer to it, use it, or adapt it for their own usage (Langellier, 1989). It has been used in researching patients' stories in consultations (Clark & Mishler, 1992) and for our purposes, it seems an evidence-based starting point for making sense of authentic personal stories – the type that most patients will be telling in consultations (Easton, 2017). Here is a brief description of each of the main stages in Labov's model (Easton, 2017):

1. Abstract [Opening]

This is a short summary of what is to come. In medical settings, the abstract might be 'I've got this rash doctor, and I think it's spreading. I've tried putting antiseptic cream on it but it just isn't going away'. We know that patients often prepare these abstracts before seeing the doctor or health professional – what Neighbour called 'opening gambits' (Neighbour, 2004).

2. Orientation [Details]

This section provides the 'who, what, when and where' information. It sets the scene. This stage is sometimes left out or provided much later in the story. Sometimes there is a lot of detail here which can distract from the main story: 'It was while I was out walking the dog, in Lemoin Park, just by the playground there, do you know it? Anyway, I was talking with my friend Claire, who teaches at the primary school, and suddenly she noticed the rash ...'.

3. Complicating Action [Main Events]

This is really reflecting the 'rising action' in a classic story, or Act 2 of the 3-act structure. It is where someone tells you the sequence of events, and how it has affected them and others. It may clarify the main character's goals and motivations, and any struggles or conflict getting in the way. If it doesn't, that can be a helpful focus for a therapeutic conversation. For example: 'First I didn't know what it was and thought it would go away. But it didn't. It just got worse and spread to my lower leg. The cream didn't work. It was getting really itchy so I couldn't sleep ....' And so on.

4. Resolution [Ending, or denouement]

This is the telling of the final key event of a story. Patients may come to the doctor looking for some resolution to their illness story, and it's the doctor's job to help to find some sort of acceptable resolution with the patient. This isn't always a happy ending; but some sort of resolution is usually required. If there has already been an ending ('the rash has disappeared now doc'), then the healthcare professional's role may be to clarify what sort of resolution or ending to the story the patient is looking for.

5. Evaluation [Meaning]

This section of the model makes the point of the story clear. Labov has described evaluation as 'perhaps the most important element in addition to the basic narrative clause' (Labov, 1972) and Riessman calls it the 'soul of the narrative', telling us what the point of the story is, as well as showing us how the narrator wants to be understood (Riessman, 2002). This is a crucial part of the patient's story, and often the part that doctors and health professionals have to tease out of the patient if it is not forthcoming. In medical education, we often refer to establishing the patient's Ideas, Concerns and Expectations (ICE); we might equally refer to it as clarifying the meaning, or evaluation, of the patient's story.

6. Coda [Hand-back]

This is a signal that the patient's story has ended, and it is now our tun to take the baton. An example might be: 'My wife said I should come because it's gone on so long, but I am not sure there is really anything you can do doc?' It's important that doctors/healthcare professionals recognise these end-of-story hand-backs – that's how patients tell us that it's our turn to speak.

Patients' stories are not always neat and linear as portrayed in Labov's diagram. Labov himself acknowledges that the evaluations – in other words the narrator's explanations about what the story means – are often spread over the entire story, not just at the end. As most health professionals will be aware , patients might start a story in the middle, or at the end, or even tell two or three concurrently. What is useful is to have a clear idea of the key elements and how they are important in telling an authentic personal story (Easton, 2017).

Some may have misgivings about this structured approach to storytelling – focused on *what* people say rather than *how* they say it, which does not preclude a deeper analysis of *how* people tell their stories in consultations. In fact, more in-depth consultation skills such as picking up on cues and paying attention to body language or paralanguage (meaning the non-lexical component of communication by speech, for example intonation, pitch, speed of speaking, and hesitation noises), may start to make more sense in the context of greater narrative structural understanding (Easton, 2017).

Narrative consultation skills

Table 3.3 highlights some generic examples of how healthcare professionals can make practical use of this narrative understanding of a consultation. John Launer, a general practitioner and family therapist, describes a useful conceptual framework for thinking about a narrative-based approach, called the seven Cs (Launer, 2002), outlined in Table 3.3.

Table 3.3 Questions and prompts useful in narrative-based practice

Questions and prompts useful in narrative-based practice
Exploratory questions and prompts: • Tell me about it • Tell me more • Is this something else? • Is there something that you are worried about? • What is worrying you most? • Has this ever happened before? • What else was happening at that time? • What do you think about ...? • What do others think about ...? • How do you feel [or react] when ....? • What does this mean for you? • What do you think might be causing ...? • How would you describe? • How do you explain?
Questions and prompts inviting change? • How else might you explain ...? • Are there any other possibilities? • Suppose ... • What would happen if ...? • If you had a magic want, what would you do? • What needs to happen for the situation to change? • If the situation did change, what would happen then? • What will happen if nothing changes?
(Zaharias, 2018; Adapted from Launer, 2002)

Table 3.3 Continued

Questions and prompts useful in narrative-based practice
Seven Cs (Launer, 2002) • Conversations Conversations can be used to describe and create reality. Launer argues that communication skills can elicit 'conversations that invite change', exploring connections, differences, new options and new realities. • Curiosity Curiosity can invite patients to reframe and reconstruct their stories. Curiosity also extends to the healthcare professional's own person – the exploration of one's own feelings, emotions and reactions to the patient's story. • Contexts Curiosity can be focused in this area. This is pertinent to the story and is often captured in the question 'why has this patient presented at this moment with this problem?' • Circularity This contrasts the traditional linear concept of cause and effect and unchangeable problems and instead helps the patient to focus on meanings. It acknowledges complexity and an awareness of the interconnectedness of things in order to counter fixed notions of cause and effect. This might involve circular questions (perhaps based on the words that patients use and using questions which promotes a descriptive rather than explanatory worldview). • Co-construction The aim to create a story with the patient that makes sense and gives meaning to their experience. • Challenge and caution Considers the importance to challenge the patient and one's self to consider new ideas and alternate explanations and to contemplate change and how that might be about realistically. It is also necessary to have an awareness of one's limitations and be sensitive to the patient and their needs, including willingness to go into unexplored areas and readiness for change. • Care Launer argues that 'nothing can be achieved if the practitioner does not genuinely care about the patient'.

Whilst these examples can be helpful to consider with most of the healthcare population, those with atypical communication are likely to require different strategies. Storyboarding can be a helpful technique and in simple terms is a graphical representation of how a story unfolds, event by event. Whilst its use has generally been confined as a pre-production tool for directors and playwrights, new evidence suggests merit in its application with atypical communicators. For those unable to or struggling to verbally articulate their story with its accompanying emotions and feelings, drawing pictures can help visualise the patient's experience and focus one's story in terms of specific events and the timing of those events. Storyboarding can be a creative tool to help patients pinpoint the sequence of events that led them to hospital or to explain the next steps. Additionally, using visual images such as a clock (changing the hands of the clocks) or a timeline can help the patient explain a sequence of events or thoughts.

Pictorial health information is another useful strategy to consider when having conversations with atypical communicators. The large majority of health information is verbal or written, however words alone have been shown to not be the most effective way to communicate health issues (Schubbe et al., 2018). Pictorial superiority is a term used to describe the tendency to understand information more easily when it is presented as pictures rather than words (Hockley et al., 2011). Furthermore, those with atypical communication and attention are shown to better respond to faces, objects, and pictures. Pictures can be used to explore patients' experiences and visceral responses such a pain, mood or motivation.

Health infographics are being increasingly used given the time pressured environment we often find ourselves in. They can be an effective way to capture in a concise manner the most salient health information or to summarise key recommendations or evidence. Examples can be found at the *British Medical Journal* (see weblink: www.bmj.com/infographics). Collectively employing these strategies can further help in creating a space and avenue for those with atypical communication to express their healthcare stories and experiences.

Storytelling and the challenges of Covid-19

The 'how' of storytelling is every bit as important as the 'what'. In fact, the non-verbal aspects of storytelling are more than half the story; research suggests that as much as 90% of communication is non-verbal – either how we use our voice, or through our body language (Lorié et al., 2017). During the Covid-19 pandemic, personal protective equipment (PPE) including face masks became the norm in healthcare. This physical barrier to facial and body communication also became an important obstacle to communication in healthcare (Hampton et al., 2020), including the telling and listening to patients' stories. In addition, the rapid move to remote and virtual consultations, either by telephone, or video, posed significant challenges to effective storytelling as maintaining eye contact became a complex skill on screen, and normal non-verbal cues disappeared.

In the last 20 years or so there has been mounting evidence of a close relationship between doctors' (or more broadly speaking healthcare professionals') non-verbal communication (in the form of eye contact, head nods and gestures, position, and tone of voice) with outcomes such as patient satisfaction, patient understanding, physician detection of emotional distress, and physician malpractice claim history (Silverman & Kinnersley, 2010). Non-verbal communication becomes most significant when there is a mismatch between verbal and non-verbal signals (Hall et al., 1995). In one fascinating observational study from Poland, doctors' tone of voice and degree of eye contact were particularly associated with patients picking up signs that their doctors seemed uninterested in them (Marcinowicz et al., 2010). In another detailed observational study of the effects of doctors' non-verbal behaviour on their patients, researchers found that eye contact and the posture of the doctor were influential in determining what the patient revealed in the consultation (Byrne & Heath, 1980). It is not hard to see how PPE, masks, and online or phone consultations can therefore block much of the vital signals in storytelling – whether someone is really interested in what you are saying, and therefore how much you are willing to reveal.

Non-verbal behaviour is also considered the most important medium for expressing empathy; in particular, the direction of gaze and body orientation (Brugel et al., 2015). It is clear now that empathic consultations, or doctors, can have important positive outcomes for patients from greater satisfaction to concrete physical outcomes such as better diabetic control or pain control. As online consultations and PPE-based consultations became the norm, expressions of empathy while sharing stories with patients became much more problematic. On screen, on the phone, or wearing face masks means it is much more difficult to read direction of gaze and body orientation – so harder to pick up on expressions of empathy, or to read non-verbal cues from patients which might signal an appropriate moment to express empathy.

One observational study established some of the significant obstacles to turn-taking during online consultations (Seuren et al., 2021), which impacted on telling and hearing stories in both directions. The researchers highlighted the importance of joint attention that involves getting camera angles and body position just right and working hard at maintaining appropriate gaze. They observed the need for increased verbalisation in turn taking to compensate for the reduction of verbal cues on screen.

Finally, for people with hearing impairment, face masks were a disaster for communication; both patients (Maru et al., 2021) and healthcare teams (for example in operating theatres (Hampton et al., 2020)) found hearing human voices particularly challenging. The implications for effective storytelling for the 1 in 6 of the UK population (and 1 in 2 over the age of 70) with hearing impairment are clear to see (Maru et al., 2021).

Conclusion

Healthcare deals with human beings. The consultation between healthcare professional and patient can be seen as a meeting of stories. Human life is more complicated than the science of the body alone and it is therefore important in healthcare to view the patient as a whole person rather than simply a list of symptoms to be fixed. A narrative understanding of what goes on during a consultation can offer new insights into the healthcare professional–patient encounter and may encourage a more patient-centred, collaborative approach. There are several practical techniques and principles that can guide practitioners in making the most of this narrative perspective in the consultation, including existing consultation models and skills designed to help patients tell their stories and to co-create a satisfactory shared story. Another potentially helpful tool is the model structure of personal narratives suggested by Labov, which offers practitioners a way to identify and engage with authentic narratives and their key elements.

References

Brugel, S., Postma-Nilsenová, M., & Tates, K. (2015). The link between perception of clinical empathy and nonverbal behavior: the effect of a doctor's gaze and body orientation. *Patient Education and Counseling, 98*(10), 1260–1265.

Bruner, J. (1986). *Actual minds, possible worlds.* Cambridge, MA: Harvard University Press.

Bruner, J. (2002). *Making stories.* New York: Farrar, Strauss, & Giroux.

Byrne, P. S., & Heath, C. C. (1980). Practitioners' use of non-verbal behaviour in real consultations. *The Journal of the Royal College of General Practitioners, 30*(215), 327–331.

Cambridge Dictionary Online link: https://dictionary.cambridge.org/dictionary/english/story (accessed 27 May 2022).

Charon, R. (2009). Narrative medicine as witness for the self-telling body. *Journal of Applied Commununication Research, 37*(2), 118–131.

Charon, R., Hermann, N., & Devlin, M. J. (2016). Close reading and creative writing in clinical education: teaching attention, representation, and affiliation. *Academic Medicine, 91*(3), 345–350.

Clandinin, J., Cave, M. T., & Cave, A. (2011). Narrative reflective practice in medical education for residents: composing shifting identities. *Advanced Medical Education Practice, 2*, 1–7.

Clark, J. A., & Mishler, E. G. (1992). Attending to patients' stories: reframing the clinical task. *Sociology of Health & Illness*, 14(3), 344–372.

De Silva, D. (2012). *Evidence: helping people share decisions.* London: The Health Foundation.

Easton, G. (2017). Stories in the consultation. In: C. Robertson and G. Clegg (Eds.), *Storytelling in medicine: how narrative can improve practice* (pp. 19–40). Boca Raton, FL: Taylor & Francis.

Glatch, S. (2020, May 21). *The 5 elements of dramatic structure: understanding Freytag's pyramid.* Retrieved from https://writers.com/freytags-pyramid

Hall, J. A., Harrigan, J. A., & Rosenthal, R. (1995). Nonverbal behavior in clinician–patient interaction. *Applied and Preventive Psychology, 4*(1), 21–35.

Hampton, T., Crunkhorn, R., Lowe, N., Bhat, J., Hogg, E., Afifi, W., … & Sharma, S. (2020). The negative impact of wearing personal protective equipment on communication during coronavirus disease 2019. *The Journal of Laryngology & Otology, 134*(7), 577–581.

Haven, H. (2007). *Story proof: the science behind the startling power of story.* Westport, CT: Libraries Unlimited.

Hockley, W. E., & Bancroft, T. (2011). Extensions of the picture superiority effect in associative recognition. *Canadian Journal of Experimental Psychology, 65*, 236–44.

Klitzman, R. (2007). *When doctors become patients.* New York, NY: Oxford University Press.

Labov, W., & Waletsky, J. (1967). Narrative analysis: oral version of personal experience. In: J. Helm (Ed.), *Essays on the verbal and visual arts.* Seattle, WA: University of Washington Press, 12–44.

Labov, W. (1972). *Sociolinguistic patterns.* Philadelphia, PA: University of Pennsylvania Press.

Langellier, K. M. (1989). Personal narratives: perspectives on theory and research. *Text and Performance Quarterly, 9*(4), 243–276.

Launer, J. (2002). *Narrative-based primary care: a practical guide.* Abingdon, UK: Radcliffe Publishing.

Launer, J. (2013). Narrative-based supervision. In *Clinical uncertainty in primary care* (pp. 147–161). New York, NY: Springer.

Launer, J. (2018). *Narrative-based practice in health and social care: conversations inviting change.* London: Routledge.

Lorié, Á., Reinero, D. A., Phillips, M., Zhang, L., & Riess, H. (2017). Culture and nonverbal expressions of empathy in clinical settings: A systematic review. *Patient Education and Counseling, 100*(3), 411–424.

Marcinowicz, L., Konstantynowicz, J., & Godlewski, C. (2010). Patients' perceptions of GP non-verbal communication: a qualitative study. *British Journal of General Practice, 60*(571), 83–87.

Maru, D., Stancel-Lewis, J., Easton, G., & Leverton, W. E. (2021). Communicating with people with hearing loss: COVID-19 and beyond. *BJGP open, 5*(1). https://doi.org/10.3399/BJGPO.2020.0174

McWhinney, I. R. (1995). *Patient centred medicine. transforming the clinical method.* Thousand Oaks, CA: Sage Publications.

Mishler, E. (1984). *The discourse of medicine: dialectics of medical interviews.* Norwood, N.J: Ablex.

Myers, K. R. (2008). A perspective on the role of stories as a mechanism of meta-healing. In: P. L. Rudnytsky & R. Charon (Eds.), *Psychoanalysis and narrative medicine* (pp. 199–208). Albany, NY: State University of New York Press.

Neighbour, R. (2004). *The inner consultation: how to develop an effective and intuitive consulting style* (2nd ed.). Abingdon, UK: Radcliffe Medical Press.

Ofri, D. (2015). The passion and the peril: storytelling in medicine. *Academic Medicine, 90*(8), 1005–1006.

Patterson, W. (2008). Narratives of events: Labovian narrative analysis and its limitations. In: M. Andrews, C. Squire & M. Tamboukou (Eds.), *Doing narrative research* (p. 176). Thousand Oaks, CA: Sage Publications.

Polkinghorne, D. E. (1996). Narrative knowing and the study of lives. In J. E. Birren (Ed.), *Aging and biography: explorations in adult development* (pp. 77–99). New York: Springer Publishing.

Polkinghorne, D. E. (1988). *Narrative knowing and the human sciences.* Albany, NY: SUNY Press.

Riessman, C. (2002). Narrative analysis. In A. Huberman & M. Miles (Eds.), *The qualitative researcher's companion.* Thousand Oaks, CA: Sage Publications.

Roter, D., & Hall, J. (2006). *Doctors talking with patients/patients talking with doctors: improving communication in medical visits* (2nd ed.). Westport, CT: Praeger.
Scholes, R. (1982). *Semiotics and interpretation.* New Haven, CT: Yale University Press.
Schubbe, D., Cohen, S., & Yen, R, W., et al. (2018). Does pictorial health information improve health behaviours and other outcomes? A systematic review protocol. *British Medical Journal Open*, *8*, e023300.
Seuren, L. M., Wherton, J., Greenhalgh, T., & Shaw, S. E. (2021). Whose turn is it anyway? Latency and the organization of turn-taking in video-mediated interaction. *Journal of pragmatics*, *172*, 63–78.
Silverman, J., & Kinnersley, P. (2010). Doctors' non-verbal behaviour in consultations: look at the patient before you look at the computer. *British Journal of General Practice*, *60*(571), 76–78.
Sinnott, C., McHugh, S., Browne, J., Bradley, C. (2013). GPs' perspectives on the management of patients with multimorbidity: systematic review and synthesis of qualitative research. *British Medical Jouornal Open*, *9*(3), e003610.
Sobel, R. J. (2000). Eva's stories: Recognizing the poverty of the medical case history. *Academic Medicine*, *75*(1), 85–89.
Zaharias, G. (2018). What is narrative-based medicine? Clinical review. *Canadian Family Physician*, *64*: 176–180.

Technology and atypical communication

A healthcare context

Yasmin Elsahar, Sijung Hu, David Kerr, and Kaddour Bouazza-Marouf

Chapter contents:

Introducing augmentative and alternative communication (AAC)

Verbal communication is an integral aspect of a typical healthcare setting. It enables patients to freely voice their individual needs through the explanation of their symptoms and the clarification of their health concerns. Difficulties arise when medical conditions are compounded with speech impairments, limiting a patient's ability to communicate with the healthcare providers. Such conditions can become restrictive and frustrating, as they prevent the patient from engaging in conversations to express their health-related concerns. Hodge (2007) explains that individuals with differing degrees of speech, language, and communication needs (SLCN) potentially suffer from extreme marginalisation in several aspects of their lives. Under the umbrella of assistive technologies (ATs), AAC techniques work to address the shortfall in speech production by complementing or replacing speech for persons with communication impairments. AAC methods encompass a variety of tools, mechanisms, and communication means, aiming to enable individuals

DOI: 10.4324/9781003142522-6

with SLCN to engage with their surroundings. AAC has been introduced for use in the healthcare context, as it has the potential of creating new paths through which the patients may reconnect with their professional healthcare consultants and carers.

In the context of AAC, 'speech' is usually used to describe the rapid motor movements involving the coordination of muscles to produce spoken words; whereas 'language' refers to the cognitive skill that is not confined to verbal communication (Cook & Polgar, 2015). A common attribute of modern AAC solutions tends to rely on the translation of a user's language into speech via speech-synthesis (Garcia et al., 2017; Kerr et al., 2016). AAC methods are classified into three categories depending on the level of technological complexity of the given solutions. These include no-tech AAC (interpretation of sign language, facial expressions, and body movements to deliver non-verbal messages), low-tech AAC (utilisation of books or board displays to communicate messages), and medium-high-tech AAC (use of powered electronic devices for assisted communication). Devices falling under the category of high-tech AAC integrate hardware and software in the design of solutions serving patients with SCLN. This expands to include the use of mobile devices, portable electronic devices, or specialist equipment specifically developed to produce digitised or synthesised speech to support the communication processes (Communication Matters, 2020). This chapter outlines the current AAC technologies and provides an overview of the benefits and challenges pertaining to predominant technological AAC tools used in the context of healthcare.

Failures of communication between patients and healthcare providers may be linked to severe medical missteps, increased treatment costs, and deteriorating health conditions (Blackstone & Pressman, 2011). Patients with communication disabilities are more likely to experience adverse medical events if the communication process between the patient and the healthcare provider is poor (Hemsley & Balandin, 2014). To overcome this problem, AAC tools are usually introduced. However, the diverse realm of AAC solutions and the range of disabilities encountered by healthcare professionals introduces a set of challenges when it comes to the management of successful patient–healthcare provider communication.

In terms of disabilities, the complex composition of the human body means that speech and communication impairments requiring a form of AAC intervention, result from diverse medical conditions (Communication Matters, 2020; Smith & Delargy, 2005). These include (but are not limited to) autistic spectrum disorder (ASD), strokes, learning disabilities, locked-in syndrome, head and neck cancers, and brain injuries. This also expands to include patients with progressive diseases, such as Parkinson's disease, and amyotrophic lateral sclerosis (National Institute of Neurological Disorders and Stroke, 2020; Communication Matters, 2020).

Rehabilitation aids might support a range of users in regaining some communication functions (Smith & Delargy, 2005). For example, high-tech AAC is currently seen as having the potential to aid the communication process of individuals with SLCN in intensive care units (ICUs; Ju, Yang, & Liu, 2020). However, the diverse medical conditions requiring the use of an AAC intervention mean that generic AAC tools may not be ideal for efficient patient–provider communication, specifically within a hospital environment. Waller (2019) explains that AAC systems need to be flexible and adaptable given the increased and diverse severity levels of disabilities in combination with increasing human life expectancy. Fager et al. (2020) similarly demonstrates that a potential need exists for the personalisation of AAC systems to meet the specific and individual requirements of the assistive communication user.

Ideally, the development of an AAC solution needs to be guided by AAC users, carers of the users, healthcare consultants, and speech and language therapists to tailor the AAC development to serve its specific user's needs, as schematically displayed in Figure 4.1. The interplay between these key contributors is essential to design solutions benefiting the users and optimising the performance of AAC platforms through regular feedback and ongoing

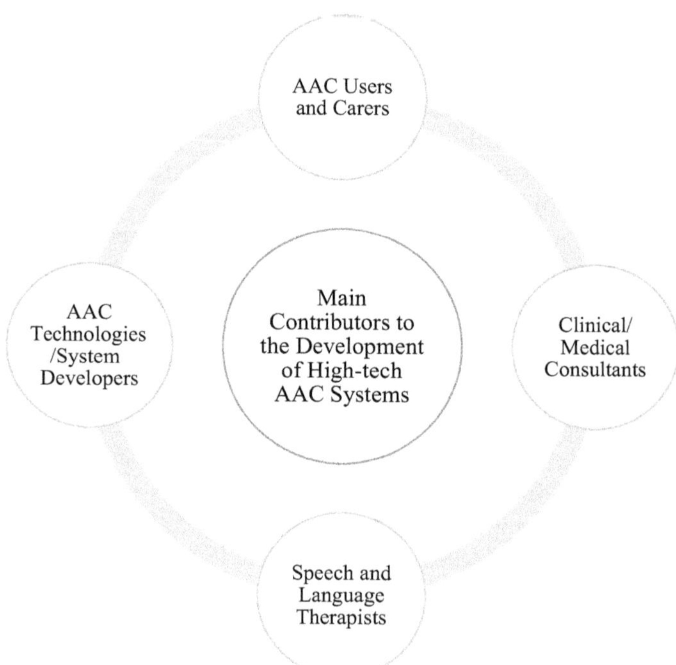

Figure 4.1 Main contributors to the development of effective high-tech AAC systems

observation and monitoring. Uthoff et al. (2021) highlights that along with the knowledge about AAC and the communication between contributors, the facilitation of collaborations is subject to a set of factors. These principally comprise of adequate time resources and planning of the necessary finances to support such collaborations.

Several frameworks have been introduced in the literature to model the relationships between the person and the environment, such as the Canadian Model of Occupational Performance and Engagement (CMOP-E) and the Person Environment Occupation and Performance (PEOP) (Cook & Polgar, 2015). In the specific context of the interaction with AT, the Human Activity Assistive Technology (HAAT) model presented by Cook & Polgar (2015) highlights the key interactions between four essential components of communication with individuals with complex communication needs (CCN): the activity, the human, the context, and the AT.

Common healthcare settings where AAC technologies are used include clinics, emergency rooms, ICUs, and acute care hospitals (Blackstone & Pressman, 2011). Nonetheless, Cook and Polgar (2015) explain that the context of intervention use goes beyond the physical environment, encompassing a broader range of external factors (e.g., social, institutional, and cultural) affecting a person's use of AT over a length of time. In this sense, the correct governance of AAC interventions in the healthcare context could have a direct impact on the quality of care and medical outcomes. The optimisation of such an interaction is consequently necessary to ensure a good patient experience (Blackstone, 2009).

Given the diverse nature of the users of communicators with CCN and the requirement to help groups of patients with different abilities to communicate, research efforts have been redirected to establish AT systems tailored to respond to individual users' needs, rather than off-the-shelf solutions. At the core of this concept, the healthcare provider (in collaboration with AAC specialists) may need to assess the condition of the user to determine which AAC tools are likely to be of benefit for the patient. For example, interventions needed for pre-treatment and post-treatment scenarios may differ. For the latter, AAC use during recovery and rehabilitation may allow the patients more time to select, trial, and learn how to effectively use an AAC system for communication. For the former, it may be the case that a rather different kind of AAC is needed, particularly one that does not require a lengthy training process to use.

Although low-tech AAC solutions (e.g., display boards, books with lexicons of images and phrases) are still widely used due to their affordability and availability, high-tech AAC possesses the potential to provide user-tailored solutions if the process is correctly managed. The next section outlines the current predominant high-tech AAC solutions and discusses these technologies in terms of the benefits and challenges in the healthcare context.

Technological AAC interventions in the healthcare context

Present high-tech AAC applications

High-tech AAC devices can be activated through a variety of purposeful signals generated by the human body. The signals represent a measured variation corresponding to specific body movements, such as purposeful gestures, eye movements, respiratory patterns, or brain activity signals. The systems' interfaces are programmed to respond to the signals and output specific communicative responses. Figure 4.2 shows common high-tech AAC systems, including eye gaze systems, portable devices activated via advanced switches or touchscreens, breath activated systems, and brain computer interface (BCI) systems.

Most of the listed AAC modalities could be used either in a standalone format and/or in combination with one another as an AAC system. For example, several commercial solutions combine eye gazing, touch screens, and advanced switch capabilities for a multimodal device access for the accommodation of individual needs. Utilising ATs, and specifically AAC solutions, could have potential benefits to improve the communication of individuals with CCN; however, tailoring optimised solutions to the individual needs of patients in the healthcare context is subject to an additional set of challenges.

Benefits of high-tech AAC in healthcare

Ensuring swift communication between the patient and the healthcare provider comes with an extensive set of benefits. In the typical setting of a healthcare consultation, a patient's free expression helps in the process of diagnosis and adherence to the prescribed regimens of treatment (Blackstone & Pressman, 2011). Such benefits also expand to include several other aspects in relation to the broader context of communication in the healthcare setting. In terms of the physical settings, AAC could provide means of communication

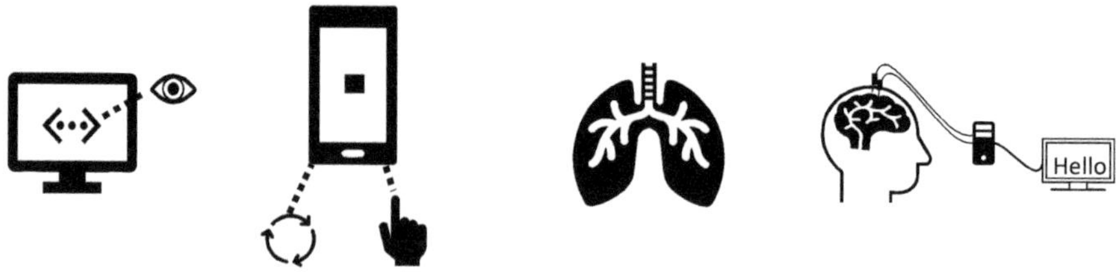

(a) Eye gaze systems (b) Switch scanning and touch-based devices (c) Breath activated solutions (d) Brain computer interface

Figure 4.2 Common activation methods of high-tech AAC devices, (BCI image source: Williams, 2021)

for patients in doctors' offices, medical care units, ICUs, rehabilitation hospitals, long-term care facilities, as well as home care. However, communication with the help of an AAC tool is subject to several technical and contextual challenges, thus requiring further management.

For successful patient–provider communication, the assessment of individual user requirements and the challenges related to the use of the intended technology within a specific context are essential (Gosnell, Costello, & Shane, 2011). Simion (2014) explains that individuals benefiting from AAC interventions can be classified into three major groups based on their medical conditions and/or the intended use of the AAC aid. These three user categories are:

1. Alternative-language users: users who lack the abilities to produce articulated words and understandable phrases but have a well-established cognitive understanding of language and speech.
2. Augmentative-language users: users who have difficulties both in understanding speech and in conversing. To be able to use an AAC device, augmentative-language users need assistance in the re-categorisation of their surroundings into labels they can comprehend and could hence integrate to form a communication language.
3. Temporary AAC users: users who require AAC interventions for a limited time, e.g., children with developmental conditions and adults who require transient speech assistance following surgical intervention or while in a medical state prohibiting oral communication.

The assessment of the patient's conditions and capabilities to determine a suitable AAC intervention is crucial. This includes aspects of whether the patient has any experience of using an AAC device and the specific context in which the intervention is required. In the Venn diagram in Figure 4.3, the overlap of technical and contextual challenges of using AAC devices in the healthcare setting is depicted. Balancing solutions for the challenging

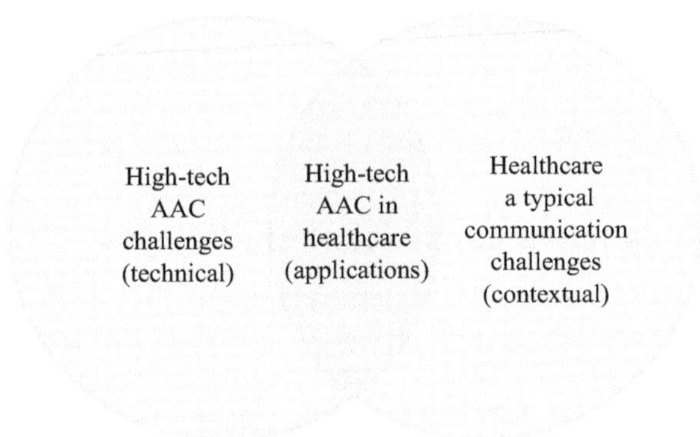

Figure 4.3 Overlap of technical and contextual challenges of using AAC devices in healthcare applications

aspects of user requirements, the capabilities of the deployed AT, and the context in which the device is used is essential to ensure effective patient–provider communication. Tackling both the technical and contextual challenges related to high-tech AAC in healthcare allows for the development of optimised AAC applications.

Tackling technical challenges

As demonstrated in Figure 4.3, numerous means of activation of high-tech AAC devices are used by individuals with CCN. Nevertheless, a set of technical challenges is still apparent in the general area of high-tech AAC for communication. Lindsay (2010) demonstrates that viewing technology as a cure alongside the increased complexity of the devices could be among the first technical barriers for communication, especially for children. The adaptability of the solutions to respond to individual user's needs is also variable. 'Off-the-shelf' devices still lack this and might require cumbersome efforts and/or extensive user training to effectively utilise an AAC intervention. Moreover, instances have been reported where system developers might prioritise the needs of the technology over the needs of the patient. In other words, some high-tech AAC systems may still lack hardware and software functionalities to address the real patient's requirements. This results in drawbacks in terms of continuous use of the AAC system, user satisfaction, and might even lead to device abandonment and user frustration (Hodge, 2007). Table 4.1 displays commonly used high-tech AAC activation modes from a technical point of view, including their associated benefits and challenges. The listed device activation methods include eye gazing, advanced switching, touchscreens, breath activation, and BCI.

In the technical sense, the general usability of high-tech AAC devices is highly interconnected with the ease of acquisition of user-generated control signals together with the technical robustness of the control interfaces. For example, a continuous need to calibrate an AAC device (e.g., eye gaze) or the necessity of extensive assistance to operate a system (e.g., BCI) could result in user frustration or reduced usage. Maintaining a balance between the maximisation of signal information content and minimal activation requirements introduces a bandwidth of beneficial usability features (Elsahar et al., 2019).

Tackling healthcare contextual challenges

In addition to the technical barriers related to high-tech AAC devices, healthcare professionals may be affected by social and contextual factors when assessing which AAC devices may be suitable for a patient. Blackstone (2009) explains that the healthcare setting poses an extra layer of communication challenges between the patient and the healthcare provider, given that the situations are often tense, at a fast pace, and the interacting parties are generally strangers. This is further complicated by the linguistic,

Table 4.1 Benefits and technical challenges of predominant high-tech AAC devices activation modes, adapted from Elsahar et al. (2019)

High-tech AAC modes	*Benefits*	*Technical challenges*
Eye gazing devices	• Non-invasive. Infrared is also invisible to the user's eyes. • Require minimal voluntary control of muscles. • Can be used with patients requiring mechanical ventilation.	• High cost. • Require complex data processing and programming. • Need extensive calibration and training.
Scanning switches and mechanical keyboards	• Require minimal motor control. • Provide an instant feedback mechanism.	• Slow.
Touchscreens	• Require minimal pressure for activation. • Widely available (common portable devices).	• No direct feedback mechanism (need to append auditory/sensory feedbacks).
Breath activated devices	• Involve minimal voluntary control of muscles.	• Slow conversational rates depending on the way breathing is encoded.
Brain computer interface (BCI)	• Can be activated with minimal body movements.	• • Highly complex systems. • Require extensive assistance from carers and healthcare professionals.

cultural, and behavioural barriers precluding the establishment of meaning between the patient and the healthcare professional. In this context, O'Halloran, Hickson, and Worrall (2008) show that the attitudes of healthcare providers towards individuals with CCN play an integral role in facilitating or impeding the communication process. The authors also demonstrate that healthcare providers need to be aware of the influences of communication disabilities and their impact on the interaction with specific patients. The environmental aspect within the context of healthcare itself might also introduce a layer of challenges. For example, Jansson et al. (2019) demonstrate that due to the nature of physical and medical conditions of patients in ICUs, healthcare professionals may need to optimise the facilitation of communication using a variety of tools to respond to the unique needs of each specific medical case.

To establish meaning, it is essential for healthcare professionals to match a user's real capabilities with the correct high-tech AAC systems for the specific context of usage. There also exists a need to segregate the disabilities of individuals with CCN to optimise the necessary communication skills and AAC tools required to deal with a specific disability. This also includes the need to monitor all changes related to the patient's medical conditions which may alter the communication requirements of the patient, for instance, during recovery (Santiago et al., 2020).

Steps for action for optimised AAC applications in healthcare

The maximisation of the quality of patient–provider communication is subject to the management of the interactions between the people within the context of healthcare provision (Clancy, Povey, & Rodham, 2018). For AAC to be successful, healthcare providers need communication training and patients need access to an arsenal of communication tools and strategies, including some simple, easy-to-use AAC approaches (Blackstone, 2009). Successful patient–provider communication revolves around three main areas, namely the specific user needs, the AAC intervention being used, and the training aspect related to the usage of the technology for the governance of the communication process. The main components constituting this process are shown in Figure 4.4.

The multidimensional nature of the training required for all communication parties to attain optimal results from the use of AAC interventions remains a challenging process for efficient patient provider communication. However, the establishment of training protocols and unified strategies to overcome this challenge has been receiving increasing research efforts within the healthcare context. For example, the communication partner training (CPT) strategy to support individuals with aphasia is reported to potentially aid in the establishment of a more accessible environment for patients with aphasia within a hospital context (Heard, Anderson, & Horsted, 2020).

The patient, the healthcare provider, and the carer/communication partner are all key players in the process of jointly establishing meaning during

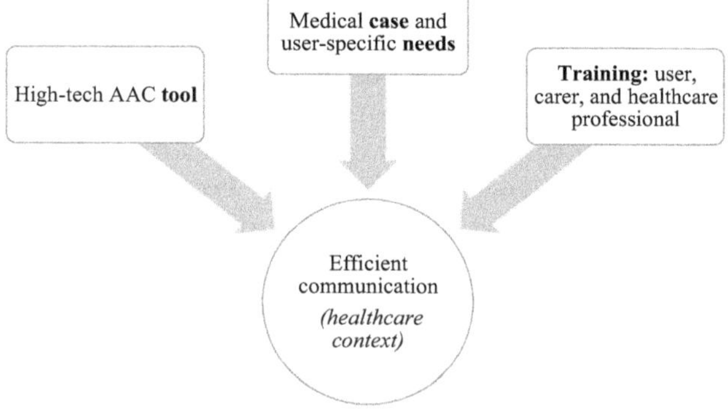

Figure 4.4 The basic components governing the communication process of individuals with CCN in the healthcare context

patient–provider interactions. Depending on the specific context of usage and the situational challenges that may impede successful communication, training protocols for patients to utilise an AAC intervention and for healthcare providers and communication partners to support this process are essential. A study by Simmons et al. (2019) shows that a group of nurses reported limited knowledge with regards to AAC usage, but expressed a strong desire to support their patients through AAC. Heard, Anderson, & Horsted (2020) similarly reported that providing nurses dealing with patients with adequate background information and arrays of AAC interventions and/or resources might result in improved communication within a hospital environment. Evidence increasingly suggests that appropriate training and tools availability play a major role in successful patient–provider communication. Improved communication improves the safety of patients with SLCN who are critically ill, forming a pressing need from healthcare professionals to learn, use, and apply the appropriate AAC strategies (Handberg & Voss, 2018).

Future AAC in healthcare

Given the complexity of the user base, and the escalating need for AAC solutions to serve diverse groups of individuals with speech disabilities, current research efforts are being redirected towards the establishment of assistive systems that are suited to respond to the personal user's needs and capabilities (Elsahar et al., 2019). In terms of assisting communication, research shows that the technical hurdles are often centred on the need for further research when it comes to non-typical conversation based on the user's past experiences, preferences, and communication patterns (Waller, 2019). Extended benefits based on state-of-the-art applications in the area of artificial intelligence (AI) could assist individuals with CCN. For example, Gibson et al. (2020) demonstrate that simple mobile applications, such an interface allowing patients utilising AAC to select their symptoms prior to the medical consultation process, could be beneficial for improved patient–provider communication. It aids in supporting the messages the patient wants to communicate and in turn shows that solutions could be sought to health conditions that may have otherwise been overlooked by the healthcare provider.

Other examples of utilising AI with high-tech AAC include the deployment of technology to label the objects in the vicinity of the user. This allows the prediction of the environment of use and the customisation of the AAC tool in accordance with the surroundings of the patient.

Decision algorithms are also being utilised to match a patient's abilities with suitable AAC interventions (Istanboulian et al., 2020). In this sense, customising solutions powered by AI could be beneficial for improved patient–provider communication. However, as demonstrated throughout this chapter, ensuring that AAC technologies are adapted to respond to the unique needs of the user remains an essential component for efficient device utilisation. The subsequent case studies provide further illustrations of how ACC technologies can be utilised in a patient-centred manner.

Case study 4.1 Sanjev

A 29-year-old male, PhD student, and lecturer in psychology was suddenly admitted to hospital with a tumour on the brainstem. The patient suffered limited vision, loss of motor control in all limbs, and Anarthrica (he could no longer generate any speech sounds). However, he had some low power thumb adduction and a small amount of rotation of his head was possible. He was in an ICU, where a specialist AAC team assessed his needs. The patient had a good level of support and was highly motivated to carry on with his studies. A paper-based AAC system was provided. His communication partner would read letters of the alphabet and look at his moves to select those letters. Next, two thumb buttons were provided. These were placed in his hands using polymorph, a mouldable plastic that firms up after heating. This allowed him to scan and select items on a computer running specialist software. The AAC team next taught him Morse code as an efficient method of using his two buttons. Technology was sought that allowed the patient to enter text to any system and write in this way.

Case study 4.2 Matthew

Matthew, an 11-year-old boy with cerebral palsy suffered a condition affecting his motor control in all four limbs and his ability to be understood by others. Cognitively, he was on par with his peers. The patient was observed to have difficulty coordinating his limbs but had good head control and could eyepoint to items in the room. He used this efficiently to access a paper-based communication book to point to symbols. Head-operated mice were explored to aid communication, but this was sometimes difficult to control, overshooting items on the display screen. Switches were then assessed as suitable to be controlled at the left and right side of his head. He made few mistakes selecting items on a screen, but the process was effortful and slow. Eye gaze equipment was trialled and was observed as having potential as he could target and select items on a screen. He made some mistakes but learned quickly how to pause and resume the system. Despite having access to equipment and being cognitively able, the patient and his school still required significant training and support as to how to integrate this technology for activities such as writing, maths, and art.

Communication guidelines

I. Collaboration is required between healthcare providers to ensure patients with CCN are adequately supported. Collaborations between speech and language therapists, clinicians, and nurses to identify AAC interventions suitable for patients and the best means of establishing communication are of paramount importance.

II. Generic AAC devices may not be ideal for efficient patient–provider communication. The customisation of AAC devices to serve the specific needs of the patient would result in improved communication by matching a patient's capabilities with the corresponding high-tech AAC system.

III. Training is an essential component for effective communication when utilising AAC technologies. Protocols and strategies need to be implemented for specific contexts and individual groups of users. Efficient training of the patient, the provider, and the communication partner increases the benefits of utilising AAC tools by establishing a well governed communication process.

IV. The attitude of healthcare providers towards individuals with CCN plays an important role in facilitating or impeding the communication process, given that the situations of AAC use in healthcare settings are often tense. Supporting patients through optimised protocols and efficient training helps create a more accessible communication environment.

V. The degree of engagement and successful communication using high-tech AAC interventions may vary across groups of patients suffering the same disability as a result of individual conditions and challenges. Specialised AAC professionals may help in the process of providing communicative solutions and the customisation of AAC interventions to suit the needs of the patients for improved communication.

Summary

Training protocols and effective patient–provider communication strategies are integral aspects of efficient communication for individuals with CCN in the healthcare context. Diverse user conditions and unique user requirements indicate that the customisation of AAC interventions is essential for the establishment of meaning. Similarly, the development of protocols governing the use of AAC interventions within different contexts, such as pre-treatment and post-treatment is essential for improved patient–provider communication. Collaborations between healthcare providers and AAC specialists, high-tech AAC developers, and communication partners enrich and enhance the atypical communication process and form an integral aspect for future AAC in healthcare.

Acknowledgement

The authors would like to acknowledge the support of the ACE Centre for the provision of the case studies, as well as the support of Loughborough University in this research.

References

Blackstone, S. (2009). Clinical news. *Augmentative Communication News, 21*(2), 1.

Blackstone, S., & Pressman, H. (2011). *Providing communication access: converging solutions to effective patient–provider communication*. Retrieved 8 March 2022, from www.patientprovidercommunication.org/files/Providing Communication Accessfinal for posting.pdf

Clancy, L., Povey, R., & Rodham, K. (2018). 'Living in a foreign country': experiences of staff–patient communication in inpatient stroke settings for people with post-stroke aphasia and those supporting them. *Disability and Rehabilitation, 42*(3), 324–334.

Communication Matters. (2020). What is AAC? | *Communication Matters*. Retrieved 21 February 2020, from www.communicationmatters.org.uk/page/what-is-aac

Cook, A., & Polgar, J. M. (2015). *Assistive technologies principles and practices* (4th ed.). New York: Elsevier.

Elsahar, Y., Hu, S., Bouazza-Marouf, K., Kerr, D., & Mansor, A. (2019). Augmentative and alternative communication (AAC) advances: a review of configurations for individuals with a speech disability. *Sensors, 19*(8), 1911.

Fager, S., Burnfield, J., Pfeifer, C., & Sorenson, T. (2020). Perceived importance of AAC messages to support communication in rehabilitation settings. *Disability and Rehabilitation: Assistive Technology, 16*(7), 796–801.

Garcia, R., Ibarra, J., Paglinawan, C., Paglinawan, A., Valiente, L., Sejera, M., Bernal, M., Cortinas, W. J., Dave, J., Villegas, M. (2017). Wearable augmentative and alternative communication device for paralysis victims using brute force algorithm for pattern recognition. In *IEEE 9th International Conference on HNICEM* (pp. 1–6).

Gibson, R., Dunlop, M., Bouamrane, M.-M., & Nayar, R. (2020). Designing clinical AAC tablet applications with adults who have mild intellectual disabilities. In *Proceedings of the 2020 CHI Conference on Human Factors in Computing Systems* (pp. 1–13). New York: ACM.

Gosnell, J., Costello, J., & Shane, H. (2011). Using a clinical approach to answer 'What communication apps should we use?' *Perspectives on Augmentative and Alternative Communication, 20*(3), 87–96.

Handberg, C., & Voss, A. (2018). Implementing augmentative and alternative communication in critical care settings: perspectives of healthcare professionals. *Journal of Clinical Nursing, 27*(1–2), 102–114.

Heard, R., Anderson, H., & Horsted, C. (2020). Exploring the communication experiences of stroke nurses and patients with aphasia in an acute stroke unit. *Speech, Language and Hearing, 25*(2), 177–191.

Hemsley, B., & Balandin, S. (2014). A metasynthesis of patient–provider communication in hospital for patients with severe communication disabilities: informing new translational research. *AAC: Augmentative and Alternative Communication, 30*(4), 329–343.

Hodge, S. (2007). Why is the potential of augmentative and alternative communication not being realized? Exploring the experiences of people who use communication aids. *Disability & Society, 22*(5), 457–471.

Istanboulian, L., Rose, L., Gorospe, F., Yunusova, Y., & Dale, C. (2020). Barriers to and facilitators for the use of augmentative and alternative communication and voice restorative strategies for adults with an advanced airway in the intensive care unit: A scoping review. *Journal of Critical Care, 57*, 168–176.

Jansson, S., Martin, T., Johnson, E., & Nilsson, S. (2019). Healthcare professionals' use of augmentative and alternative communication in an intensive care unit: A survey study. *Intensive and Critical Care Nursing, 54*, 64–70.

Ju, X.-X., Yang, J., & Liu, X.-X. (2020). A systematic review on voiceless patients' willingness to adopt high-technology augmentative and alternative communication in intensive care units. *Intensive and Critical Care Nursing, 63*, 1–10.

Kerr, D., Bouazza-Marouf, K., Gaur, A., Sutton, A., & Green, R. (2016). A breath controlled AAC system. *The Journal of Communication Matters-ISAAC(UK), 30*(3), 11–13.

Lindsay, S. (2010). Perceptions of health care workers prescribing augmentative and alternative communication devices to children. *Disability and Rehabilitation: Assistive Technology, 5*(3), 209–222.

National Institute of Neurological Disorders and Stroke. (2020). Amyotrophic lateral sclerosis (ALS) fact sheet. NIH Publication No. 16–916.

O'Halloran, R., Hickson, L., & Worrall, L. (2008). Environmental factors that influence communication between people with communication disability and their healthcare providers in hospital. *International Journal of Language and Communication Disorders, 43*(6), 601–632.

Santiago, R., Howard, M., Dombrowski, N., Watters, K., Volk, M., Nuss, R., ... Rahbar, R. (2020). Preoperative augmentative and alternative communication enhancement in pediatric tracheostomy. *The Laryngoscope, 130*(7), 1817–1822.

Simion, E. (2014). Augmentative and alternative communication: support for people with severe speech disorders. *Procedia – Social and Behavioral Sciences, 128*, 77–81.

Simmons, A., McCarthy, J., Koszalinski, R., Hedrick, M., Reilly, K., & Hamby, E. (2019). Knowledge and experiences with augmentative and alternative communication by paediatric nurses: a pilot study. *Disability and Rehabilitation: Assistive Technology, 16*(6), 567–579 .

Smith, E., & Delargy, M. (2005). Locked-in syndrome. *British Medical Journal, 330*, 406–409.

Uthoff, S., Zinkevich, A., Boenisch, J., Sachse, S., Bernasconi, T., & Ansmann, L. (2021). Collaboration between stakeholders involved in augmentative and alternative communication (AAC) care of people without natural speech. *Journal of Interprofessional Care, 35*(6), 821–831 .

Waller, A. (2019). Telling tales: unlocking the potential of AAC technologies. *International Journal of Language and Communication Disorders, 54*(2), 1–11.

Williams, S. (2021). *Brain–computer interface user types 90 characters per minute with mind.* Retrieved 29 July 2021 from www.the-scientist.com/news-opinion/brain-computer-interface-user-types-90-characters-per-minute-with-mind-68762

Part II

Practical guidance for working with children and families

5

Children and young people with atypical communication in healthcare

Mari Viviers and Louise Edwards

Chapter contents:

- Communication in context
- Cultural and diversity factors
- Legislation and governance considerations
- Supporting and empowering healthcare professionals
- The role of the multidisciplinary team in supporting communication
- Strategies for supporting communication
- Clinical case studies: optimising communication
- Resources for healthcare professionals to support communication
- Recommended resources
- References

Children and young people with atypical communication are increasingly seen in a variety of healthcare settings, and healthcare professionals may not have the skills and training needed to support this patient group. This chapter presents information on a range of atypical communication disorders, which may be linked either to congenital or to acquired conditions. We provide some strategies to support effective communication and introduce the role of the speech and language therapist in the multidisciplinary team. If children and young people are not to be restricted in their participation in educational, vocational, family, and community environments, including healthcare, their communication disorders must be addressed and their needs for support must be met. We explore the hierarchy of communication, with an emphasis on a child-led approach that is based on the child's skill rather than their age. We describe some resources available to healthcare professionals for their own learning and to support the families, children and young people that they serve. Finally, we use practical examples to empower healthcare professionals to optimise their communication to enable

DOI: 10.4324/9781003142522-8

maximum participation. The message for everyone in healthcare, but especially for those working with people who have communication disorders, is to 'make every interaction count'.

We consider children and young people with atypical communication as part of congenital or acquired conditions. These conditions include neurological problems (e.g. cerebral palsy, neuromuscular disorder), anatomical problems (e.g. cleft palate, children and young people requiring tracheostomy), chromosomal or genetic disorders (e.g. Down syndrome, 22q11 syndrome), and other acquired conditions (e.g., head injury, tumours). Recognising typical expectations of child development enables us to understand and suggest ways to respond to atypical presentations. If we expect a child aged seven to show the beginnings of logical concrete thinking, we cannot expect them to understand abstract concepts or metaphors. When explaining procedures, it is important to remember what level of understanding can be expected in order to ensure honesty in exchanges. Another example involving a child aged seven who has atypical communication needs may even need concrete language to be reinforced with other communication methods, such as modelling, visual or pictographic aids, or use of toys or gesture, to be sure of understanding and engagement.

Communication in context

Our focus will be on children and young people presenting in a healthcare setting with a range of communication abilities and needs. These abilities may co-occur with other diagnoses that then exacerbate the communication challenge, for example, a young person with a communication problem who also has ongoing speech sound errors from a previous cleft lip and palate repair (Kummer, 2018). We recognise that developmental problems can also be co-occurring in the population of children considered atypical communicators. It is important to note that poor communication by the healthcare professional can lead to compromised outcomes for the patient and family (Bell & Condren, 2016). Whilst we have included examples of diagnoses that may include atypical communication, it is important that healthcare professionals do not assume communication need or ability based on diagnosis.

Damm et al. (2015) noted that the relationships among healthcare professionals, child, and parent or carer can be complex, and indeed most of the communication is between adults. This invariably means that rich, personal, and important information that can potentially be gleaned from children and young people may be missed or misunderstood. A basic understanding of speech and language development may benefit healthcare professionals. The communication pyramid that many healthcare professionals may be familiar with (shown in Figure 5.1) is a loose representation of the typical hierarchical bottom-up pattern of communication development ('Language pyramid', n.d.). It is important for healthcare professionals to note that

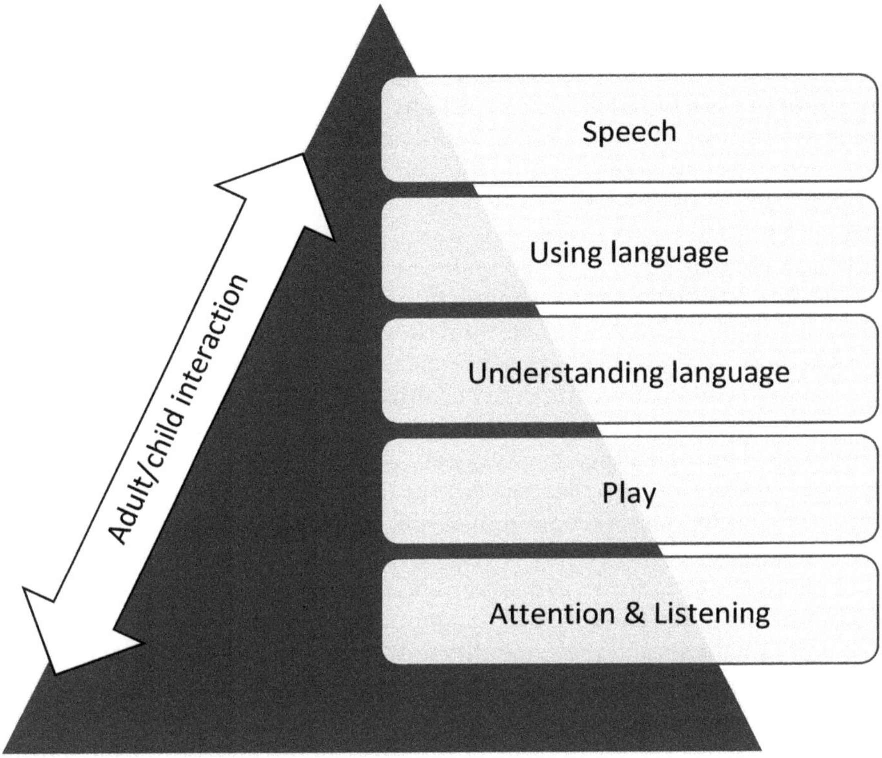

Figure 5.1 Communication pyramid (original source unknown, n.d.)

this is not a strict hierarchy of needing one building block completely in place before progressing to the next (Morgan & Dipper, 2018). However, it is paramount to understand that atypical communication development is not necessarily linear and can present a mixed picture of ability and need. For example, a child who has a cleft palate repaired in infancy experiences attention, listening and comprehension difficulties due to glue ear in early development (Gani et al., 2012; Skuladottir et al., 2015). Furthermore speech sound development may be disrupted secondary to articulation and nasality issues (Russell & Albery, 2017). Moreover, this pattern can change, for instance, if the child has tympanostomy tubes or hearing aids placed for persistent glue ear, improved attention, listening and understanding may result.

Cultural and diversity factors

As physical environments are adapted to meet the needs of those with physical disabilities, it is important that healthcare professionals also promote health equality by ensuring the communication environment is accessible (Simeonson et al., 2012). There are daily barriers to accessible information and support for children and young people with communication impairments (Communication Access UK, 2020; DCB1605 Accessible Information, 2016). Contextual factors, especially environmental and social factors such as attitudes of professionals, family members, and society at large can create barriers to accessing information and support for communication impairment. In addition, personal factors, including children and young people's attitudes, socio-economic status and culture can further influence how communication is accessed and viewed (Moorcroft et al., 2019).

Atypical communication should be understood by healthcare professionals within the context of cultural, linguistic, ethnic, gender, economic, health, and religious diversity. Difference and diversity does not equate to atypicality. Culturally competent healthcare professionals recognise and celebrate the rich, global diversity of children, young people, and families they work with. Healthcare professionals should strive to always provide culturally effective care that reaches the desired outcome while respecting cultural distinctions. As 'communication is a fundamental part of healthcare' (Sharkey et al., 2016), it is crucial for healthcare professionals to get communication right the first time. The risk of not getting it right during healthcare interactions can lead to communication breakdown, distrust on the part of patients and their inability to take advice or follow recommendations. Additionally, it can affect obtaining informed consent, effectiveness of treatment, and the 'buy in' by children and young people in treatment. Healthcare professionals should ensure that the information being relayed is provided at a level that can be understood, to ensure patient safety as well as to keep children and young people engaged in their own medical care and decision making at every contact with the healthcare system (Bell & Condren, 2016).

Legislation and governance considerations

All healthcare professionals' training should include opportunities to develop skills in communicating with children and young people, and in particular atypical communicators. Within the realm of healthcare, professionals may work with children and young people who have complex medical problems. Respecting the communication rights of the child and the right to access their own healthcare information should be at the forefront of practice. In line with considering the wider functioning and needs of children and young people (Simeonson et al., 2012), participation is achieved by effective patient–provider communication (De Beule, 2017). It is also the responsibility of healthcare professionals to understand their role in ensuring access to communication for those children and young people with atypical communication. Since the global Covid-19 pandemic of 2020, healthcare professionals are more aware of the impact of personal protective equipment (PPE) on effective communication. With the evolving pandemic came guidance on how to support communication amongst healthcare professionals and patients. This was even more pertinent to communication with vulnerable children and young people such as those with hearing impairments where communication may normally be augmented through lip-reading and facial expression.

The UN Convention on the rights of the child implies a requirement that healthcare professionals provide whatever adaptations are necessary to support communication access during healthcare interactions. Healthcare professionals should be familiar with the rights of the child, to afford children and young people entering healthcare settings the required communication dignity and the assurance that their needs are prioritised, and their voices are listened to. In the United Kingdom the General Medical Council (GMC) gives clear guidance to medical staff on supporting communication exchanges with children and young people (GMC, 2007/2018). This is echoed in the Royal College of Nursing (RCN) guidance on supporting children and young peoples' communication needs in a way that is accessible to the individual (RCN, 2021). Additionally, in the United Kingdom, the Health and Care Professions Council notes in the document titled 'standards of conduct, performance and ethics' (HCPC, 2016) the importance of healthcare professionals ensuring 'arrangements are made to meet service users' and carers' language and communication needs'.

Supporting and empowering healthcare professionals

In professional clinical training, learning how to support children and young people with communication difficulties is typically limited to on-the-job practice. Here we offer practical guidance and support to inform and empower healthcare professionals when working with children and young people with atypical communication. But how do healthcare professionals adapt to the needs of children and young people, especially when they are likely to have other needs, or are in pain or displaying anxieties in a healthcare environment?

It is known that the somatic experience of pain can starkly influence children and young people's communication abilities, even in the absence of any communication needs. Johnson (2020) noted that pain can impact a child/ or young person's ability to communicate their needs effectively. This can result in miscommunication, misinterpretation, and communication breakdown. Children and young people with atypical communication may need additional support and effective access to help them to express themselves, communicate wants and needs, ask questions, give consent, and explore the implications of assessment and treatment of their health-related conditions.

The healthcare professional is responsible for adapting and responding to these needs in a flexible, accessible manner. Furthermore, it's important to consider how the clinical environment may further impact children and young people's ability to engage in communication, for example with busy clinic rooms, additional observers or difficult procedures (blood and dental work). It is therefore useful to consider the support that is available in the clinical context, for example access to play therapists, therapy assistants, clinical psychologists, and other healthcare professionals or support workers. It is helpful to check whether there are optimal links with different supportive services, such as learning difficulties support teams, advocates, intermediaries, and clinical nurse specialists. De Beule (2017) found that alternative and augmentative communication (AAC) improves children and young people's activity and participation, enhances patient–provider communication and completion of medical procedures. In addition, this author's systematic review of AAC use found that the consistent use of AAC (whether paper-based, technology based, or even scaffolding) resulted in a decrease in anxiety, stress, or pain at some point of the medical procedure.

Health literacy has been defined by the Institute of Medicine and National Library of Medicine in the United States as 'the degree to which individuals have the capacity to obtain, process, and understand basic health information and services needed to make appropriate health decisions' (Bell & Condren, 2016). Limited health literacy skills have been associated with poorer health knowledge, aversive health behaviours, and increased healthcare costs (Bell & Condren, 2016). Health literacy includes a variety of skills beyond reading and writing, including numeracy, listening, and speaking. Whilst our focus is obviously on children and young people with atypical communication, an opportunity arises to also support family members or carers where communication impairments may also exist. Supporting health literacy in children and young people and their families to allow for engagement is important, especially for those with chronic healthcare needs. Providing medical information that children and young people can understand may increase adherence, decrease adverse effects, and increase knowledge (Bell & Condren, 2016).

The healthcare professional must allow for not only the adult caregiver's health literacy, but also for that of the child, which is evolving as the child develops. Children and young people with atypical communication are likely to need ongoing adjustments and accommodations to support access to health literacy. If we expect these children and young people to be more involved and take an active role in their own health, it is imperative that healthcare professionals ensure that health literacy skills are supported from an early age (Bell & Condren, 2016). Whether children and young people are able to communicate verbally or through other non-verbal means such as sign language or AAC, they should be supported in an environment conducive to communication opportunities, such as minimising background noise or offering information in different visual formats. Whilst interactions may be slow, the healthcare professional must be mindful of the impact of completing a young person's utterances for them: respecting the voices of children and young people is vital.

The role of the multidisciplinary team in supporting communication

There are some roles recognised within the healthcare setting that offer enhanced support for interaction and communication. Speech and language therapists specialise in the assessment, diagnosis, and treatment of atypical communication. They are employed across different sectors for example, community settings, private practice, charitable organisations, education, and within hospital settings. It is important to highlight that not all atypical communicators need specialist level assessment and treatment. Some children and young people with atypical communication needs may cross settings, for example a child with vocal fold palsy may be supported by a local service where the family lives as well as a specialist speech and language therapist in an ear, nose, and throat service. Due to the likely impact of vocal fold palsy on how the child may sound and the clarity of their voice, there may be the need to implement strategies and structures in an education setting to ensure access and participation in the curriculum, for example answering questions and working with peers.

Healthcare professionals would benefit from consulting with speech and language therapists to explore speech and language needs and how best to support individual communication access. Speech and language therapists provide child- and family-centred support for goal setting that is relevant for their individual healthcare journey, ensuring that children and young people are included in discussions. Asking 'how is it best to communicate with [name]' is important to optimise inclusion. Healthcare professionals should appropriately support access to decision making, rehabilitation options, discharge planning, and continued care post discharge, particularly at key points such as transitioning to adult services.

The healthcare professional may be the first to notice atypical communication presentation, and if this is the case it is especially important to signpost to advice and refer to other services where appropriate. Examples of such services may include joint assessment in cochlear clinics, working with primary care healthcare professionals on early communication access and working with the neuro-rehabilitation team to support children and young people in their reintegration to home life, education and community participation.

Healthcare professionals should be encouraged to liaise with speech and language therapists where available, to empower and support the skills healthcare professionals bring to the interaction. Healthcare professionals should consider liaising with speech and language therapists to develop communication resource packs for each healthcare environment that may contain resources such as pictures of feelings and pain scales, whiteboard and pen, alphabet board, familiar objects, action pictures, or word boards. A communication resource pack can then be an easily accessible, central resource to facilitate easy access for all healthcare professionals to support communication. In addition, play specialists, psychologists, therapy assistants or technicians, nursery nurses and healthcare assistants can all be part of the core 'communication team' around children and young people and their families. Healthcare professionals offer vital support to ensure flexibility and consistency of communication in a variety of contexts.

Strategies for supporting communication

In this section we share practical ideas and strategies that can be used by healthcare professionals to empower themselves in adding supportive communication strategies to their toolkit of skills.

It is important when supporting children and young people with atypical communication to pre-empt communication breakdown. For example, asking the question 'how do you prefer to communicate?' may minimise confusion or frustration. Additionally, involving children and young people in their own healthcare journey through the development of story or picture books that explain a procedure may help them to be more prepared for their healthcare visit, including offering opportunities to talk about feelings in an accessible way.

- A strategy to support children and young people should focus on discussion. To minimise distractibility, it is useful to say their name before instructions are given. Conversely, saying a child's name after or during an instruction may mean they miss this information and fail to respond or respond incorrectly. Offering commentary rather than questions gives children and young people opportunities to respond without pressure if they want to. This is an important consideration where initiation of communication is difficult, or direct questioning results in non-response.
- Use of simple language and non-verbal communication strategies supports better understanding and may help children and young people visualise what is happening. For example, saying 'more please', rather than 'give me more of that one over there please' is a clearer request. Adding a gesture, for example pointing may improve understanding and response.
- In this digital age, children and young people usually have access to a tablet or smartphone, so accessing some of the standard functions on a device (such as jotter/notes pages, texting) may support communication. Paper/whiteboard can be substituted if this technology is not available, or to include family members if appropriate.

- If children and young people are unable to make choices or understand the written word, consider pictures, and if they are unable to choose or identify pictures, consider using objects. For some children, objects of reference are used to help understanding of routine or interventions, as well as enabling choices, for example a flannel to indicate washing or a cup to indicate drinking.
- A visual timetable using pictures helps to create a schedule of events that supports children and young people in understanding what is happening now and in the future. This strategy helps avoid ambiguity, clarifies the sequence of events ensures no surprises and enables transitions between events. Similarly, song signifiers can be used to support children and young people in anticipating what is going to happen next (Binns et al., 2019). A specific song can be used as a signal or alert, at the start or end of an activity, supporting children and young people in understanding events.
- Some children and young people with atypical communication needs may access interactions via a communication system such as AAC. This may be paper-based or digital technology, for example an alphabet board or device keyboard. Healthcare professionals may consider using different background colours, for example yellow paper to support those with visual impairments. Both technology and paper-based support require patience and understanding of the system.
- Strategies that add additional cues may further support understanding for children and young people with atypical communication needs. For example, sign aided languages offer visual cues where signs are used alongside the spoken word; tactile signing systems or on-body signing may also be used. Typically, every word is not signed. Examples of sign aid language include baby sign, Makaton, and Sign-a-Long and an example of an on-body signing approach is 'tactile signing for sensory learners' (TaSSeLs).
- Healthcare professionals should also ensure that interactions with children and young people promote active listening and display greater interactivity so that they are engaged with the information that is being shared. Age-related developmental stages and diagnoses related challenges must be considered when creating accessible communication opportunities for children and young people.

Healthcare professionals can also consider implementing some of the following strategies in daily practice with children and young people and their families. According to Bell and Condren (2016), the following additional strategies optimise the communication environment:

- Use of icons and images that convey health information.
- Use of plain language principles.

- Encouraging retelling of the relevant information to check understanding
- Creating a shame-free care environment
- Using the ASK ME 3-strategy: (1) What is my main problem? 2) What do I need to do? 3) Why is it important for me to do this?).
- Limit the number of messages by taking out the 'nice to know' and keeping the 'need to know'.
- Make visuals culturally relevant and sensitive information.

Clinical case studies: optimising communication

The following two cases will give a brief illustration of the possible application of some of the strategies discussed in this chapter to support children and young people with atypical communication.

Case 5.1 Gabriel

Gabriel (4 years old) was admitted to critical care to receive treatment for acute respiratory distress. Gabriel has Down Syndrome and was therefore considerable vulnerable in regard to his communication needs. He was ventilated for a week and was extubated successfully. The use of PPE by healthcare professionals due to Covid-19 coupled with Gabriel's existing communication vulnerability resulted in a number of communication breakdowns occurring. Gabriel became distressed and displayed challenging behaviour. As part of Gabriel's admission, the medical team gathered a detailed case history, including information about his communication needs and abilities. Gabriel's family advised he didn't say any words but babbled, pointed at things, and used some signs. He became easily distressed when his parents were not present or when the routine changed. They reported Gabriel had been discharged from a local speech and language therapy service due to non-attendance. To support Gabriel's communication needs following his discharge from hospital, he was re-referred to his local speech and language therapist.

The speech and language therapist provided strategies based on parental reports, observations and communication assessments to support healthcare professionals' interactions with Gabriel. This included using a picture book to explain why staff were wearing PPE, picture pain charts, and some simple Makaton signs, for example 'stop', 'pain', 'mummy', 'daddy', 'sleep', and 'look'. Parents reported Gabriel enjoys music and so a song signifier was introduced to reduce Gabriel's anxieties and help him understand blood pressure monitoring and blood tests. Whilst these strategies addressed immediate challenges in the hospital context, longer term communication support post discharge was still needed.

Case 5.2 Aaliyah

Aaliyah (15 years old) attended a nurse-led outpatient clinic following a recent broken wrist. She attended with her mum. The medical notes highlighted that she had a severe brain injury at 7 years of age following a road traffic accident. Her mum reported that Aaliyah was now fully recovered and had no follow up, although is often off school and struggles in the classroom and with schoolwork. The clinic was busy and extremely noisy, with the door propped open. Although the nurse asked how Aaliyah was managing with her wrist at school and with physical activity, Aaliyah only responded with yes or no answers. She was distracted by her phone and was unable to answer longer, more abstract questions. She appeared to look to her mum to answer.

The nurse queried whether Aaliyah's history of brain injury may have impacted on her ability to communicate effectively. To support Aaliyah's focus and engagement, the nurse closed the door to create a quieter environment and asked Aaliyah to put her phone away. The nurse used a model of a wrist and some pictures to explore how Aaliyah was recovering. The nurse gave Aaliyah choices regarding treatment options and used simple language with short sentences. With more focus and less distraction, Aaliyah was able to explain her level of wrist pain and comfort in different situations using the pain scale and making choices. Finally, the nurse asked Aaliyah to explain what she understood about their discussion. The nurse advised them that a referral back to the brain injury clinic may be useful. She advised that whilst Aaliyah's brain injury was a long time ago, her communication and cognitive skills may benefit from further assessment and support to ensure she can access and participate in social and educational experiences.

Resources for healthcare professionals to support communication

Healthcare services should consider adjustments and materials for children and young people including:

- Creating a picture dictionary of medical terms with simple definitions for diseases, instruments, medicines, and other health-related items.
- Access to a website with a section on various kinds of injections, with images, videos, quizzes and simple texts, walking children and young people through the process.

- A place where children and young people can post their stories or messages about their experiences.
- An advice page for caregivers or parents, for example covering topics such as how to explain to children and young people what will happen whilst in hospital and how to comfort them.

Healthcare professionals are encouraged to access additional training within their organisations on topics related to communication skills. Links to resources that healthcare professionals may find useful are included below to support their understanding of some atypical communication conditions. In addition, practical support and information are shared in these resources for healthcare professionals to explore.

Recommended resources

Websites

- Ausmed: www.ausmed.com/cpd/guides/communication-skills – offers guidance on communicating with children and young people, acknowledging this to be one of the most challenging aspects of healthcare.
- The Children's Trust Brain Injury Hub: www.thechildrenstrust.org.uk – charity supporting rehabilitation, education, and skilled teams. The brain injury hub provides resources around brain injury.
- The Child Brain Injury Trust: www.childbraininjurytrust.org.uk – charity offering emotional, practical support, information and learning resources for childhood brain injury.
- ICAN 'helps children communicate': https://ican.org.uk/ – consortium of communication charities with access to tools, resources and frameworks supporting speech, language and communication needs.
- Cleft Lip and Palate Association: www.clapa.com/ – charity supporting, connecting and empowering those affected by cleft lip and palate.
- Down Syndrome International: www.ds-int.org – organisation committed to improving quality of life for people with Down syndrome, promoting their right to be included on a full and equal basis.
- Royal College of Speech and Language Therapists: www.rcspeech and language therapist.org/ – the professional body of speech and language therapists in the United Kingdom with access to communication resources and guidance.
- American Speech-Language-Hearing Association: www.asha.org – the professional body of American speech and language pathologists access to communication resources and guidance.
- Video of therapeutic communication in action – aimed at nurses but applicable to wider healthcare professionals workforce: https://study.com/

academy/lesson/therapeutic-communication-in-nursing-examples-techniques.html
- Me First: www.mefirst.org – a website offering training modules and resources co-designed by children and young people to support communication skills of healthcare professionals, including having difficult conversations.

*Mobile applications (apps)**

- iCommunicate for (iOS)
- iConverse (iOS)
- QuickTalk AAC (iOS/Android)
- LetMeTalk (iOS/Android)
- Predictable App (iOS/Android)
- The Conversation Therapy app from Tactus Therapy Solutions (iOS/Android)
- DAF Pro app from Speech Tools (iOS/Android)
- My Talking Tom (iOS/Android)
- Voice4U (iOS/Android)
- Dragon Naturally Speaking (iOS/Android).

*This list of applications is by no means exhaustive and the authors have not done an in-depth review regarding the functionality of the suggested applications. This resource list is just an example showcase of what is currently available for use to support children and young people with atypical communication.

Signing resources

- Makaton: www.makaton.org
- Singinghands: www.singinghands.co.uk via YouTube, Twitter, and Facebook
- Isabella signs: www.isabellasigns.com/ and via YouTube, Twitter, and Facebook
- Makaton with Lucinda: via YouTube, Twitter, and Facebook
- Sign Language: Sign to hear (Irish Sign Language) – via Instagram, YouTube, Twitter, and Facebook).

Conclusion

The take home messages from this chapter are as follows.

1. Actively engage with children and young people rather than fixate on their diagnostic labels.

2. Provide opportunities for the children and young people to participate.
3. Follow the children and young people's leads in communication.
4. Use a total communication approach.
5. Anticipate and be flexible to the communication needs of children and young people.

Healthcare professionals should consider access to communication resources that support specific clinical settings. This may include pre-made communication boards, whiteboard, alphabet charts, and quick tips on supporting communication. It is our hope that this chapter has provided a window into supporting atypical communication in children and young people and their families when interacting with the healthcare system. We hope that healthcare professionals will now know where to access support for successful communication. Healthcare professionals should feel empowered to use a child-led approach to communication that is based on skills and needs, rather than age. The signposting to resources can be referenced in everyday practice to support the participation for children and young people with atypical communication.

References

Bell, J., & Condren, M. (2016). Communication strategies for empowering and protecting children. *The Journal of Pediatric Pharmacology and Therapeutics*, *21*(2), 176–184.

Binns, A., Hutchinson, L. R., & Oram Cardy, J. (2019). The speech-language pathologist's role in supporting the development of self-regulation: A review and tutorial. *Journal of Communication Disorders*, 78, 1–17.

Communication Access UK (2020). Retrieved from https://communication-access.co.uk/register/

Damm, L., Leiss, U. Habeler, U., & Ehrich, J. (2015). Improving care through better communication: continuing the debate. *The Journal of Pediatrics*, *167*(2), 501–502.

De Beule, K. (2017). The use of communication aids with children in health care and the outcomes for the child's functioning based on the ICF-CY: A systematic literature review. Jonkoping University. Master's Thesis.

DCB1605 Accessible Information (2016, updated 2017). *Accessible Information Standard including Specification and Guidance.* Retrieved from www.england.nhs.uk/ourwork/accessibleinfo/

Gani, B., Kinshuck, A. J., & Sharma, R. (2012). A review of hearing loss in cleft palate patients. *International Journal of Otolaryngology*, Article ID 548698, https://doi.org/10.1155/2012/548698

General Medical Council (GMC, 2007, updated 2018). 'Communication' in 0–18 years: guidance for all doctors, pp. 8–10. Retrieved from www.gmc-uk.org/-/media/documents/0_18_years_english_0418pdf

Health & Care Professions Council (Healthcare Professionals, 2016). *Standards of conduct, performance and ethics.* Retrieved from www.healthcare professionalsc-uk.org/globalassets/resources/standards/standards-of-conduct-performance-and-ethics.pdf

Johnson, E. (2020). Supporting communication vulnerable children to communicate their pain. In: V. Y. Waisundara (Ed.), *Pain management*. London: IntechOpen.

Kummer, A. (2018). *Cleft palate and craniofacial conditions: a comprehensive guide to clinical management* (4th ed.). Burlington, MA: Jones & Bartlett Learning.

'Language Pyramid'. Retrieved from https://dl.acm.org/doi/abs/10.1145/1871437.1871520

Morgan, S., & Dipper, L. (2018). Is the communication pyramid a useful model of language development? *Royal College of Speech & Language Therapists Bulletin*, 2018 (May), 26–28. Retrieved from www.rcslt.org/wp-content/uploads/media/Project/Bulletins/May-2018---AtE.pdf?la=en&hash=752F7EC88E9A2A3A4013745E321CCD6800FBA283

Moorcroft, A., Scarinci, N., & Meyer, C. (2019). A systematic review of the barriers and facilitators to the provision and use of low-tech and unaided AAC systems for people with complex communication needs and their families. *Disability and Rehabilitation: Assistive Technology*, *14*(7), 710–731.

Royal College of Nursing (RCN, 2021). Children and young people's nursing: a philosophy of care: RCN guidance for nursing staff. RCN, retrieved from www.rcn.org.uk/-/media/royal-college-of-nursing/documents/publications/2021/january

Sharkey, S., Lloyd, C., Tomlinson, R., Thomas, E., Martin, A., Logan, S., & Morris, C. (2016). Communicating with disabled children when inpatients: barriers and facilitators identified by parents and professionals in a qualitative study. *Health Expert*, 19, 738–750.

Skuladottir, H., Sivertsen, A., Assmus, J., Remme, A. R., Dahlen, M., and Vindenes, H. (2015). Hearing outcomes in patients with cleft lip/palate. *The Cleft Palate-Craniofacial Journal*, *52*(2), 23–31.

Russell J., & Albery L. (2017). *Practical intervention for cleft palate speech*. London: Routledge.

Simeonson, R. J. , Bjorck-Akesson, E., & Lollar, D. J. (2012). Communication, disability, and the ICF-CY. *Augmentative and Alternative Communication*, *28*(1), 3–10.

United Nations General Assembly. (1989). UN Convention on the Rights of the Child (www.unicef.org/crc). New York: United Nations.

Communicating with children and young people with speech, language, and communication needs

James Law, Penny Levickis, and Linda Jose

Chapter contents:

- Functional difficulties and diagnostics: speech, language, and social communication difficulties
- Comorbidities and associations
- Considering what successful communication looks like
- Involving children and families in decision making
- Sensitivity to the child's age and developmental stage
- Considering where children with SLCN are encountered
- Clinical practice recommendations
- References

In this chapter we consider the communication skills of children where the primary concern is their speech and language difficulties. These children are described in several ways, but most commonly in the United Kingdom's educational system they are described as having speech, language, and communication needs (SLCN). These individuals may also have difficulties in other areas of their development. In societal terms this group of children is of particular concern precisely because their difficulties may not be obvious and health practitioners may find it challenging to recognise them. Clearly, recognising these difficulties warrants close attention, and we begin with a brief introduction to the diagnostic categories used for these children and the functional difficulties that they can experience. In practice, diagnosis may be less important than the appropriate response to the children's functional difficulties.

Key to understanding what children and their families need is to ask them, and in this chapter, we include a section on how parents and the children themselves can be involved in decision making. The fact that they have communication difficulties will affect the way practitioners respond to other

DOI: 10.4324/9781003142522-9

aspects of their needs. Thus, if a child visits a practitioner because they have hurt themselves or because the parent wants advice about a special educational need, understanding the child's communication needs will be central to any decisions that the practitioner makes about them. Age, and perhaps more importantly, the child's developmental level is also key to understanding the needs of the child. The decisions made about the involvement of the child will vary depending on their age but also their ability to understand what is being proposed by the practitioner. The more they are engaged, the better their response is likely to be. As we have indicated, the children covered by this chapter primarily have communication difficulties but, of course, some will also have other developmental (cognition/motor) or sensory (hearing/vison) difficulties that warrant further exploration. We consider some of the areas where communication skills and other developmental conditions are most related, and touch on the association between the environments in which the children are raised and their language abilities. We then look at the locations where practitioners are most likely to encounter children with SLCN and the role that the context plays in how best to communicate with them. Finally, we provide five clinical practice recommendations which are critical to understanding the needs of children with communication difficulties.

Functional difficulties and diagnostics

Children potentially come into contact with a wide variety of practitioners in health and education services, especially in their early years. Primary care clinicians and early educators are often the first point of contact for children with speech and language delay (Sunderajan & Kanhere, 2019). Speech and language therapists and other professionals may use a range of terms to describe different types and/or combinations of SLCN. Although these terms are sometimes used interchangeably by both parents and practitioners who are not specialists in the area, they indicate distinct problems even if they can have similar effects on the listener – i.e., difficulty understanding fully what the child is trying to say. It is often quite simple to identify a child with unintelligible speech but other difficulties with talking and communication can be hidden and are not always as easy to spot. It is important when attending to a child's communication skills to pay attention to other aspects of their development though that will not be our main focus here (Asmussen, Law, Charlton, Acquah, Brims, Pote, McBride 2018).

Speech difficulties

By the time most children start school their speech is clear and intelligible to others. Some children take longer to develop speech sounds, but their speech difficulties are often short-lived and may resolve spontaneously or in response to intervention. For other children their speech difficulties persist or are more severe. Approximately 3.8% of children have speech difficulties that persist into school (Shriberg, Tomblin, & McSweeney, 1999) and the most recent UK data suggests that as many as 8% of children will be experiencing SLCN at school entry (Norbury, Gooch, Wray, Baird, Charman, Simonoff, Vamvakas, & Pickles, 2016).

Speech difficulties may include difficulties with:

- **Phonology** – Delay in acquiring phonemes (sounds) of a language so speech is typical of a younger child and marked by speech sound error patterns not appropriate for age (delay), or they have difficulty acquiring or organising the sound system of speech and speech is characterised by delayed and unusual sound error patterns (phonological disorder) (Dodd, 2005).
- **Articulation** – Atypical production of speech sounds characterized by substitutions, omissions, additions, or distortions that may affect intelligibility (ASHA, 2004).
- **Fluency** – Interruption to the flow of speech, such as unusual rate, rhythm, and repetitions in sounds, syllables, words, and phrases. This may be accompanied by excessive tension and other secondary mannerisms (e.g. blinking, grimacing) (ASHA, 2004). Stammering or stuttering is a fluency disorder.
- **Voice** – Atypical production and/or absences of vocal quality, pitch, loudness, resonance, and/or duration, which is incongruous with an individual's age and/or sex (ASHA, 2004).

Considering a child's age, it is important to consider the impact of a child's speech difficulty on how they talk to others. Persistently unintelligible speech may affect behaviour, social confidence, and self-esteem (Lindsay & Dockrell, 2000). The sound awareness skills required for speech also affect the development of reading and spelling skills, so school age children with speech sound difficulties may also have difficulties in these areas (Holm, Farrier, & Dodd, 2008; Raitano, Pennington, Tunick, Boada, & Shriberg, 2004).

Several terms are used to describe speech difficulties, such as phonological disorder, speech sound disorder, speech delay, and developmental dyspraxia. Each of these describes a specific diagnostic category of speech disorder that requires its own type of intervention that a speech and language therapist will determine after assessment.

Speech difficulties may be secondary if they are associated with a medical diagnosis such as cerebral palsy, hearing impairment, or global developmental delay. There is a high comorbidity of ear infections and mental disorders and other health related conditions in children with speech disorders (Keating, Turrell, & Ozanne, 2001). However, many children have primary speech difficulties that occur with no apparent cause, and that may be a result of a complex interaction between the social environment in which the child learns to talk and their biological maturation (Shriberg et al., 2003).

Key strategies for communicating with a child with speech difficulties are outlined below:

- If a child who stammers, speak slowly. Use short sentences and simple language to reduce the communication demands on the child. Make sure you give them time to understand and process what you have said and to work out their response. Do not interrupt or finish sentences for them.
- If a child's speech is unintelligible ask them to show you what they mean in another way e.g., writing, drawing, or showing a gesture. You could ask closed questions (i.e., questions that require a yes/no response) to try and clarify what they mean.

Language difficulties

Language difficulties can affect what a child understands (receptive language) and/or what they can produce (expressive language) in both verbal and written forms. These difficulties may be accompanied by other SLCN and are often associated with difficulties learning to read and write. The total prevalence of children with a language disorder of any kind is estimated to be approximately 9.9% (Norbury et al., 2016). Lack of awareness or understanding can lead to children not being identified or being misdiagnosed. Approximately 50% of children with developmental language disorders in the United Kingdom are not receiving the help they need (Norbury et al., 2016). If a child's language is following the typical developmental pattern but at a slower rate it is said to be delayed. Language delay can be an isolated delay where the child's other areas of development are normal or may form part of a more general developmental delay. There may be a range of possible causes or associated factors for language delay, including environmental factors (e.g., lack of language stimulation), genetic factors and physical factors (e.g., early fluctuating hearing loss) (Sunderajan & Kanhere, 2019). The term 'delayed' is usually used when referring to younger children and implies that their speech and language development will catch up.

However, there are children who have difficulties with language who are not following the typical developmental pattern of language acquisition and their language appears disordered. For example, they have difficulty learning vocabulary and understanding or using complex sentences. Until recently, a range of terminology was commonly used to describe children who have difficulties with expressive and/or receptive language skills that impact on everyday life, including: 'specific language impairment', 'language disorder', and 'developmental language impairment' (Bishop, Snowling, Thompson, Greenhalgh, CATALISE Consortium, 2016).

An international group of 57 experts (the CATALISE panel) reached consensus on the criteria used for children's language difficulties in 2016 (Bishop et al., 2016). 'Language disorder' (LD) was the term the panel agreed on to refer to children with "language difficulties that create obstacles to communication or learning in everyday life and is associated with poor prognosis". The LD may be associated with other medical diagnoses or conditions such as autism spectrum disorder (ASD), brain injury, genetic conditions (e.g., Down's syndrome), and sensorineural hearing loss. 'Developmental language disorder' (DLD) was the agreed term for when the LD is a primary disorder and thus not associated with a known condition such as those mentioned above.

There are a variety of reasons children may have difficulties with comprehension or expression. These may include difficulties with:

- Maintaining attention and listening.
- Processing language (this may be very slow).
- Memory (holding spoken language for long enough to be able to work out the meaning).
- Word knowledge: concepts (words that tell us about location, i.e., next to/behind), size (i.e., big/little), time (i.e., yesterday/tomorrow), prepositions (i.e., on/under) and sequential language (e.g., first, last) and vocabulary (the number of words they are familiar with) may not be in line with typical development.
- Remembering or retrieving vocabulary they know when they need to use it (word finding difficulties).
- Morphology or word structure (e.g., may misuse or misunderstand word endings such as possessives or verb tenses).
- Syntax or sentence structure (their sentences are shorter and less complex).
- Sequencing their thoughts and ideas (e.g., they may tell stories that are jumbled or hard to follow).

Children may become frustrated if they cannot understand or are not understood by others. Research shows children with DLD are at risk of long-term behavioural and psychiatric problems (Conti-Ramsden, Durkin, Mok, Toseeb, & Botting, 2016; Law, Rush, Schoon & Parsons, 2009). Children may develop an awareness of their own difficulties, which impacts on confidence and self-esteem (Conti-Ramsden & Botting, 2004; Durkin et al., 2017). These issues may have an impact on the child's motivation to interact with others and affect our capacity to understand their true ability.

Social communication difficulties

Speech and language are the foundation for our verbal and non-verbal communication. Whilst grammar, syntax, vocabulary, pronunciation, and phonology are all important aspects of speech and language, they are subordinate to another important concept called pragmatics. Pragmatics describes how language is used in context. Children with a social (pragmatic) communication disorder (SCD), sometimes known as a pragmatic language impairment, have difficulty using verbal and non-verbal communication appropriately in social situations (APA, 2013). According to the diagnostic criteria for SCD detailed in the *Diagnostic and Statistical Manual of Mental Disorders*, 5th Edition (DSM-5) (APA, 2013), primary difficulties are in social interaction, social cognition, and pragmatics. children with SCD may have difficulties with the following.

- Following conversational rules (going 'off topic' or 'one sided' conversation).
- Using appropriate language based on the listener or situation (too little or too much information, adjusting language appropriately to the situation with friends, familiar and unfamiliar adults, etc.).
- Extracting salient points from a conversation, story, or information.
- Understanding jokes, idioms, metaphors, and sarcasm (resulting in literal interpretation).
- Understanding and using non-verbal communication, for example, eye contact (too much or too little), facial expression, and gesture.
- Reading comprehension.
- Prediction, inferencing, and narrative skills.
- Organisational skills.
- Intonation (speech is monotone or lacks variation).

Children with SCD may say inappropriate or unrelated things during conversations or use unusual language and vocabulary. However, their expressive language is often age appropriate in terms of sentence structure and grammar, so is clear and fluent.

Children with SCD have a pattern of characteristics that are often mistaken for ASD (Mandy, Wang, Lee, & Skuse, 2017). However, children with SCD do not meet all the diagnostic criteria for ASD. Children with ASD also have social communication impairments but in addition they have *significant* repetitive behaviours, narrow interests, or ritualistic or compulsive behaviours (APA, 2013). Whilst SCD cannot co-occur with ASD, it can co-occur with other conditions such as attention deficit hyperactivity disorder (ADHD), and intellectual disability and traumatic brain injury.

Strategies to support communication of children with SCD include:

- As with language difficulties, be clear and concise and use visual support where appropriate when giving information.
- Taking account that the child may have literal understanding and may not be able to infer meaning from what you say: you need to be explicit.

- Help a child to understand what to expect and what is expected of them. Social Stories (short descriptions of a particular situation, event or activity, which include specific information about what to expect in that situation and why (Gray, 2015) and comic strip conversations (Gray, 1994) (simple visual representations of a conversation) may be helpful. These may also be helpful for younger children.

Comorbidities and associations

While it is always possible to address the needs of children and young people from a specific professional perspective (such as when a child is attending a GP for fever, audiology for hearing tests, child psychology for a mental health assessment, or physiotherapy for a physical ability assessment) it is always important to consider their communication skills and be aware that communication skills are often associated with other aspects of the child's development and their experiences. If other problems of development are apparent, they are known as comorbidities. Communication disabilities commonly co-occur with other neuro-developmental conditions. For example, although it is quite possible for a child to have difficulties only with speech and language, it is always important to consider the possibility of associated learning disabilities. These may be general and associated with broader cognitive difficulties, such as poor memory or processing skills, but they may also be specific, such as dyslexia or dyscalculia.

Some children will also have associated social and emotional difficulties. We commonly see a child with ADHD having associated communication difficulties. Unfortunately, practitioners often focus on the immediate problem, in this case, usually the child's conduct or hyperactivity, but we need to be especially vigilant about this child's communication skills which may be part of an underlying neurodevelopmental disability. It is sometimes argued that the communication disability leads to the social or emotional difficulty and of course it is possible for the frustration over not being understood or being able to express oneself effectively to lead to behavioural difficulties. In practice it can be difficult to tease the relationship between communication and behaviour apart. Problems with one need not lead directly to problems with the other, they simply overlap and need to be considered together.

Another neurodevelopmental condition that has attracted considerable attention in recent years has been ASD. All children with ASD experience some form of communication disability. These children often present with unusual behaviours and their communication problems may not be immediately obvious. Children, until recently described as having Asperger's syndrome (after Austrian psychiatrist Hans Asperger) but now regarded as being on the autism spectrum. perform relatively well on formal language tests. However, they often use an unusual vocabulary and have difficulty interacting with others, being unable to take turns and often misunderstanding their conversation partner.

A third type of comorbidity is associated with sensory difficulties, particularly hearing loss. Given the relationship between hearing and language, it is hardly surprising that children that have difficulty hearing commonly have difficulty acquiring language at the same rate as their hearing peers. This is most marked in cases of children with severe sensory-neural hearing loss. Even if children are given cochlear implants soon after birth, they may still have difficulty acquiring language at the normal rate. It is important to acknowledge that deaf children with deaf parents commonly communicate using sign language, which shares many of the characteristics of spoken language in terms of its creativity, although it is clearly understood only by those who are proficient in it. A less certain relationship between hearing loss and language development occurs for children with conductive hearing losses. For most children these are intermittent and have little lasting effect, but language delays are common for some children with persistent glue ear and otitis media with effusion (OME) leading to grommet insertion. Recently this has been investigated further and it appears that those with language difficulties associated with OME were more likely to have grommets inserted rather than the reverse causal relationship.

Another consideration which warrants careful attention is the relationship between the child's linguistic experience (i.e., what they hear around them and how it is communicated to them) and their communication skills. Like many aspects of child health and development, there is a marked social gradient in children's language development, children from more socially disadvantaged backgrounds having on average lower levels of language performance. Some have argued that what has become known to campaigners in the field as the 'big word gap' is a function of the linguistic input that the children receive, essentially the less the child is spoken to the less proficient they are in their linguistic abilities. However, the phenomenon may not be as linear as it appears. For example, there may be a genetic component, with parents of these children being less competent themselves. Nevertheless, at the extreme end there are undoubtedly children who are raised in harsh environments who are actively discouraged from speaking, especially those who have been abused or more likely, actively neglected.

There may also be issues associated with multilingualism, where the child uses two or more languages and may be less proficient in the one being assessed by mainstream services. Multilingualism is, of course, the norm for a substantial proportion of children worldwide. Parents are often concerned about their child's development in one or another language and teachers may also see this as a focus of concern. In fact, the process by which children learn language is extremely robust and learning more than one language at a time is very unlikely to become a problem. It is true, of course, that children, especially when young, will switch between their languages mid-sentence. Generally, being multilingual is a tremendous advantage to most children, but the few for whom language learning is difficult usually manifest their problems in every language they speak. There are children who are exposed to different levels of a range of different languages, and it would be reasonable to expect that this would be reflected in their language performance generally.

Considering what successful communication looks like

Communication among health professionals, children, and families is critical to health care and ensuring that treatments and interventions are effective. Successful communication involves not only considering the child's developmental stage, but also establishing rapport with the child to help increase their level of comfort and engagement (Bell & Condren, 2016). Children can feel discomfort and become disengaged due to previous negative episodes of care, such as medical procedures and hospitalisation. It can be emotionally threatening and even psychologically traumatising for all children whether or not they have a communication difficulty (Lerwick, 2016). As a result of their developmental level and limited cognitive development, children may use behaviour, instead of words, to communicate their emotions. Thus, they may present with anxiety, aggression, anger, and similar expressions of emotion (Lerwick, 2016) A child with SCLN may be more likely to feel emotionally threatened in a healthcare situation and use behaviour instead of words. This highlights the importance of addressing the child's anxiety and reducing feelings of helplessness by building rapport and empowering them. Below are some strategies to assist communication with children with speech and language difficulties.

We look first at strategies to help children who have difficulties with speaking, since they are generally easier to identify than those who have difficulty understanding what is being said to them.

- If you have difficulty understanding the child's message, ask questions to clarify what they are talking about – who, what, where, why, how? The last two are often especially difficult for young children and those with language difficulties.
- Use closed questions (ones that require yes/no or other short responses) rather than open questions, to reduce the demand on them to produce language.
- Build rapport and reduce anxiety by getting down to the child's level and facing them (towering over them can be intimidating). Maintain a calm, gentle, unhurried, and open manner (Bell & Condren, 2016) and use a soft and gentle tone of voice.

- Show that you are paying attention by maintaining eye contact if possible (but recognise that eye contact may be difficult for children with ASD or some who are very anxious).
- Try to maintain relaxed, fluid movements with your hands and friendly, open facial expressions.

A child's failure to understand is not always obvious, but there are steps we can take to help.

- Speak clearly and slowly, using short, simple sentences. Be clear and concise.
- Emphasise key words when giving information.
- Use visual support when giving information – gestures or pictures.
- Some children need extra time to process information, so leave a pause (10 seconds) if the child does not immediately respond.
- If a child has not understood, repeat what was said rather than rephrasing. Rephrasing can increase the language load for a child who is already struggling.

Involving children and families in decision making

Historically, children and families were often seen as passive recipients of 'help'. Decision making regarding speech and language therapy was made on behalf of, rather than by children and young people with SLCN. However, it is now widely recognised that children have the right to express their views on what they think should happen when adults are making decisions that affect them and that their views need to be considered (United Nations, 1989). Not only do children's rights mean that they deserve to be actively involved in their own decision making but listening to and valuing a child's views can promote their engagement with interventions and lead to better outcomes. Although children's direct involvement in their health care is expected to be beneficial, research demonstrates that in practice, children have little meaningful involvement in their health care consultations (Cahill & Papageorgiou, 2007). While parents and health care practitioners are typically the primary decision makers in treatment decisions for children, in instances where treatment was in the best interest of the child, research shows children have been content for adults to make the major decisions, trusting their parents and seeing the healthcare professional as the expert regarding treatment of their disease (Coyne et al., 2014). Ensuring that information is shared with the child, at a level that they can understand, ensures patient safety, encourages child engagement in their medical care and can support the child's involvement in decision making (Bell & Condren, 2016).

Practitioners may determine a child's views or preferences indirectly, from observation or by consulting a parent. However, research shows that children do not always share the perspectives of adults such as parents or speech and language therapists (Owen, Hayett, & Roulstone, 2004). While it is acknowledged that all individuals have the right to express their views and have them heard, especially regarding decisions that will affect them, children, and young people with SLCN are at an increased risk of not being given a voice due to their communication difficulties. By simply providing developmentally appropriate choices, anxiety can be reduced, and a child can feel empowered. Power through choice giving in a medical setting may seem arduous to healthcare professionals at first, but it is easy to put in place when the goal to empower patients and their families (to provide psychological control of the environment) is clear. A few extra seconds to allow for choices can reduce anxiety and in the long term improve patient cooperation and set up expectations for future episodes of care (Lerwick, 2016).

There is a growing body of research involving children and young people with SLCN, examining their perspectives on communication, speech-language therapy, and decision making (Merrick & Roulstone, 2011; Lyon & Roulstone, 2017). Findings from a UK-based project involving 54 children between the ages of 7 and 16 with a range of SLCN resulted in a variety of recommendations in how best support and involve children and young people with SLCN in decision making (Roulstone, Harding, & Morgan, 2016). This report provides suggestions of good practice and recommendations that can be helpful to health professionals working with children and young people with SLCN and their families across different settings and contexts (Roulstone, Harding, & Morgan, 2016):

- The use of objects and supporting materials: having access to the actual objects or paperwork that are being discussed, rather than just using symbols or pictures, can provide a supporting context to help children and young people with SLCN remember the right words and remind them of the activity or event.
- The use of dynamic activities to support engagement: including physical actions and dynamic activities that reflects the verbal activities, such as choosing stickers to indicate preferences, sorting cards for voting or indicating choices or moving counters to indicate a score on a scale can support children and young people's engagement with the decision-making process.
- Knowledge of children and young people's role in decision making: to support children's involvement in making decisions, use accessible, relevant, and interactive materials to convey information; information should include the process of involvement, the expectation and possibility that children and young people play an important role and clear information about how they can express their preferences and needs.

- Relevant decisions: it is important to identify the most appropriate level of involvement in decision making for any individual child or young person. Therefore, the health professional and parents need to understand the different levels of involvement in decision making to select the most appropriate in consultation with the child or young person and their parent.
- Responsive to children and young people's preferences: the child or young person's preferences should be taken into account regarding their level of involvement in decision making; action and physical movements should be included in processes of involvement to support their level of engagement in decision making.

Research demonstrates repeatedly that parents play a major role in children's development, especially in the early years of childhood. Parents are best placed to provide health practitioners with an indication of their child's communication skills/stage of development. Observing the parent and child interacting may also provide an insight into the child's communication skills and strategies that support them. Health professionals can serve children with SLCN best by working in collaboration with their parents. However, whilst there are clear benefits to health professionals in involving parents in decision making, this can often be a challenge to both parties (Klatte et al., 2020). To empower parents to be actively involved in shared decision making, health professionals not only need to support parents' development of understanding, but also need to address the power imbalance, whereby the health professional may be perceived to hold all responsibility for decision making (Reeder & Morris, 2020). Ideally, shared decision making will involve health professionals, parents, and children and young people with SLCN.

One area that is of particular concern to those delivering services to children is the need to obtain their opinions on the services they receive, especially as they get older. This process can be a challenge for many groups but particularly for those with SLCN (including most children with neurodevelopmental disabilities). This needs to be handled with care. Although it is common for services to tick the box of engagement by putting out an iPad and asking children to press a button, in practice this rarely gets to the problems faced by those with communication difficulties. It is not just the literacy skills needed to read the text but the fact that it often takes work to encourage the children to express themselves in this way.

The need for sensitivity to the child's age and developmental stage

Collaborating with children and young people with speech and language difficulties means engaging with them in meaningful participation by establishing a good understanding of their ability to communicate and process information (Owen, Hayett, & Roulstone, 2004). To do this successfully, it is important to consider not only the age of the child or young person, but also their developmental level. Child development drives both what the child can understand and how their parents respond to them, and it is critical that all practitioners are aware of how this might affect the interaction between the professional and young person whatever their age. It is useful to know what children should be doing at different ages and stages to support their communication and identify when they may be struggling to communicate or understand.

Children develop at different rates, and it may be difficult to identify whether they have SLCN in the very early years. It is important to be aware that for most children, language continues to develop throughout the school years and into adulthood. Young people who are experiencing communication difficulties will often have associated literacy and social difficulties and will find it hard to develop more sophisticated language without support (Hartshorne, 2011). The Communication Trust has produced a series of booklets for anyone working with children and young people that show where children should be with their communication skills at different ages and stages from birth to age 18 (see Universally Speaking in additional readings). Below is a table derived from the Universally Speaking resources that shows key milestones for what children should be doing at different ages. It is important to remember that children reach different milestones at different ages.

Considering where children with SLCN are encountered

The prevalence rates of SLCN is high (about 10%) and it is likely that professionals will encounter individuals with these needs in their own professional context (i.e. because they have a difficulty with their communication skills and perhaps parents are expressing concerns) or because their difficulties are associated with some other conditions. These messages are important for health visitors, foster carers, early years workers, teachers, school nurses, child and adolescent health workers, and those working in centres for young offenders.

It is likely healthcare professionals will meet children with SLCN wherever they work, whether in primary, secondary, or tertiary healthcare environments and in all educational and community settings. The key is for all those who work with children to pay attention to their communication skills and not assume that the children they see can understand what is being said to them or that they can explain their needs without assistance. As we know all too well, parents may attend a clinic for one aspect of their child's life but then ask professionals about other concerns. Parents may be concerned

Age	*Communication and language milestones*
By 6 months of age	Makes cooing, gurgling, and babbling sounds Smiles and laughs when others smile and laugh Makes noises to get your attention
By one year	Says first word/s Recognises the names of familiar objects Takes turns in 'conversations', babbling back to an adult
By 18 months	Understands simple words and short phrases Recognises and points to familiar objects when you ask them Says up to 20 words, usually things they hear a lot, e.g., doggy, bye-bye, more
By two years	Uses over 50 single words Asks simple questions, such as, "what that?" Understands simple questions and instructions
By three years	Understands simple 'who', 'what', and 'where' questions Puts four or five words together to make a simple sentence Refers to something that has happened in the past
By four years	Describes events that have already happened Listens to longer stories and answers questions about a story they have just heard
By five years	Takes turns in much longer conversations Uses talk to help work out problems to organise their thinking and take part in activities Understands more complicated language such as 'first', 'last', 'might', 'maybe', 'above', and 'in between'
By seven years	Understands complex 2 to 3 part instructions Uses newly learnt words in a specific and appropriate way Uses sound and letter links to read and spell unfamiliar words
By nine years	Uses a wide range of verbs to express their thoughts, or explain cause and effect Uses a whole range of regular and irregular grammatical word endings, with few errors being made
By eleven years	Begins to appreciate sarcasm when it's obvious Uses long and complex sentence structures including more sophisticated connectives to join ideas together in conversation

Figure 6.1 Key milestones in speech and language

about their child's speech and language skills and commonly look for advice, regardless of the clinic they are attending.

Healthcare professionals will encounter children with recognised or unrecognised SLCN, regardless of their role in the healthcare system. Children with SLCN have a wide range of strengths, difficulties, and needs. These can have a wide-ranging impact on their everyday functioning, including their ability to access and make choices about their healthcare. Children with SLCN and their families require added patience, flexibility, and (like all children) regulation for their ever-changing emotions in their healthcare process. Children's primary needs are to know they are safe, be given age-appropriate and developmentally appropriate information and to feel empowered by being heard, given choices, and involved as far as possible in joint decision-making processes about their healthcare. This chapter includes a range of principles and strategies to help practitioners meet these needs. Healthcare professionals have a valuable opportunity to provide positive healthcare experiences and have meaningful conversations with children with SCLN, by employing strategies that promote the child's understanding, their ability to express themselves and to make choices about the care that they receive. Below are key clinical practice recommendations and suggested recommended reading and resources.

Clinical Practice Recommendations

- Listen to children and their families. This can be especially important if the children and young people do not have good communication skills.
- Distinguish between the way that a child speaks (sometimes described as articulation, phonology, fluency, or voice), what they are saying (how well they can use vocabulary, string sentences together into a narrative), and how well they interact with others (listening, taking turns etc).
- Always consider what the child or young person understands by what you are saying. If in doubt check back with them or with their parent/carer as appropriate but don't take for granted that they understand what you are saying. This applies to written and spoken language. Check that they understand written instructions (on medicines for older children) but also leaflets, handouts, etc.
- See the children and young people's needs in terms of the developmental level of the child. It is not just how old they are but also what they can do relative to children of their own age.
- Consider using pictorial representations of what you are communicating with the young person.

Five key resources

1. Universally Speaking: The Communication Trust has produced a series of booklets, which are for anyone who works with children and young

people. The booklets show where children should be with their communication skills at any given age: www.thecommunicationtrust.org.uk/resources/resources/resources-for-practitioners/universally-speaking.aspx (Accessed 22.2.2021).

2. *ICAN Resources for professionals* ICAN is one of the key charities supporting children with SLCN in the UK and their produce excellent resources for parents and professionals. For example they produce this leaflet for professionals Supporting children with SCLN (ican.org.uk) but equally it is important that professionals are able to point parents to summaries of key information which can be found on the same site (Accessed 22.2.2021) Parents of bilingual children are often looking to find out whether their children have additional SLCN and again ICAN produce relevant material on this issue supporting-children-learning-english-as-an-additional-language.pdf (ican.org.uk) (Accessed 22.2.2021).
3. This reference guide which was developed by Orygen, the National Centre of Excellence in Youth Mental Health (Orygen) and Speech Pathology Australia (SPA), provides strategies and tips for mental health clinicians to support young people with SCLN to navigate mental health settings: www.orygen.org.au/Training/Resources/Neurodevelopmental-disorders/Clinical-practice-points/Reference-guide-How-to-support-young-people-with/Support-YP-with-speech-language-communication-need.aspx?ext= (Accessed 22.2.2021).
4. AFASIC is a UK charity specifically for children with SLCN and produces helpful materials on the provision of services and how best to make sure that they receive the right services https://www.afasic.org.uk/ (Accessed 22.2.2021).
5. Some children have pronounced difficulties and there is a real interest in campaigning for their needs to be met. There is a website with this specific focus called Raising Awareness of Development Language Disorders providing useful information and opportunities to get engaged. https://radld.org/ (Accessed 22.2.2021).

References

American Psychiatric Association (APA). (2013). *Diagnostic and statistical manual of mental disorders: DSM-5* (Vol. 5). Washington, DC: American Psychiatric Association.

American Speech-Language-Hearing Association (ASHA). (2004). *Preferred Practice Patterns for the Profession of Speech-Language Pathology [Preferred Practice Patterns]*. Retrieved from www.asha.org/policy

Asmussen, K., Law, J., Charlton, J., Acquah, D., Brims, L., Pote, I., & McBride, T. (2018). *Key competencies in early cognitive development: Things, people, numbers and words.* London: Early Intervention Foundation. Research Summary London: Early Intervention Foundation.

Bell, J., & Condren, M. (2016). Communication strategies for empowering and protecting children. *The Journal of Pediatric Pharmacology and Therapeutics, 21*(2), 176–184.

Bishop, D. V., Snowling, M. J., Thompson, P. A., Greenhalgh, T., & Catalise Consortium. (2016). CATALISE: A multinational and multidisciplinary Delphi consensus study. Identifying language impairments in children. *PLOS one, 11*(7), e0158753.

Cahill, P., & Papageorgiou, A. (2007). Triadic communication in the primary care paediatric consultation: a review of the literature. *British Journal of General Practice, 57*(544), 904–911.

Conti-Ramsden, G., & Botting, N. (2004). Social difficulties and victimization in children with SLI at 11 years of age. *Journal of Speech, Language, and Hearing Research*, 47(1), 145–161.

Conti-Ramsden, G., Durkin, K., Mok, P. L., Toseeb, U., & Botting, N. (2016). Health, employment and relationships: Correlates of personal wellbeing in young adults with and without a history of childhood language impairment. *Social Science & Medicine, 160*, 20–28.

Coyne, I., Amory, A., Kiernan, G., & Gibson, F. (2014). Children's participation in shared decision-making: children, adolescents, parents and healthcare professionals' perspectives and experiences. *European Journal of Oncology Nursing, 18*(3), 273–280.

Dodd, B. (2005). *Differential diagnosis and treatment of children with speech disorder.* Chichester, UK: John Wiley & Sons.

Durkin, K., Toseeb, U., Botting, N., Pickles, A., & Conti-Ramsden, G. (2017). Social confidence in early adulthood among young people with and without a history of language impairment. *Journal of Speech, Language, and Hearing Research, 60*(6), 1635–1647.

Gray, C. (1994). *Comic strip conversations: Illustrated interactions that teach conversation skills to students with autism and related disorders.* Arlington, TX: Future Horizons.

Gray, C. (2015). *Social stories.* Retrieved from http://best-practice.middletownautism.com/approaches-of-intervention/social-stories/

Hartshorne, M. (2011). *Speech, Language and Communication in Secondary Aged Pupils.* I CAN Talk Series – Issue 10. London: ICAN.

Holm, A., Farrier, F., & Dodd, B. (2008). Phonological awareness, reading accuracy and spelling ability of children with inconsistent phonological disorder. *International Journal of Language & Communication Disorders, 43*(3), 300–322.

Keating, D., Turrell, G., & Ozanne, A. (2001). Childhood speech disorders: Reported prevalence, comorbidity and socioeconomic profile. *Journal of paediatrics and child health, 37*(5), 431–436.

Klatte, I.S., Lyons, R., Davies, K., Harding, S., Marshall, J., McKean, C. and Roulstone, S. (2020), Collaboration between parents and SLTs produces optimal outcomes for children attending speech and language therapy: gathering the evidence. *International Journal of Language & Communication Disorders, 55*, 618–628.

Law, J., Rush, R., Schoon, I., & Parsons, S. (2009). Modeling developmental language difficulties from school entry into adulthood: literacy, mental health, and employment outcomes. *Journal of Speech, Language, and Hearing Research,* 52(6), 1401–1416.

Lerwick, J. L. (2016). Minimizing pediatric healthcare-induced anxiety and trauma. *World journal of clinical pediatrics*, *5*(2), 143.

Lindsay, G., & Dockrell, J. (2000). The behaviour and self-esteem of children with specific speech and language difficulties. *British Journal of Educational Psychology*, *70*(4), 583–601.

Lyons, R., & Roulstone, S. (2017). Labels, identity and narratives in children with primary speech and language impairments. *International Journal of Speech-language Pathology*, *19*(5), 503–518.

Mandy, W., Wang, A., Lee, I., & Skuse, D. (2017). Evaluating social (pragmatic) communication disorder. *Journal of Child Psychology and Psychiatry*, *58*(10), 1166–1175.

Merrick, R., & Roulstone, S. (2011). Children's views of communication and speech-language pathology. *International Journal of Speech-Language Pathology*, *13*(4), 281–290.

Owen, R., Hayett, L., & Roulstone, S. (2004). Children's views of speech and language therapy in school: consulting children with communication difficulties. *Child Language Teaching and Therapy*, *20*(1), 55–73.

Norbury, C., Gooch, D., Wray, C., Baird, G., Charman, T., Simonoff, E., Vamvakas, G., & Pickles, A. (2016). The impact of nonverbal ability on prevalence and clinical presentation of language disorder: evidence from a population study. *Journal of Child Psychology and Psychiatry*, *57*(11), 1247–1257.

Raitano, N. A., Pennington, B. F., Tunick, R. A., Boada, R., & Shriberg, L. D. (2004). Pre-literacy skills of subgroups of children with speech sound disorders. *Journal of Child Psychology and Psychiatry*, *45*(4), 821–835.

Reeder, J., & Morris, J. (2020). Becoming an empowered parent. How do parents successfully take up their role as a collaborative partner in their child's specialist care? *Journal of Child Health Care*, 1367493520910832.

Roulstone, S., Harding, S., & Morgan, L. (2016). Exploring the involvement of children and young people with speech, language and communication needs and their families in decision making-a research project. London: Communication Trust.

Shriberg, L. D., Kent, R. D., Karlsson, H. B., Mcsweeny, J. L., Nadler, C. J., & Brown, R. L. (2003). A diagnostic marker for speech delay associated with otitis media with effusion: backing of obstruents. *Clinical linguistics & phonetics*, *17*(7), 529–547.

Shriberg, L.D., Tomblin, J.B., & McSweeney, J.L. (1999). Prevalence of speech delay in 6-year-old children and comorbidity with language impairment. *Journal of Speech, Language, and Hearing Research*, *42*(6), 61–81.

Sunderajan, T., & Kanhere, S. V. (2019). Speech and language delay in children: prevalence and risk factors. *Journal of Family Medicine and Primary Care*, *8*(5), 1642.

United Nations (1989). Convention on the Rights of the Child, retrieved from www2.ohchr.org/english/law/pdf/crc.pdf, accessed 14 Dec 2020.

Conversing with families of atypical communicators

Rosalind Pawar and Gavriella Simson

Chapter contents:

Considering the role of families

A communication impairment has the potential to have far-reaching consequences for both the atypical communicator and their family. Due to the impact of a communication impairment on activity and social functioning, the family of an atypical communicator often adopts a caregiver role (Brown et al., 2012; World Health Organization, 2013). This is likely to include facilitating communication with healthcare professionals. Establishing and maintaining effective communication with the family of an atypical communicator is therefore essential to delivering patient-centred care. Using two case studies, this chapter explores the barriers to communication between the atypical communicator, their family, and healthcare professionals. Recommendations for clinicians communicating with atypical communicators and their families are also discussed.

DOI: 10.4324/9781003142522-10

For the purposes of this chapter, an atypical communicator refers to an individual who has a communication impairment that impacts on their activity and social functioning (WHO, 2013). Some atypical communicators may be able to communicate independently with modifications such as the use of writing or a communication aid. However, other atypical communicators may need the assistance of others to facilitate communication or communicate on their behalf. Many people live with communication difficulties, and common causes include stroke, various cancers, traumatic injuries, degenerative neurological disorders, and cerebral palsy. There are an estimated 350,000 individuals living with aphasia in the UK, with the most common aetiology being stroke (Simmons-Mackie et al., 2010; Stroke Association, 2020). A third of stroke victims experience aphasia and in some cases the communication impairment will be chronic (Stroke Association, 2020).

Dysphonia and dysarthria are a common consequence of head and neck cancer (HNC) treatment, with up to 70% of patients experiencing chronic communication difficulties, which in turn limit their social interactions (Ringash et al., 2017). Due to an increase in five-year survival, years lost to disability are growing in the HNC population (Breen et al., 2017). This has negative financial, social, and psychological implications (Breen et al., 2017). The increasing prevalence of human papillomavirus related oropharyngeal cancer results in communication problems for more adults of working age, who may also have young children (Ringash et al., 2017). Conditions such as traumatic brain injury may lead to chronic changes in communication while neurodegenerative conditions such as motor neuron disease results in a progressive loss of verbal communication (Mackenzie et al., 2016).

Irrespective of the cause of the communication disorder, it has the potential to negatively impact on activity, participation, and psychosocial well-being (Northcott et al., 2016). Research has demonstrated that family involvement plays an essential role in optimising treatment outcomes (Bond et al., 2016; Northcott et al., 2016; Ringash et al., 2017). Clinicians should therefore ensure that their communication supports both the patient and their family.

Communication and families

Communication, our interface with the world, is essential in all facets of life. However, society is laden with communication barriers (Money, 2016). The Royal College of Speech and Language Therapists (RCSLT) is committed to raising awareness of these communication barriers through its advocacy of inclusive communication (Money, 2016). RCSLT have defined inclusive communication as an "approach to communication which enables as many people as possible to be included in an interaction" (Money, 2016). Inclusive communication seeks to facilitate the creation of environments that allow everyone, including those with communication disorders, to communicate (Money, 2016). It is incumbent on clinicians to ensure that their communication meets the needs of both the atypical communicator and their family. Investment in and from family members is essential in the management of long-term communication disorders (Bond et al., 2016; Mackenzie et al., 2016). Family often forms the link between the patient and the healthcare system when atypical communicators need treatment or advice for any health problem. Also, where the individual has additional care needs, family members may be vital caregivers (Bond et al., 2016). For example, in the HNC population, family support is essential to facilitating self-management, maximising therapy compliance, and implementing care regimens (Bond et al., 2016).

Family members of atypical communicators often demonstrate flexibility and an ability to adapt and facilitate communication (Mackenzie et al., 2016). They offer stability and a sense of familiarity to the atypical communicator. However, family members may sometimes be a barrier to good communication, speaking for the patient and assigning them a passive role in social interactions and in activities of daily living (Northcott et al., 2016). It is the responsibility of healthcare professionals to ensure that the family of the atypical communicator are provided with the skills to facilitate communication opportunities.

Case studies

This section presents two case studies. The first is of a young female with post-stroke aphasia and the second is of a middle aged, male patient with HNC.

Case study 7.1 Andrea

Andrea was in her forties and leading a team in a busy job when she suddenly suffered a large left hemisphere stroke. Three months after the stroke her verbal communication remained limited to an unreliable yes/no response and reflexive swearing. Andrea maintained her gregarious personality and preferred pointing and gestures to technological communication aids. Andrea was close to her sister, and through a program of communication partner training, facilitated by a speech and language therapist, they modified their exchanges with both reporting positive outcomes in terms of communicative success. The training also helped her sister to facilitate communication at health consultations. Through this approach, focusing on successful interactions and strategies, whilst dealing with the profound physical, cognitive, and communication changes, Andrea and her sister were able to engage in premorbid and new leisure activities to progress towards a goal of living well with aphasia.

Case study 7.2 Joe

Joe, a seventy-year-old Croatian man, and his wife Mary were enjoying their retirement. Ten years previously, Joe had been diagnosed with a base of tongue (BOT) tumour which was treated with radical radiotherapy. When Joe presented to the HNC team, there was evidence of recurrence in the BOT. Joe underwent a hemiglossectomy, leaving him severely dysarthric and dysphagic. Following discharge from hospital, Mary adopted a caregiver role which included, due to Joe's speech impairment, communicating with the HNC team on Joe's behalf. She was provided with a key worker contact. Shortly after surgery Joe began to deteriorate. Using communication strategies developed together with the speech and language therapist, Mary was able to identify the deterioration and promptly raised it with the HNC team. Further assessments revealed that Joe had residual disease, which meant that palliative care was most appropriate. The team maintained regular contact with Mary and were able to ascertain when she was no longer able to continue with her role as Joe's primary carer. Joe was referred to his local hospice, where end of life (EOL) care was provided. The hospice provided Mary with counselling which she continued to access following Joe's death.

Guidance for clinicians

Treating the patient in the context of family life

This section provides recommendations for clinicians when communicating with families of atypical communicators. Table 7.1 provides a summary of the most salient communication strategies discussed. National Institute for Health and Care Excellence (NICE) Guidance: '*Patient experience in adult NHS services: Improving the experience of care for people using the NHS services*', provides communication recommendations for clinicians. The guidance stipulates that clinicians 'develop an understanding of the individual, including how the condition affects the person and how the person's circumstances and experiences affect the condition and treatment' (NICE, 2012). Included in a patient's 'circumstances' is their family. A patient's diagnosis, treatment, treatment side effects, rehabilitation, and prognosis have direct implications for their family. Further, as illustrated in the case studies, family members often play an essential caregiver role (Parker et al., 2016; Ringash et al., 2017).

Prior to involving family members in a patient's care, the clinician must gain consent from the patient. If the individual cannot indicate consent, family members or carers should be kept appropriately informed (Mental Capacity Act, 2005). The clinician must be mindful of their duty of confidentiality (NICE, 2012).

The impact of a condition on an individual's family has been well documented (Bond et al., 2016; Marra et al., 2020; Northcott et al., 2016; Ringash et al., 2017). Increased tension and disharmony have been reported between stroke survivors and their families, particularly when the individual has aphasia (Northcott et al., 2016). Research has demonstrated a shift in marriage roles following a stroke, which often causes friction and marital strain (Northcott et al., 2016). Some family members report assuming greater responsibilities and becoming informal carers, 'sometimes that gets really tough … it's having a support network for the carer' (Brown et al., 2012). Additionally, family caregivers report a lack of support for themselves (Ringash et al., 2017). The consequences of a HNC diagnosis and its subsequent treatment are also felt by the patient's family (Bond et al., 2016). Communication impairments as a result of HNC treatment impact on the individual and their family, as one family member expresses in a qualitative study: 'I worry about ever being able to speak again' and 'it was tough when she could not speak; she used sign language that was hard to understand at first' (Sterba et al., 2017). Families frequently report worry and a lack of confidence when performing specific caregiver tasks such as maintaining breathing and feeding tubes (Sterba et al., 2017). This lack of confidence in meeting their new caregiver role often leaves family members feeling isolated (Sterba et al., 2017). Families of HNC survivors frequently report reduced psychological wellbeing associated with the disease and treatment, with up to 70% experiencing depression and 39% reporting anxiety (Parker et al., 2016).

When managing the care of an atypical communicator, family members should be actively engaged. This includes ensuring that families can attend appointments. When this is not possible, clinicians should contact the family following consultations. This is essential, as atypical communicators may be unable to relay information provided during consultations. It is recommended that the patient and their family are provided with a key worker within the multidisciplinary team, with whom they can raise concerns. Failure to maintain communication with an individual's family increases the risk of miscommunication which may impact on the quality of the care provided and the wellbeing of the patient and their family (Parker et al., 2016). Furthermore, family members play a key role in facilitating communication between the atypical communicator and the clinician. This is demonstrated in case study 7.1, where Andrea's sister was able to facilitate communication during consultations as a result of her participating in communication partner training. Clinicians are responsible for educating the patient and their family about the implications of a diagnosis and treatment for both the patient and their family. This includes educating the family on specific caregiver roles such as administering supplements through a feeding tube. Clinicians should also verbally acknowledge the burden of adopting a caregiver role and its likely psychological implications (Bond et al., 2016; Ringash et al., 2017; Sterba et al., 2017). This includes recognising specific changes in family roles because of a communication impairment (Brown et al., 2012; Ross & Wedcliffe, 2001). It is important to identify the unique and specific needs of family members as part of the relationship dynamic (Brown et al., 2012). Research has demonstrated that there is distinction between support and sympathy, only the former of which was welcomed (Brown et al., 2012). Psychological support should be offered when required. This will reduce the risk of carer burnout and distress (Bond et al., 2016).

The importance of active engagement with a patient's family is highlighted in case study 7.2. As Joe's disease progressed, Mary adopted the role of his primary caregiver, a role which she was determined to maintain. Joe's diminishing ability to communicate and his increasing care needs placed considerable strain on their relationship and impacted on Mary's well-being. The team maintained regular contact with Mary, acknowledging the enormity of her caregiver role. Regular contact also allowed the team to identify when Mary was no longer able to sustain her role as Joe's caregiver. This enabled a timely referral to their local hospice and initiation of counselling for Mary.

Providing families with training to facilitate communication with atypical communicators

It is important to recognise that the term 'atypical communicator' is not synonymous with being unable to communicate. It is the responsibility of the clinician to facilitate communication wherever possible (Sterba et al., 2017). Adopting a holistic view of the communication disorder includes considering the context in which an individual is communicating. This often includes the individual's family. The family should therefore be educated on how best to facilitate communication. To do this, it may be necessary to offer some training to family members.

In some instances, formal communication training for the family may be indicated. In case study 7.1, Andrea's sister engaged in communication partner training, a program specifically designed for caregivers of individuals with aphasia (Simmons-Mackie et al., 2010). Research has demonstrated that individuals with aphasia have said that the use of communication strategies is important for living successfully with their communication impairment (Brown et al., 2012). Evidence suggests that communication partner training is effective for improving communication and participation for people with aphasia and traumatic brain injury (Simmons-Mackie et al., 2010; Sim, Power, & Togher, 2013). Educating family members on facilitating communication of an atypical communicator is not integral to the role of all clinicians. However, clinicians are responsible for identifying the need for communication intervention and referring and/or signposting patients and their families to the appropriate services.

When managing the dysarthria and dysphonia associated with MND, the focus is primarily on the use of assistive communication devices (Mackenzie et al., 2016). The rapidly degenerative nature of this disease means that impairment-based therapy would not increase activity and participation for the individual and would therefore add little value to their quality of life (Mackenzie et al., 2016).

In aphasia treatment, one intervention model proposes focusing on supporting individuals and their families to live successfully despite their communication disability (Brown et al., 2012). This approach involves working with the individual and those around them to identify positive factors, personal strengths, and opportunities for participation in meaningful and rewarding activities in order to enable independence and wellbeing (Brown et al., 2012; Cruice, Worrall, & Hickson, 2006). Emphasis is given to relationships, and the need for a couple to work as a 'united front' and have 'love and respect' (Brown et al., 2012). There is evidence that families of individuals with aphasia may have their own aphasia-related rehabilitation goals which need to be identified and recognised (Howe et al., 2012).

It is important that clinicians adopt a family-centred approach to communication therapy. The severity of impairment is a factor in the impact of aphasia on an individual's life; however, individual contexts vary. Whilst some family members perceive aphasia to have little impact on their relationships, for others it results in large changes (Brown et al., 2012). Enabling individuals to be empowered and have control of key decisions in, finance, legal, and health related matters has been recognised as important for living well with aphasia (Brown et al., 2012; Cruice et al., 2006).

In the case of dementia, where a cognitive decline often occurs simultaneously with a language disorder, family may also require guidance on adopting alternative modes of communication. This may include the use of sensory modalities (Johnson, Kelch, & Johnson, 2017). For example, family may be encouraged to show the individual pictures of people pertinent to the conversation to provide context to the conversation (Johnson et al., 2017).

For some patients and their families, an informal process of learning by trial and error may be adopted. Members of the families of atypical communicators often demonstrate flexibility and adaptability and may develop their own strategies to facilitate communication. For example, family members of individuals with MND, especially children, were reported to be the most common source of technological ideas and advice (Mackenzie et al., 2016). In case study 7.2, Mary developed her own strategies to facilitate Joe's communication. This included encouraging Joe to write and use gestures rather than communicating verbally. However, Mary required professional guidance with regards to providing Joe with sufficient time to answer questions and checking that she had understood Joe's communication.

Mind the gap

When engaging with family it is important that clinicians ensure that their communication facilitates a patient's care rather than becoming a barrier (Maguire & Pitceathly, 2002). Clinicians should adapt their communication so that it meets both the needs of the patient and their family (Mistraletti et al., 2020). They should take care to explain any unfamiliar terms (Maguire & Pitceathly, 2002; Mistraletti et al., 2020), and should demonstrate that they are listening to the patient and their family by summarising the information they receive from them. The patient and their family should be provided with the opportunity to correct any misunderstandings (Maguire & Pitceathly, 2002).

Moreover, to focusing on their own communication, clinicians should be mindful of the gap a communication disorder can create between a patient and their family. Family, friends, and carers are an invaluable source of support and information, but it is also important to recognise their limitations (Northcott et al., 2016). For people living with aphasia, it has been demonstrated that family members and friends rate the patient's quality of life, physical functioning, health, pain, and vitality lower than the individual themselves (Cruice et al., 2005). This was mirrored in the HNC population with family caregivers reporting more treatment side effects than the patient themselves at six-months post treatment (Richardson, Morton, & Broadbent, 2016). Therefore, family cannot always be relied upon as a source of information on the patient's quality of life (Cruice et al., 2005). These differences in perception can lead to misunderstandings in personal and professional relationships. It is important for all parties to identify and discuss their opinions (Cruice et al., 2005).

Alternative modes of communication

Consultations remain the primary mode of communication with the atypical communicator and their family. However, clinicians should be familiar with alternative methods used to supplement information provided during consultations (Mistraletti et al., 2020). This may include, but is not limited to, written information, pictures, pertinent objects, symbols, large print, and resources in different languages (Money, 2016). An open conversation with the patient and their family may highlight which alternative forms of communication are useful and preferred by the individual and their family. It should be noted, however, that alternative modes of communication are not a replacement for effective dialogue.

The effectiveness of employing alternative modes of communication to supplement information provided during consultations was demonstrated by Parker et al. (2016). These authors developed a DVD to explain the laryngectomy procedure and its consequences to both the patient and their partner/family. The DVD was used in addition to, not in place of, face-to-face consultations. A laryngectomy, surgical removal of the voice box, is an unfamiliar procedure to most patients and their families. However, its functional implications are profound for both the patient and their family, with speech, breathing and the ability to eat and drink affected. Use of alternative modes of communication such as the DVD can be used to reinforce information provided during consultations (Parker et al., 2016). Before meeting with a patient and their family, clinicians should consider the practicalities of the appointment. Appointments with atypical communicators and their families are likely to require extra time, adequate time should therefore be allocated. Appointment letters, text messages, phone calls or emails should outline consultation expectations in an accessible format. This will enable the patient and their family to prepare for the appointment.

To maximise patient autonomy and reduce caregiver burden, clinicians should, where possible, facilitate communication for the atypical communicator during consultations. For example, clinicians encouraged Joe (case study 7.2) to use writing, as he was unable to communicate verbally. This ensured that Joe's needs and wishes were understood and respected. This was demonstrated when discussing palliative care. Joe was able to communicate via writing that he did not wish to have any further treatment. The use of written communication maximised Joe's autonomy and relieved Mary of the burden of having to make EOL decisions on Joe's behalf. To identify what strategies to use, patients themselves should be encouraged to identify what methods facilitate/inhibit their communication.

Access to healthcare if English is not the first language

A professional trained interpreter should be arranged if the patient and/or their family are not English speakers. If possible, the interpreter should be present; however, remote access via telephone or video link may be arranged. While some patients and their families may speak some English, information provided during consultations may be complex and sensitive and should therefore be delivered in the primary language of the patient and their family. In the event that the atypical communicator is English speaking, but the family are not, an interpreter should be arranged as the atypical communicator may not be able to relay information to their family. However, in this instance patient consent for arranging an interpreter may be required. Family should not be required to interpret for the atypical communicator, particularly when distressing and sensitive information is being shared. A consultation requiring an interpreter is likely to be time consuming and the healthcare professional should therefore ensure that adequate time has been allocated (Hadziabdic & Hjelm, 2013).

Prior to the consultation, the appointment aims, plan, and content should be discussed with the interpreter. The interpreter should be encouraged to ask the healthcare professional questions during the consultation to ensure that accurate information is communicated. Unfamiliar terms should be explained to the interpreter prior to the consultation (Hadziabdic & Hjelm, 2013). At the start of the consultation the clinician should explain their own and the interpreter's roles and emphasise that the consultation is confidential. The use of jargon should be avoided, and any unfamiliar terms explained. Throughout the consultation, the healthcare professional should direct verbal and non-verbal communication to the patient and family to optimise natural communication. At the conclusion of the consultation the clinician should give the patient and their family an opportunity to ask questions, and then check that they have understood everything communicated (Hadziabdic & Hjelm, 2013).

Communication during EOL care

The NICE Guidance, *End of life care for adults*, outlines the importance of involving the individual's carer, including their family, in EOL care decisions (NICE, 2019). Inclusion of the carer in EOL care decisions improves the quality of the care provided by the carer and reduces carer burnout (NICE, 2019). In addition to adopting a caregiver role, family members are often responsible for facilitating communication between the atypical communicator and clinicians (Keeley, 2017). Atypical communicators may be unable to communicate their wishes and family may therefore play an essential advocacy role.

When planning EOL care, an individual's cultural background becomes particularly important. The family of the atypical communicator are likely to be an invaluable source of information regarding the individual's cultural and religious beliefs and how these would be taken into consideration when planning EOL care. There is a need for clinicians to recognise that heterogeneity that exists within and between cultural groups (Keeley, 2017). It is important to consider that the cultural and religious beliefs within a family may not be homogenous. It is the role of the clinician to ensure that the values of the patient are actively considered when planning EOL care. Clinicians working in EOL care should try to engage with diverse groups about values and beliefs associated with EOL (Keeley, 2017). Clinicians should be mindful that their communication is sensitive to the cultural and religious beliefs of the patient and their family (Keeley, 2017). This may include clarifying the correct pronunciation of names and providing diet recommendations which are considerate of an individual's religious and cultural values (Keeley, 2017). This can be achieved through open communication with the individual's family. There is a need for culturally sensitive resources to be developed. This may include but is not limited to video explanations, online resources, written information, and pictures. Resources should be translated and provided to both the patient and their family (Keeley, 2017).

Research has demonstrated that members of the families of terminally ill patients often struggle to transition from hope for a particular outcome (e.g. cure for cancer) to a more broadly defined hope (e.g. good death or no pain). Families often require the guidance of clinicians when transitioning to a generalised hope (Koenig Kellas et al., 2017). Clinicians should ensure that their communication is sensitive without setting unrealistic expectations. This will help to ensure that EOL care is initiated in a timely manner, reducing unnecessary hospital admissions, and preventing the provision of aggressive treatment when it is no longer appropriate (Koenig Kellas et al., 2017).

The impact of COVID-19 on communication with families

The COVID-19 pandemic suddenly and drastically changed the way clinicians communicated with families (Marra et al., 2020; Mistraletti et al., 2020). This extreme situation has provided an opportunity for healthcare staff to reflect on how they communicate with families and facilitate communication between atypical communicators and their families. This change was most evident on intensive care units where large numbers of patients were unable to communicate with their families due to the severity of their illness. In addition, most acute hospitals prohibited or significantly restricted visitors (National Health Service, 2021). Contact with families was limited to telephone and video calls (Marra et al., 2020). As a result, non-verbal communication, which is of immeasurable value in sensitive situations, was significantly reduced (Marra et al., 2020). The importance of communication in intensive care has been well documented, with many families reporting that communication skills are as important as clinical skills (Marra et al., 2020). Communication with families requires honesty and sensitivity. Hope should be communicated; however, it is important that realistic expectations are conveyed.

When communicating with families in isolation there are facilitating strategies clinicians can employ. Where possible clinicians should use video calls to maximise non-verbal communication. Clinicians should also focus on the non-verbal communication that remains available such as the tone of voice, pause and inflection (Marra et al., 2020). In addition to facilitating social calls for patient wellbeing, it is important for clinicians to maintain regular contact with the patient's family to provide clinical updates. It is recommended that clinicians make daily contact with the individual's family when relatives are isolated. In the event that an individual is deteriorating, the family should be contacted more frequently. Whenever possible, the same clinician should make the calls. When transferring to another clinician is necessary, adequate handover should be provided (Mistraletti et al., 2020). The clinician should be sure to be adequately prepared before contacting a patient's family for a clinical update. This includes checking that they have the correct names for the patient and their family, up-to-date information regarding the patient's current clinical condition and plans for treatment. During the call, family members should be provided with one piece of information at a time, with communication being adapted to meet their needs. The use of jargon should be avoided and interruptions from the family member accepted. Clinicians should be mindful of and verbally acknowledge the psychological implications for the family (Mistraletti et al., 2020). Research has demonstrated that rates of post-traumatic stress disorder, anxiety, and depression in relatives of critically ill patients were 57%, 80%, and 70%, respectively (Marra et al., 2020). Psychological support should be offered when indicated. Clinicians should facilitate religious assistance when requested. Written information, for example via email, can be used to supplement verbal communication (Mistraletti et al., 2020).

Table 7.1 Key clinical recommendations

Tip	*Explanation*
Make communication a team effort	Delivery of effective care for an atypical communicator is a team effort. Included in this team is the patient's family. Where possible, with the patient's consent, family members should be invited to consultations to reduce the risk of miscommunication, facilitate communication between the patient and the clinician, and to relay information regarding care. One family member should be nominated as the primary contact with the healthcare team. This will reduce the risk of miscommunication between the healthcare team and the family. Likewise, the family should be provided with the contact details for a key worker within the healthcare team with whom they can raise queries or concerns.
Be patient	Caring for an atypical communicator is likely to be distressing for the family. Adopting a caregiver role, particularly in the context of a communication disorder is likely to strain family relationships and impact on family wellbeing. When communicating with an individual's family, clinicians should ensure that their communication is sensitive to the family's circumstance. Sufficient time should be allocated to consultations so that information can be clearly communicated, and the patient and their family feel valued. Engagement with healthcare professionals may be impacted if patients and their families begin to sense that the healthcare professional is time pressured. This may have significant consequences for the quality of the care delivered and psychological well-being. If at first communication is unsuccessful, try again, sometimes it's just not the right time.

Table 7.1 (Continued)

Tip	*Explanation*
Establish the family's knowledge base	When managing an atypical communicator, family often adopt a caregiver role. This may include assuming the role of the patient's primary contact with the healthcare team. Clinicians should therefore establish the family's understanding of the healthcare system and the patient's condition. Communication should then be modified to meet the family's needs.
Avoid technical language	Where possible the clinician should avoid using technical language and always explain unfamiliar terms.
Reveal competence	The family of the atypical communicator may be the primary point of contact between the patient and clinicians. However, it should not be assumed that the patient cannot communicate using alternative forms of communication, for example via email, writing or an assistive communication device. A communication impairment is not synonymous with a cognitive impairment. Whenever possible the patient should be encouraged to communicate with the healthcare team. This will maximise patient autonomy and reduce family caregiver burden.
Acknowledge the family's burden	Living with and/or caring for an atypical communicator has been shown to have negative psychological implications for the family. Clinicians should acknowledge the enormity of the caregiver role. Psychological support and signposting to appropriate services and support should be offered to the family when indicated.

Building upon the two illustrative case studies, this chapter highlighted the role family members play in the clinical management of atypical communicators. The importance of adapting communication to meet not only the needs of atypical communicators but their family members has been explained. Practical communication recommendations for clinicians working with atypical communicators and their families were presented. Recommendations focused on adopting a family-centred approach to communication through actively involving the atypical communicator's family in their care. Clinicians are encouraged to use alternative forms of communication to supplement verbal communication.

References

Bond, S. M., Schamuchaer, K., Sherrod, A., Dietrich, M. S., Wells, N., Lindau III, R. H., & Murphy, B. A. (2016). Development of the head and neck cancer caregiving task inventory. *European Journal of Oncological Nursing, 24*, 29–38.

Breen, L. J., O'Connor, M., Calder, S., Tai, V., Cartwright, J., & Bailey, J. M. (2017). The health professionals' perspective of support needs of adult head and neck cancer survivors and their families: a Delphi Study. *Support Care Cancer, 25*, 2413–2420.

Brown, K., Worrall, L. E., Davidson, B., & Howe, T. (2012). Living successfully with aphasia: A qualitative meta-analysis of the perspectives of individuals with aphasia, family members, and speech-language pathologists. *International Journal of Speech-Language Pathology, 14*(2), 141–155.

Cruice, M., Worrall, L., Hickson, L., & Murison, R. (2005). Measuring quality of life: Comparing family members' and friends' ratings with those of their aphasic partners. *Aphasiology, 19*(2), 111–129.

Cruice, M., Worrall, L., & Hickson, L. (2006). Perspectives of quality of life by people with aphasia and their family: suggestions for successful living. *Topics in Stroke Rehabilitation, 13*(1), 14–24.

Hadziabdic, E., & Hjelm, K. (2013). Working with interpreters: practical advice for use of an interpreter in healthcare. *International Journal of Evidence-Based Healthcare, 11*, 69–76.

Howe, T., Davidson, B., Worral, L. Hersh, D., Ferguson, A., Sherratt, S. & Gilbert, J. (2012). 'You needed to rehab...families as well': family members' own goal for aphasia rehabilitation. *International Journal of Language & Communication Disorders, 47*, 511–521.

Johnson, C., Kelch, J., Johnson, R. (2017). Dementia at end of life and family partners: A symbolic interactionist perspective on communication. *Behavioural Sciences, 7*(3), 42.

Keeley, M. P. (2017). Family communication at the end of life. *Behavioural Sciences, 7*(3), 45.

Koenig Kellas, J., Castle, K. M., Johnson, A., & Cohen, M. Z. (2017). Communicatively constructing the bright and dark sides of hope: family caregivers' experiences during end of life cancer care. *Behavioural Sciences, 7*(2), 33.

Mackenzie, L., Bhuta, P., Rusten, K., Devine, J., Love, A., & Waterson, P. (2016). Communication technology and motor neuron disease: An Australian survey of people with motor neuron disease. *JMIR Rehabilitation and Assistive Technologies, 3*(1), e2, retrieved from https://rehab.jmir.org/2016/1/e2/authors

Maguire, P., & Pitceathly, C. (2002). Key communication skills and how to acquire them. *The British Medical Journal 7366*(325), 697–700.

Marra, A., Buonanno, P., Vargas, M., Iacovazzo, C., Ely, E. W., & Servillo, G. (2020). How COVID-19 pandemic changes our communication with families: losing nonverbal cues. *Critical Care, 297*(24), https://doi.org/10.1186/s13054-020-03035-w

Mental Capacity Act. (2005). Mental Capacity Act. TSO.

Mistraletti, G., Gristina, G., Mascarin, S., Lacobone, E., Giubbilo, I., Bonfanti, S., Fiocca, F., Fullin, G., Fuselli, E., Bocci, M. G., Mazzoh, D., Giusti, G. D., Galazzi, A., Negro, A., De Iaco, F., Gandolfo, E., Lamiani, G., Del Negro, S., Monti, L., Salvago, F., Di Leo, S., Gribaudi, M. N., Piccinni, M., Riccioni, L., Giannini, A., Livigni, S., Maglione, C., Vergano, M., Mariangela, F., Lovato, L., Mezzetti, A., Drigo, E., Vegni, E., Calva, S., Aprile, A., Losi, G., Fontanella, L., Calegari, G., Ansaloni, C., Pugliese, F. R., Manca, S., Orsi, L., Moggia, F., Scelsi, S., Corcione, A., & Petrini, F. (2020). How to communicate with families living in complete isolation. *BMJ Supportive & Palliative Care, 0*, 1–12.

Money, D. (2016). *Inclusive communication and the role of speech and language therapy royal College of speech and language therapy position paper.* Royal College of Speech and Language Therapists. Retrieved from www.rcslt.org

National Institute for Health and Care Excellence. (2012). *Patient experience in adult NHS services: improving the experience of care for people using adult NHS services.* Retrieved November 9, 2020, from www.nice.org.uk/guidance/cg138/chapter/1-guidance

National Institute for Health and Care Excellence. (2019). *End of life care for adults.* Retrieved February 19, 2021, from www.nice.org.uk/guidance/qs13/resources/end-of-life-care-for-adults-pdf-2098483631557

National Health Service. (2021). *Visiting someone in hospital.* Retrieved February 19, 2021, from www.nhs.uk/nhs-services/hospitals/going-into-hospital/visiting-someone-in-hospital/

Northcott, S., Moss, B., Harrison, K., & Hilari, K. (2016). A systematic review of the impact of stroke on social support and social networks: associated factors and patterns of change. *Clinical Rehabilitation*, *30*(8), 811–831.

Parker, V., Bennett, L., Bellamy, D., Britton, B., & Lambert, S. (2016). Study protocol: Evaluation of a DVD intervention designed to meet the informative needs of patients with head and neck cancer and their partners, carer and families. *BMC Health Service Research*, *670*(16). Retrieved from www.ncbi.nlm.nih.gov/pmc/articles/PMC5118897/

Richardson, A. E., Morton, R. P., & Broadbent, E. A. (2016). Changes over time in head and neck cancer patients' and caregivers' illness perception and relationship with quality of life. *Psychology & Health*, *31*(10), 1203–1219.

Ringash, J., Bernstein, L. J., Devins, G., Dunphy, C., Giuliani, M., Martiono, & McEwen, S. (2017). Head and neck cancer survivorship: learning the needs, meeting the needs. *Seminars in Radiation Oncology*, *28*, 64–74.

Ross, E., & Wecliffe, T. (2001). The psychological effects of traumatic brain injury of the quality of life a group of spouses/partners. *South African Journal of Communication Disorders*, *48*, 77–99.

Sim, P., Power, E., & Togher, L. (2013). Describing conversations between individuals with traumatic brain injury (TBI) and communication partners following communication partner training: using exchange structure analysis. *Brain Injury*, *27*(6), 717–742.

Simmons-Mackie, N., Raymer, A., Armstrong, E., Holland, A., & Cherney, L. R. (2010). Communication partner training in aphasia: a systematic review. *Archives of Physical Medicine and Rehabilitation*, *91*, 1814–1837.

Sterba, K. R., Zapka, J, LaPelle, N., Garris, T. K., Buchanan, A., Scallion, M., & Day, T. (2017). Development of a survivorship needs assessment planning tool for head and neck cancer survivors and their care givers: a preliminary study. *Journal of Cancer Survivorship*, *11*, 822–832.

Stroke Association. (2020.). What is aphasia. Retrieved November 9, 2020, from www.stroke.org.uk/what-is-aphasia

World Health Organization. (2013). *How to use the ICF: A practical manual for using the International Classification of Functioning, Disability and Health (ICF).* Retrieved August 8, 2021, from https://cdn.who.int/media/docs/default-source/classification/icf/drafticfpracticalmanual2.pdf?sfvrsn=8a214b01_4

Communicating with people with tracheostomies and head and neck cancers

Anne Hurren, Kirsty McLachlan, and Nick Miller

Chapter contents:

- Guidelines for working with patients who have a tracheostomy
- Clinical relevance for tracheostomy patients
- Guidelines for working with those who have HNC
- Clinical relevance for HNC patients
- A: non-specialist clinical settings
- B: specialist clinical settings
- Clinical case studies
- Cultural considerations
- Recommended resources
- References

This chapter looks at why and how people with a tracheostomy and/or head and neck cancer (HNC) experience altered communication. These two groups are not mutually exclusive; some, but not all, patients with HNC will require a tracheostomy, but most tracheostomy procedures are performed for reasons unrelated to local carcinoma. The first part of the chapter relates to communication issues in tracheostomy regardless of aetiology and we then take a closer look at the population of people who have HNC without a tracheostomy. It is important to highlight a critical distinction between types of patients who breathe via a visible neck stoma. Whilst some have undergone a tracheostomy, others have had a total laryngectomy which involves very different changes to anatomy and communication and is carried out almost entirely due to laryngeal cancer. For these reasons, total laryngectomy will be discussed in the HNC (second) section. In the final section we provide two case studies, then examine cultural issues and the implications of changes for anyone who

DOI: 10.4324/9781003142522-11

interacts with people in this population. We conclude with guidelines for optimising communication and minimising any negative impacts and list key resources for those who would like to learn more about issues concerning this population.

Guidelines for working with patients who have a tracheostomy

Tracheostomy involves creating an opening in the front of the neck, leading directly into the trachea, and fitting a tube to maintain an open stoma. This is a lifesaving procedure when the upper-airway is occluded or critically narrowed by trauma, structural failure, or disease and/or when the individual is unable to protect their airways from aspiration and possible blockage due to ingress of nasal-oral secretions. A tracheostomy permits access to the lower airways to suction excess secretions and fluid arising from infection and disease (e.g., cystic fibrosis) and in conditions where chest muscle weakness or paralysis means the person is unable to cough forcefully enough to clear their own airways. An individual may be able to breathe under their own volition through the tracheostomy; if not, it can serve as a port for mechanical ventilation.

There are many reasons why someone may need a tracheostomy. Temporary tracheostomy may be necessary when acute trauma or acute respiratory failure (e.g. from infection, inhalation of toxic substances, sepsis) compromises the airways and ability to deliver oxygen to the lungs. Short-term tracheostomy may be required when surgery temporarily blocks the airways, and/or impedes the individual's ability to breathe voluntarily, and/or renders them unable to clear their own airways, and where mechanical ventilation may be required for a period. Exact duration is dependent on the underlying condition, recovery mechanisms (e.g. resolution of oedema, wound healing), and response to interventions. The period may range from hours to days or weeks. A longer-term or permanent tracheostomy may be employed when surgery and/or chemo+/-radiotherapy has irrevocably altered the airways, where infection or trauma has left permanently damaged tissues or structures, and in neurological conditions that have left the individual unable to adequately support their own respiration – a possible scenario, for instance, in severe brainstem stroke, and at some stage in several degenerative neurological disorders.

Whilst the procedure is lifesaving, it does mean that, because breathing now bypasses the larynx, speech is not possible. This can have serious consequences for social, psychological, and affective quality of life, both for the person with the tracheostomy and their carers. It also represents a significant variable in delivery of optimal, patient-centred care. Consideration of these issues needs to be to the fore in the care of people with tracheostomy.

Clinical relevance for tracheostomy patients

Where there may be a degree of choice in when or whether a tracheostomy is created and how long it will remain in situ, the resultant loss of voice and its potential consequences constitute an important topic of discussion between patients and the healthcare team who are supporting informed consent and planning for future needs (McGrath et al., 2016; McRae et al., 2020; Santiago et al., 2020). Ideally, patients make a choice, having been able to fully weigh up the gains in terms of prognosis for safe respiration and survival balanced against restrictions in or impossibility of speaking and all the social, psychological, affective, and care implications this has. Where delay in creating a tracheostomy was not an option, promptly establishing adequate and reliable means of communication constitutes an essential aim during recovery.

Speaking is especially likely to be impossible when the inserted tube has a cuff that inflates inside the trachea to aid the airtightness of the seal and as added protection against aspiration of secretions. Some individuals may tolerate brief spells when the cuff is (partially) deflated; such periods are also part of weaning off mechanical ventilation (McGrath et al., 2016: Pandian et al., 2019a, 2020). A deflated cuff enables air to flow via the larynx, thereby offering the possibility of some phonation. Typically, to maximise airflow via the larynx to drive the vocal cords, the stoma opening is temporarily shut off by a valve. Some cases may have a tube without a cuff that permits phonation because some air can still pass between the vocal cords. With some devices a speaking valve allows more or less permanent opportunity for speech. Sometimes it is possible for the individual simply to occlude the stoma with their finger to maximise airflow via the larynx, though the longer-term advisability of this raises questions (Pandian et al., 2019a, 2019b).

For many, though, risk of hypoxia means cuff-deflation is not an option. They must permanently use an alternative to speech for communication. Even when there is some passage of air through the larynx, conversing can remain effortful, tiring, frustrating and/or run the risk of respiratory distress. Without sufficient air, utterance length is short. There are large gaps in the flow of speech while the person inspires enough air to speak. Rapid fatigue means lengthy conversations may not be feasible. Prolonged disuse of the vocal cords can lead to atrophy and weakness, meaning voice, even if realised, remains faint. Dry mouth or excessive saliva may hamper speech for some. The tube and stoma require careful maintenance. Ill-fitting tubes and valves, cuffs inflated to the wrong pressure, tubes blocked by secretions, an insufficiently humidified trachea, all increased risk of infection, pain, and breakdown of tissue that can make speaking uncomfortable and disagreeable.

For the person wishing to communicate with individuals with a tracheostomy, important knowledge includes what type of tube and valve are fitted, what opportunities and what toleration the person might have for oral breathing and how viable and for how long phonation may be possible. Timespan may be limited by the danger of becoming hypoxic and/or from the more general consequences of their underlying condition (e.g. level of consciousness, orientation, pain, fatigue). Most communication may therefore be confined to the person with the tracheostomy expressing themselves using an augmentative or alternative means of communication (AAC) (Mobasheri et al., 2016; Santiago et al., 2020). Referrals to the speech and language therapy service are advised for their expertise as part of the multidisciplinary team if a tracheostomy patient has a communication difficulty. AAC options range from low-tech writing pads and finger pointing to an ABC chart up to highly sophisticated intelligent synthetic voice devices (Chapter 4). However, when speech is not possible, it is not just a matter of exchanging speaking for AAC. The nature of AAC communication totally alters the dynamics of interactions. It is an acquired skill both for the person using AAC and for those interacting with them. Moreover, the underlying condition that has imposed the need for a tracheostomy is likely to set constraints on which AAC is possible, how easy it is to deploy and how easy and for how long communication can last.

Level of arousal and consciousness play a part. Attention level and span exercise an influence. Presence of cognitive changes may limit or preclude AAC choices and restrict what the person is able to understand from others as well as formulating their own replies. Availability of physical stamina is a factor. Impaired motor control of fingers, hands, and arms may dictate choice of AAC and its effectiveness. Degree of voluntary eye movement, head control, lying and sitting posture and balance may need consideration. For longer-term AAC use, acceptability and usability of the device/method in the contexts where the person wants or needs to communicate become important variables in the ease, satisfaction, and success of communication. A person may employ multiple means according to context, interlocutor, and topic.

Whatever the situation, the presence of AAC should not become, consciously or unconsciously, a cause for excluding the patient from interactions. Ideally, a healthcare worker who needs to communicate with someone via AAC should inform themselves on the scope and methods of the communication device, what is readily feasible and what adjustments to their interactions and expectations might be required to facilitate optimum communication. The impact of a tracheostomy and loss of speech is not confined to physical and cognitive–linguistic matters. It is also associated with potentially profound psychological and social risks. The impact of dependence on AAC or restricted speech on conversational dynamics was also already mentioned. In common with all other causes of restricted communication, tracheostomy imposes social limitations on participation in society – whether this be the confines of the ward or family or broader intercourse in the community.

Just because some degree of spoken communication is possible and/or the individual has become adept at deploying their AAC method does not necessarily mean psychosocial issues are solved. Even when communication is relatively uncomplicated by impaired level of consciousness and cognitive and severe physical constraints, people with a tracheostomy who have restricted communication report ongoing psychosocial issues (Freeman-Sanderson et al., 2016, 2018; Pandian et al., 2020). Freeman-Sanderson et al. (2016) found that people with a tracheostomy felt that managing some speech brought relief and greater cheerfulness. However, it did not automatically increase their confidence in communicating, their sense of outgoingness and optimism, nor their sense of anger and frustration at and with impaired communication.

For some people, implementation of rehabilitation to achieve AAC or use what restricted speech capability they possess is affected by factors not confined to the mechanics of device use or speaking. For some, against the relief of being alive, of surviving, any other considerations, including investment of time and energy into acquiring new communication means, become minor issues. People may have priorities more important to them than speaking – e.g. eating and drinking, pain relief, sexual relationships. Sometimes, after the struggle to survive, there exists a degree of 'battle fatigue' that causes the person to have no inclination or energy for continued efforts to communicate. Presence of post-traumatic stress disorder (PTSD) cannot be discounted. If the individual's outlook for their shorter or longer-term survival is, or is perceived to be, curtailed, this may engender a sense of resignation or hopelessness. This in turn can undermine their motivation to acquire any new means of communication or even to communicate at all. Such issues emphasise the broader context of conversations and decision making about rehabilitation or palliative management that may impinge on forward planning, and psychosocial and spiritual care.

For someone who has undergone a tracheostomy due to sudden onset of a condition, loss of communication arrives at a time when they have vital questions and anxieties over their situation – what has happened, why, what will happen now, what are my choices; how my family are, pets, friends; will I die; how can I make my fears and worries known. For someone who has reached this stage in the deteriorating course of their illness, limitations on communication come at a time when they may wish to commune with family and friends more than ever, perhaps to express final intimate thoughts and feelings. The importance of long-term, palliative management of such cases to anticipate and prepare for this eventuality is firmly underlined. In certain circumstances here voice and message banking may be options to consider (Benson, 2021).

In some geographical areas, having a tracheostomy may pose an issue in onward destination after hospital. Nursing homes may not feel able to accept people with tracheostomy, given the necessary skills for nursing care and the risk factors associated with having a tracheostomy. Assuring knowledge and skills for self-management of stoma and tube care are also important considerations pre-discharge and in ongoing community follow-up for patients and carers. A person may have spent weeks or months totally dependent on hospital staff for all their care requirements. Quite apart from any other practical or psychosocial issues with managing aspects of the aftermath of their trauma or illness, it can be a daunting undertaking being thrust into a situation where they themselves and their family are now responsible for anticipating needs, expressing concerns, and solving problems. Hence the need for planned discharge discussions and training as well as home and community support services not just for communication but for the whole package of airway and stoma care (McGrath & Wallace, 2014).

Guidelines for working with those who have HNC

HNC may affect the structure and movement of any part of the vocal tract – these include airways, larynx and vocal cords, oro- and naso-pharynx, soft and hard palate, nasal cavities, tongue, lips, mandible, and maxilla. Cancers and surgical procedures outside the vocal tract (e.g. from the thyroid gland, salivary glands, lungs, brain, or ear) may impinge on voice and speech. Radiotherapy with or without chemotherapy can also leave patients with changes to the aforementioned structures leading to speech and voice impairments. The extent to which communication is affected depends on a complex interaction of size and site of growth, effects of treatment – including site and amount of tissue sacrificed, ability to reconstruct structures, oedema, fibrosis, and nerve damage from surgery/chemo/radiotherapy. The availability and options for speech and language therapy (SLT) support and patient choices (e.g. aiming for cure which may involve extensive removal of tissue/structures and loss of voice-speech function) also affect the communication outcome. Whilst a chemoradiotherapy option may preserve an organ (e.g. larynx), treatment effects may impact on its function, and if it fails to cure the cancer, subsequent surgery (known as salvage) is likely to be more complex. In what ways speech and voice are impacted also depends on these factors. The range of issues that individuals may experience include anything from mild hoarseness of voice, slight hypernasality, or imprecision of speech, through to inability or severe difficulty making themselves understood. Such severe difficulty may be due to aphonia from total cordectomy, extreme hypernasality from sacrifice of soft and/or hard palate, partial or total glossectomy, or restricted jaw movement. People with laryngeal cancer who require a total laryngectomy will be dependent on alternative means of communication which may include silent mouthing, an electrolarynx, or alaryngeal voice or combinations thereof. These methods are explained further, below.

Communication changes do not happen in a vacuum. They arise against a background of a life-changing, possibly life-limiting diagnosis and all that this may entail in terms of social, psychological, and spiritual adjustments (Rogers et al., 2020). Communication is always collaborative, interactive, and shared with at least one communication partner. Thus, impaired voice and/or speech impedes social discourse. One's feeling about how one speaks and communicates is intimately entwined with one's view of oneself, one's personality, character, mood, and how others perceive one. Loss or distortion of voice or speech can be as devastating and life changing as severe physical disfigurement or loss of limbs. For the person with HNC and their family, there can be devastating psychological consequences for one's lost speech and voice. All these factors contribute to the impact of HNC on communication, on the individual, on their family, and on social circles. They shape immediate questions around intervention and prognosis, about immediate and longer-term expectations, adjustments, and options. They determine the spoken and unspoken concerns of the individual and their family and how and about what they wish to communicate.

Clinical relevance for HNC patients

Communication difficulties can be a risk factor impeding an individual from receiving safe and appropriate healthcare. Pretending to understand or discounting parts of conversations that were unintelligible inevitably leaves the speaker feeling unheard. Information that was not conveyed may be of paramount importance, to the patient psychosocially or to the clinician in terms of symptoms that must be considered. Unequal power dynamics in clinical settings and/or feelings of helplessness due to repeated past communicative failures may stop patients from challenging misinterpreted or truncated discourse. Anger, frustration, tearfulness and withdrawal are other potential responses. The minimum standard of care during consultations is to enable relaxed and natural discourse that does not draw attention to altered speech or voice and allows effective assessment and treatment in the clinical setting. This requires skilful management. The guidelines in section A below outline key general issues in communication that may be encountered and how to manage breakdowns in communication. Section B summarises the more advanced knowledge needed by staff who work in more specialist HNC services.

A: Non-specialist clinical settings

The communication issues within this population can broadly be divided into those who have had a total laryngectomy and those who have other types of speech/voice impairment. Concerns relating to speech and voice are discussed first as many of the recommendations apply equally to laryngectomy, which is discussed subsequently. A key consideration is one's own non-verbal communication. This is the first thing a patient will notice. Many survivors of HNC have altered appearance. Being mindful of and controlling one's own unconscious reactions via facial expression, tone of voice, recoiling posture, or any other unconscious non-verbal cue, is essential to avoid exacerbating feelings of shame, embarrassment, negative self-identity, and 'body image distress' (Melissant et al., 2021) felt by a significant proportion of HNC patients. Conveying, even unconsciously, a negative reaction immediately raises further barriers to willingness and confidence in communicating. A concise overview of dos and don'ts when communicating with people with speech difficulties within clinical settings (Hemsley n.d.) includes a useful hyperlink to the Patient–Provider Communication website where case examples and downloadable resources such as communication charts are provided.

Those who have not had a laryngectomy face one or a combination of problems in impaired articulation, nasal resonance, or voice quality (if the vocal folds are involved). Effects on intelligibility may range from mild to severe. Degree of intelligibility should not be taken to reflect likelihood of patients' levels of distress. Someone with mild articulatory imprecision or a dysphonic voice that does not affect intelligibility may avoid social contact due to self-consciousness about their altered speech or voice, whilst another with reduced intelligibility may continue with their pre-morbid social interactions and be unperturbed by listener requests to repeat what they have just said.

To avoid disempowering and marginalising patients, it is usually helpful right at the start to ask the client how best to communicate with them, and to carefully negotiate their agreement before directing communication via other family members. The key recommendation is never to pretend you have understood. Admit this empathically and if repeated attempts still fail, switch to closed questions with only yes/no answers. Ensure the room is quiet and well lit, sit closer to the person, carefully observe their facial expressions and body language and listen to the tone of voice, as intonation may be preserved and provide insight into emotions if the larynx is unaffected. If you perceive any lack of ease in the patient around communication, enquire tentatively if this is indeed the case and again find out what may help. Gesture and pointing can be encouraged to explain symptoms, or provide pictures, models, or photographs to point to. Consultations will inevitably take longer. They should be unhurried, especially as the typical turn taking in conversations will be altered, and it is easy for a person with communication impairment to have an unequal share and miss out on what they intended to say.

Proceed diplomatically before offering an alphabet chart or pen and paper. Many with limited literacy are embarrassed to admit this. Conversely some may have functional writing and just need encouragement that even single words or drawing can convey a lot, especially when there is no judgement on their spelling or handwriting. Some may bring low technology communication aids such as photograph 'communication passports' which still rely on the skill of the participant to interpret. Allowing time for repeated attempts and employing closed questions may facilitate understanding. Some individuals may use high technology aids with pre-recorded responses or text to speech facility, but encouragement may be necessary for them to use them in clinic.

The subgroup of patients undergoing total laryngectomy will permanently breathe through a tracheostoma with no airway above the level of this stoma. Pre and post laryngectomy anatomy is shown in Figure 8.1. Unless the patient is rehabilitated with a new method of communication, their speech will be silent articulation as there are no vocal folds and no exhaled breath via the mouth. Alaryngeal communication options for SLTs to select in conjunction with the surgeon and patient are outlined below.

1. Surgical voice restoration (SVR) – this is shown in the diagram on the far right of Figure 8.1 and involves creating a tracheoesophageal puncture for a one-way silicone voice prosthesis (valve). When the stoma is occluded with a finger, exhaled air passes through the valve and into the upper oesophagus, causing the reconstructed muscles of the pharynx to vibrate to produce voice in lieu of the vocal folds. The case example of Brian (outlined below) explains some issues relating to a patient rehabilitated with SVR after total laryngectomy.
2. Oesophageal voice – patients learn techniques in pushing air from mouth to oesophagus, so its release creates short bursts of reconstructed muscle vibration.
3. Electrolarynx – a hand-held device is placed against the neck, so vibrations transfer into the oral cavity where articulation allows speech to be produced, albeit with a distinctive robotic tone and little loudness and intonation variation.

SVR is considered the gold standard (Clarke et al., 2016) as it restores the most optimal speech. However, there is considerable variation between speakers using each method. The muscle tone of the reconstructed pharynx determines the quality of voice in SVR (Hurren et al., 2019) and oesophageal voice. Patients with optimal tone have voice quality similar to laryngeal speakers with laryngitis, whilst those who undergo free flap reconstruction may have whispery or gurgly voices. High tone results in a strained and effortful voice. Similarly, some electrolarynx speakers are very intelligible whilst others with neck fibrosis find the electronic tone has a loud background buzz and limited oral transmission.

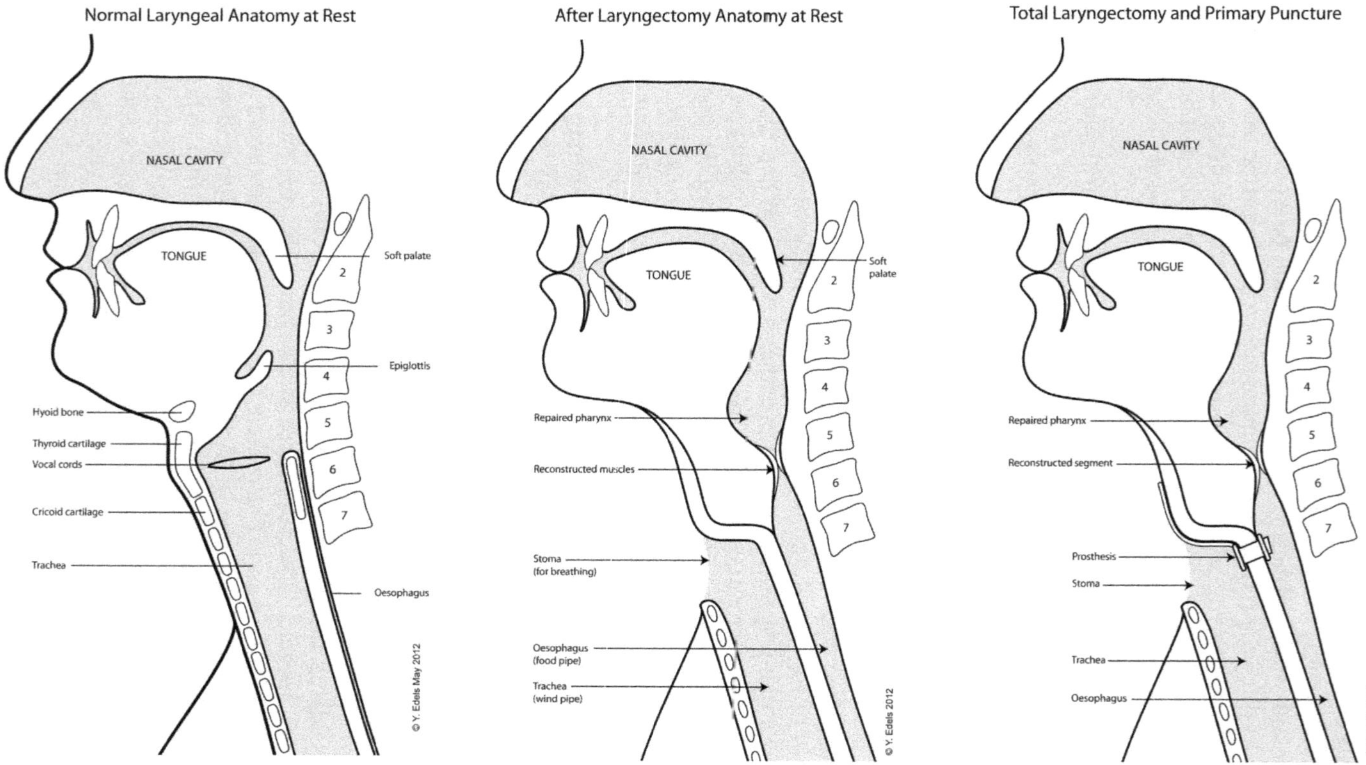

Figure 8.1 Three sagittal section diagrams of the head and neck in a row that illustrate anatomy. Copyright 2012 courtesy of Yvonne Edels.

Communication rehabilitation cannot commence until healing has occurred post-surgery and usually until effects of any adjuvant radio/chemotherapy have subsided. The same advice in dealing with limited intelligibility outlined above applies to laryngectomy speakers but it is important to be aware of potentially different needs. Patients must regularly clean their stoma and any valve or laryngectomy tube (required by some to avoid stoma shrinkage) to prevent build-up of secretions or mucus plugs. Most can self-manage this and may ask for access to a private space with a sink, mirror, and pen torch. Always ensure you have fully understood what the patient needs. All methods of communication and coughing can include loud stoma noise that can be disconcerting for unfamiliar listeners and may involve chest sputum noise or emission. If you ask yes/no questions they may be able to indicate if this noise is normal for them or if they are having difficulty breathing (e.g. if mucus crusts/plugs have started to block their trachea). If there are any concerns about their airway or breathing, get help immediately via 999. The one-way voice prosthesis (valve) used in SVR will wear out over time, resulting in fluids escaping into the trachea (leaking valve). Complications can also occur (e.g. the valve can accidentally extrude and fall into the trachea) (Lewin et al., 2017; McLachlan et al., 2022). Again, ensure you fully understand if a patient is asking for help, as their voice may be compromised by a valve difficulty. An aspirated valve requires immediate help via 999 and valve leakage needs less urgent but prompt attention via their HNC unit for a replacement to be fitted. Patients and carers are usually trained in how to access help and may carry an alert card with details.

B: Specialist clinical settings

UK National Multidisciplinary Guidelines for HNC (Humphris, 2016) specified all multidisciplinary team members should undergo communication skills training to develop consultation expertise. These skills are essential for discussing and planning cancer treatment and to ensure that the holistic needs of patients and carers are embedded in practice. Ethical care should include screening for and ameliorating any psychological distress (Deelemans et al., 2020). UK Guidelines place support and education for less serious psychosocial issues within the role of team members without mental health qualifications. Those with more serious psychological distress are referred to clinical psychology, psychotherapists, or liaison psychiatry. To achieve this, it is expected that psychology provision is integral to every team.

Several important areas need to be considered in consultations and communications with patients and carers in terms of holistic care. Fear of recurrence of cancer (known to relate to depression) is the most common concern (Humphris, 2016), and although it may not be raised overtly it is crucial to watch for it being broached covertly and deal with the issue sensitively. All consultations need careful use of language as clinicians can inadvertently generate fear of recurrence and other unhelpful, frightening mental imagery about HNC, particularly during early consultations (Lang et al., 2018). Written materials or poster images have also been observed to contribute to distress in some cases. Patients should be monitored for PTSD (intrusive thoughts, avoidant behaviour, and hyperarousal) found in 13% of a UK cohort with a further 33% with post-traumatic stress symptoms (PTSS) (Moschopoulou et al., 2018). This was not a temporary phenomenon and there was no relationship to cancer stage, site, or treatment, though younger patients were more susceptible. High rates of poor health literacy have also been observed in 47% of a HNC cohort (n = 395) in Ireland and associated with fear of recurrence, lower levels of self-management and worse HNC specific health-related quality of life (Clarke et al., 2021). It was suggested that health literacy interventions may help address self-management and fear of recurrence issues. Consultations should also screen for resilience as it is linked to enhanced quality of life. Social functioning and early resilience training interventions have been effective in other cancer populations (MacDonald et al., 2021).

It is essential to keep service users' personal agendas as a key focus in all consultations. The Patient Concern Inventory (PCI), developed and implemented by Rogers and co-workers (2009) suits this need. The 56-item patient prompt list, specific to HNC, empowers patients to select issues they wish to discuss at review appointments and which types of professionals they would like to see for physical, social, psychological, emotional, and spiritual well-being. Its use increased consultation times only by an average of approximately one minute (Rogers et al., 2021).

A final consideration concerns patients' partners and the need to communicate information that could help to alert them to potential psychological difficulties. Carers, too, can experience PTSD and PTSS. Moschopoulou et al. (2018) reported rates of 12.8% and 25.7% respectively, and these were unrelated to their partner's scores. They may also benefit from psychosocial support and information regarding how to develop protective factors in their relationship (Stenhammer et al., 2017; Gremore et al., 2020). For instance, open communication was noted as a protective factor whilst overprotective behaviour was linked to negative consequences for patients. This may be especially important when there are different illness perspectives between carer and patient. These have been found to impact negatively on patients' long-term quality of life (Richardson et al., 2016). Communication changes following chemo/radiotherapy have also been associated with negative psychosocial consequences for carers and patients (Nund et al., 2015). Sensitive education and interventions to forewarn and address these seem advisable but require further research.

Clinical case studies

Case study 8.1 Brian

Brian, aged 65, presented at the reception desk in accident and emergency but could not make himself understood. He mouthed silently and pointed repeatedly to a tracheostomy hole at the front of his neck. The junior doctor called to assess him took him to a quiet room and asked if he could speak a little more slowly. Brian calmed down and the stoma noise reduced. The doctor sat opposite Brian and carefully watched his lips as he spoke to lipread as much as possible, asked him to repeat when he could not understand and switched to closed yes/no questions if the repeat attempt was still not intelligible. He managed to clarify that Brian was not having breathing difficulties, had undergone laryngectomy not a tracheotomy, and there was a problem with a small plastic implant on the back wall of the stoma. Brian was not fully literate but wrote 'ENT please'. The doctor contacted the on-call ENT surgeon who removed the tracheoesophageal valve that had slightly dislodged and fitted a new one, allowing Brian to speak again as usual when he occluded the stoma.

Case study 8.2 Abdul

Abdul, aged 58 years, had a partial glossectomy followed by radiotherapy. This affected his articulation and he was often unintelligible without the benefit of contextual cues. He could become despondent and frustrated if not understood but did not want a communication aid as he did not want to draw attention to himself and wanted to communicate by speech. The general practitioner ensures that his appointments are not rushed by booking him in for extra time, making sure the window is shut so there is no traffic noise that may compete with his speech. He sits opposite him, giving him his full attention and not looking at the computer or typing during the consultation. If he cannot understand he calmly asks him to repeat and acknowledges he knows it is difficult and frustrating for him, but they have plenty of time and there is no hurry. During one consultation Abdul could not make the GP understand one important part of the sentence. The GP asked if he had a smart phone, then suggested Abdul could type what he was trying to explain. This quickly got the message across, and he began to use this to supplement his speech when he was unintelligible, as it did not feel like a communication aid.

Cultural considerations

Added factors potentially arise in cross-cultural contexts, in HNC as well as tracheostomy. Ability to speak English and degree of fluency may be an issue, along with how these impact on intelligibility. Working via an interpreter presents its own hurdles, but with tracheostomy, laryngectomy and use of AAC the potential risks of communication breakdown are compounded if the interpreter is unfamiliar with these modes of atypical communication. Cross-cultural factors are not confined to straightforward language competencies. Some languages (e.g. Cantonese), are tonal, where pitch inflection alone can change the meaning of a word. This means that patients who are unable to vary the intonation of their speech may have problems with intelligibility, in addition to any articulation problems with the tongue. Different cultures hold contrasting views on how and why particular health conditions may have arisen. For some cancers there may be culture-specific reasons for the prevalence of certain cancers (e.g. chewing tobacco, betel nuts). Beliefs about aetiology determine attitudes to what needs to happen to right the situation, who is responsible for that, what actions are necessary, and, vitally, what the role of the patient might be in all of this. For instance, a fatalistic acceptance of what has happened and that anything humans might do to right the situation is futile can lead to a passive or resistant attitude to rehabilitation. Cultural practices and beliefs can also colour attitudes to medical devices and use of AAC. This chapter is not the forum to elucidate all the variables that arise in cross-cultural medicine and rehabilitation, other than to underline the importance of an awareness of the factors and how they might interact with health provider roles.

We have described how structural changes to the vocal tract because of HNC or (semi)permanent tracheostomy can alter or obliterate spoken communication. SLTs take the lead in rehabilitation of speech in these cases. However, we emphasised that the challenges to communication range far beyond distorted speech and voice. Challenges encompass key aspects of non-verbal communication and all the practical issues around communicating with impaired speech and/or using AAC. These challenges cover the broader psychosocial and spiritual consequences of impaired communication in the context of a major illness episode. Vitally, solutions to challenges are found not just through rehabilitation goals for the person with altered communication, but in the communicative awareness, behaviours, and support given by the whole multidisciplinary team, and through training and support of carers. Many issues that demand awareness were covered above.

Five central messages are listed below for everyone to bear in mind in relation to this client population.

1. Communication takes time: for the person to formulate and convey their message; for the health worker to comprehend and confirm understanding. Ideally consultations allow for this.

2. Communication is more than sounds and words: facial expression, hand/arm gestures, body language all contribute to meaning. Be aware of signals from these sources; be aware what signals one conveys with one's own non-verbal messages, including unspoken 'professional in a rush', 'I've no time to listen to everything just now' insinuations.
3. Communication, especially during early rehabilitation, can be hard, embarrassing, uncomfortable, difficult to master. Appreciate this and look beyond the 'brave face' someone might be putting on. Create a relaxed, quiet, and well-lit environment conducive to maximising communicative success.
4. Carers can be as much impacted by communication changes as the person with HNC or tracheostomy. Make sure they are informed and supported too.
5. Speakers with a total laryngectomy will have a different voice quality to that of laryngeal speakers; the majority are reduced to one hand for gestures or writing as they need to hold an electrolarynx or occlude their tracheostoma to speak.

Recommended resources

1. American Speech-Language Hearing Association (ASHA), Tracheostomy and Ventilator Dependence. www.asha.org/practice-portal/professional-issues/tracheostomy-and-ventilator-dependence/
2. Doyle, P. C. (Ed.) (2019) Clinical care and rehabilitation in head and neck cancer. Cham, Switzerland: Springer.
3. Head and Neck Cancer UK (2021). http://hancuk.org/
4. Helmsley, B. (n.d.) 25 tips for communicating with people with little or no speech in clinical settings. https://bronwynhemsley.wordpress.com/about/25-tips-for-communicating-with-people-with-little-or-no-speech-in-clinical-settings/
5. Intensive Care Society (2020) Guidance for: tracheostomy care. www.ficm.ac.uk/sites/default/files/2020-08-tracheostomy_care_guidance_final.pdf
6. National Association of Laryngectomy Clubs (NALC). www.laryngectomy.org.uk/
7. National Tracheostomy Patient Safety Project (2021). www.tracheostomy.org.uk/with a sub-section including information about communication. www.tracheostomy.org.uk/healthcare-staff/vocalisation
8. Rogers, S. N., Allmark, C., Bekiroglu, F., Edwards, R. T., Fabbroni, G., Flavel, R., & Highet, V. (2020). Improving quality of life through the routine use of the patient concerns inventory for head and neck cancer patients: baseline results in a cluster preference randomised controlled trial. *European Archives Oto-Rhino-Laryngology, 277,* 3435.
9. Royal Children's Hospital, Melbourne, Australia, Clinical Guidelines (Nursing), Tracheostomy management (includes a sub-section on

communication). www.rch.org.au/rchcpg/hospital_clinical_guideline_index/Tracheostomy_management/

10. St George's Hospital Tracheostomy Guidelines, (includes a sub-section on communication). www.stgeorges.nhs.uk/gps-and-clinicians/clinical-resources/tracheostomy-guidelines/

References

Benson, J. (2021). Voice banking for people with dysarthria. In: M. Walshe and N. Miller (Eds.), *Clinical Cases in Dysarthria* (pp. 105–116). London: Taylor & Francis.

Clarke, N., Dunne, S., Coffey, L., Sharp, L., Desmond, D., O'Conner, J., O'Sullivan, E., Timon,

C., Cullen, C., & Gallagher, P. (2021). Health literacy impacts self-management, quality of life and fear of recurrence in head and neck cancer survivors. *Journal Cancer Survivorship, 15*, 855–865.

Clarke, P., Radford, K., Coffey, M., & Stewart, M. (2016) Speech and swallow rehabilitation in head and neck cancer: United Kingdom National Multidisciplinary Guidelines. *Journal Laryngology Otology, 130*, S176–S180.

Deleemans, J. M., Mothersill, K., Bultz, B. D., & Schulte, F. (2020). Ethical considerations in screening head and neck cancer patients for psychosocial distress. *Supportive Care Cancer, 28*, 617–624.

Freeman-Sanderson, A., Togher, L., Kenny, B., Elkins, M., & Phipps, P. (2016). Loss of voice in mechanically ventilated tracheostomy patients: the patient experience in ICU. *Australian Critical Care, 29*, 115–116.

Freeman-Sanderson, A. L., Togher, L., Elkins, M., & Kenny, B. (2018). Quality of life improves for tracheostomy patients with return of voice: a mixed methods evaluation of the patient experience across the care continuum. *Intensive Critical Care Nursing, 46*, 10–16.

Gremore, T., Brockstein, L., Porter, S., Brenner, T., Benfield, D., Baucom, T., Sher, & Atkins, D. (2020). Couple-based communication intervention for head and neck cancer: a randomized pilot trial. *Supportive Care Cancer, 29*, 3267–3275.

Helmsley, B. (n.d). 25 tips for communicating with people with little or no speech in clinical settings. Retrieved from https://bronwynhemsley.wordpress.com/about/25-tips-for-communicating-with-people-with-little-or-no-speech-in-clinical-settings/. Accessed March 2021.

Humphris, G. (2016). Psychological management for head and neck cancer patients: United Kingdom National Multidisciplinary Guidelines. *Journal Laryngology Otology, 130*, S45–S48.

Hurren, A., Miller, N., & Carding, P. (2019). Perceptual assessment of tracheoesophageal voice quality with SToPS: The development of a reliable and valid tool. *Journal Voice, 33*, 465–472.

Lang, H., France, E., Williams, B., Humphris, G., & Wells, M. (2018). The existence and importance of patients' mental images of their head and neck cancer: a qualitative study. *PLoS ONE, 13*, 1–20.

Lewin, J., Baumgart, L., Barrow, M., & Hutcheson, K. (2017). Device life of the tracheoesophageal voice prosthesis revisited. *Journal of the American Medicine Association Otolaryngology, 143*, 65–71.

MacDonald, C., Theurer, J. A., Fung, K., Yoo J., & Doyle, P. (2021). Resilience: an essential element in head and neck cancer survivorship and quality of life. *Supportive Care in Cancer, 29*, 3725–3733.

McGrath, B., Lynch, J., Wilson, M., Nicholson, L., & Wallace, S. (2016). Above cuff vocalisation: a novel technique for communication in the ventilator-dependent tracheostomy patient. *Journal Intensive Care Society, 17*, 19–26.

McGrath, B., & Wallace, S. (2014). The UK National Tracheostomy Safety Project and the role of speech and language therapists. *Current Opinion Otolaryngology Head Neck Surgery, 22*, 181–187.

McLachlan, K., Hurren, A., Owen, S., & Miller, N. (2022). Informing patient choice and service planning in surgical voice restoration: valve usage over three years in a UK head and neck cancer unit. *Journal Laryngology Otology, 136*, 158–166.

McRae, J., Montgomery, E., Garstang, Z., & Cleary, E. (2020). Role of Speech and language therapists in the intensive care unit. *Journal Intensive Care Society, 21*, 344–348.

Melissant, H., Jansen, F., Eerenstein, S., Cuijpers, P., Laan, E. Lissenberg-Witte, B., Schuit, A., Sherman, K., Leemans, C., & Verdonck-de Leeuw, I., (2021). Body image distress in head and neck cancer patients: what are we looking at? *Supportive Care in Cancer, 29*, 2161.

Mobasheri, M., King, D., Judge, S., Arshad, F., Larsen, M., Safarfashandi, Z., … Darzi, A. (2016). Communication aid requirements of intensive care unit patients with transient speech loss. *Augmentative Alternative Communication, 32*, 261–271.

Moschopoulou, E., Bhui, K., Korszun, A., & Hutchison, I. (2018). Post-traumatic stress in head and neck cancer survivors and their partners. *Supportive Care in Cancer, 26*, 3003–3011.

Nund, R., Rumbach, A., Debattista, B., Goodrow, M., Johnson, K., Tupling, L., Scarinci, N., Cartmill, B., Ward, E., & Porceddu, S. (2015). Communication changes following non-glottic head and neck cancer management: the perspectives of survivors and carers. *International Journal Speech-Language Pathology, 17*, 263–272.

Pandian, V., Boisen, S., Mathews, S., & Brenner, M. (2019a). Speech and safety in tracheostomy patients receiving mechanical ventilation: a systematic review. *American Journal Critical Care, 28*, 441–450.

Pandian, V., Boisen, S. E., Mathews, S., & Cole, T. (2019b). Are fenestrated tracheostomy tubes still valuable? *American Journal Speech-Language Pathology, 28*, 1019–1028.

Pandian, V., Cole, T., Kilonsky, D., Holden, K., Feller-Kopman, D., Brower, R., & Mirski, M. (2020). Voice-related quality of life increases with a talking tracheostomy tube: a randomized controlled trial. *Laryngoscope, 130*, 1249–1255.

Richardson, A., Morton, R., & Broadbent, E. (2016). Changes over time in head and neck cancer patients' and caregivers' illness perceptions and relationships with quality of life. *Psychology & Health, 31*, 1203–1219.

Rogers, S., El-Sheikha, J., & Lowe, D. (2009). The development of a patient's concerns inventory (PCI) to help reveal patients concerns in the head and neck clinic. *Oral Oncology, 45*(7), 555–561.

Rogers, S., Allmark, C., Bekiroglu, F., Edwards, R., Fabbroni, G., Flavel, R., & Highet, V. (2020). Improving quality of life through the routine use of the patient concerns inventory for head and neck cancer patients: baseline results in a cluster preference randomised controlled trial. *European Archives Oto-Rhino-Laryngology, 277*, 34–35.

Santiago, R., Howard, M., Dombrowski, N., Watters, K., Volk, M., Nuss, R., … Rahbar, R. (2020). Preoperative augmentative and alternative communication enhancement in pediatric tracheostomy. *Laryngoscope, 130*, 1817–1822.

Stenhammar, C., Isaksson, J., Granstrom, B., Laurell, G., & Ehrsson, Y. (2017). Changes in intimate relationships following treatment for head and neck cancer-A qualitative study. *Journal Psychosocial Oncology, 35*, 614–630.

Part III

Atypical communication in progressive neurological disorders

9

Atypical communication in Parkinson's disease, multiple sclerosis, and motor neuron disease

Sarah Griffiths and Nick Miller

Chapter contents:

- The nature of communication changes in PNDs and their clinical relevance
- Challenges of conversations
- Speech as identity
- Communication guidelines for working with this population
- Case studies
- Recommended resources
- References

Introduction

A person's ability to communicate may be negatively impacted as a common sequel of progressive neurological disorders (PNDs) such as Parkinson's (PD), motor neuron disease (MND) and multiple sclerosis (MS). This chapter opens with a broad outline of the motor and cognitive changes impinging on communication in PNDs, highlighting aspects of change that may not be readily apparent to listeners. The chapter then examines how health and social care workers can ensure the voices of people with communication changes are heard and understood in order to assure optimum and personalised care. We centre discussion around PD, MND and MS, however the communication changes and strategies we present could apply to a diverse range of PNDs such as multiple system atrophy, progressive supranuclear palsy, Huntington's, the dementias, and brain tumours, depending on the person and stage of condition. To close the chapter, case vignettes illustrate some key points.

Throughout, we emphasize that the roots and repercussions of communication changes spread deeper and wider than distorted pronunciation and quiet voice. Conveying one's thoughts and feelings involves more than just

DOI: 10.4324/9781003142522-13

speaking clearly: speech production is a cognitive–linguistic act; communicating is also a social act, where listeners play as important a role as speakers; speech constitutes a central component in self-identity and how others perceive us. The characterisation of communication with and for people with PNDs is severely incomplete without attention to these cognitive and psychosocial variables. Addressing the impacts of these factors requires attention from the earliest stages after diagnosis, with a long-term palliative approach to anticipate issues likely to arise as the underlying condition progresses.

The nature of communication changes in PNDs and their clinical relevance

How, when, and to what degree PNDs affect communication depends on the cause and course of the underlying neurological condition. In some conditions, impact is felt early, in others, late in the course of overall decline. Progression can be rapid, gradual, or follow a stepwise pattern. In some PNDs, communication alterations remain relatively mild. Other neurological conditions deteriorate relentlessly to produce profoundly unintelligible speech, even to familiar listeners, with subsequent need to communicate via non-verbal gestural or technological alternative or augmentative means of communication (AAC). This chapter focuses on spoken output, but PNDs can seriously restrict gesture, writing, and typing and thereby limit the options for AAC. We first turn to an overview of the impact of different neurological disorders on speech. In Parkinson's, individuals report a direct impact on communication from the start, even though speech may remain intelligible for many years, even decades (Miller, 2017; Schalling, Johansson, & Hartelius, 2017). Speech-voice changes may even have been the first sign in the prodromal period that something was amiss. By contrast, in MND, communication difficulties show themselves early and deteriorate to severe over just a few years (Yorkston, Baylor, & Mach, 2017). In MS, whether, when, and what speech changes develop depends on the sites of lesions. Nevertheless, many people with MS report from early on that cognitive–linguistic changes impair communication, even if speech/voice production sounds intact (El-Wahsh et al., 2020; Johansson, Schalling, & Hartelius, 2021; Noffs et al., 2021).

The next sections provide an overview of communication changes in these conditions, which are shared across many other PNDs. It starts with a summary of voice and speech changes but then draws attention to changes that are equally or more likely to be the root of communication breakdown.

Voice-speech changes

Voice refers to the vocal note/phonation produced in the larynx; speech refers to pronunciation of sounds made in the mouth. The two are intimately connected in speaking, but may be differentially impaired in PNDs.

Voice and respiration

Inability to control inspiration and expiration for speaking leads to overreliance on short phrases, even having to utter word-by-word. Voice may fade appreciably over the course of an utterance. The effort to take in sufficient breath and match expiration to the length of phrases makes speaking tiring. Insufficient air and/or reduced expiratory pressure lead to impaired voice quality and loudness control. Neuromuscular alterations to the vocal cords add to difficulties with phonation. Voice may sound strained, asthenic (weak) or hoarse; too soft, inappropriately loud, or with unpredictable bursts of loud voice.

Speech

Typically, the most obvious speech changes to listeners' ears concern slowed, imprecise, or slurred pronunciation. This is associated with underlying neuromuscular changes that cause loss of power to muscles, altered muscle tone, discoordination of movements, and/or problems gauging the energy/power put into achieving and maintaining the full range of articulatory movements (a prominent feature of Parkinson's). These in turn result in alterations to speed, range, and strength of movement, and placement and timing of movements of the tongue and lips.

Resonance

Sometimes soft palate movement is affected, leading to excessively nasal resonance – a frequent feature in MND.

Prosody

Problems with speech breathing and controlling the vocal cords combine to affect prosody. Prosody refers to the patterns of intonation and word/syllable stress (e.g., use of loudness/pitch/rate for emphasis) in a person's speech and the rate, fluency, and rhythm with which they speak. The person's voice may sound noticeably higher or lower pitched than previously. They may have difficulties signalling meaning contrasts that depend on raising or lowering pitch (e.g. as in the phrase 'you press this button' spoken as a question versus a command), or conveying emotional tone of voice (e.g., 'yes' spoken with definiteness, doubt, sadness, annoyance). Dysprosody can affect ability to signal contrasts between stressed and unstressed words/syllables (e.g. GREEN house/green HOUSE; THAT'S my coat/that's MY coat). When dysprosody is severe, speech may sound monoloud and monotone; a low mumble or constantly high-pitched voice; or there are inappropriate sudden swings in loudness and/or pitch.

However, as intimated above, seeing/hearing no further than distorted speech sounds and altered voice quality represents a very narrow perspective.

The following sections look at three crucial areas of breakdown that may be less apparent to listeners, but which for speakers with PNDs have potentially devastating consequences for communication.

Challenges of conversations

Engaging in conversations represents a major challenge for most people with speech changes associated with PNDs. The following factors represent key factors.

Speaking is tiring

When muscles are weak, tone is altered, movements are slow and discoordinated, and fatigue readily sets in – endeavouring to achieve anything through physical activity becomes demanding and exhausting. The physical act of speaking is no exception. Accomplishing and maintaining intelligible speech calls for sustained effort to make the movements to produce sound contrasts, to assure that the voice remains sufficiently clear and does not fade, and that stress and intonation patterns in the utterance transmit the desired grammatical and emotional meaning.

Conversations make high cognitive demands

Conversations can be problematic due to more than just physical effort. Engaging in conversations calls for adequate speed and capacity of processing, to comprehend and to compose one's responses. The discourse and cognitive–linguistic demands of conversations can be challenging.

For example, to follow and join in conversations speakers must maintain vigilance, constantly monitoring who is saying what about what topic. They must identify when a speaker is nearing the end of their turn-of-talk (in order to carry out the highly complex act of selecting oneself as the next speaker) and when a topic has shifted. They must 'read' between the lines to comprehend the unspoken content coming from speaker–listener assumptions about shared knowledge and inferences from words or turns of phrases. They have to anticipate meaning and be able to switch back if someone makes a false assumption. 'He had a spade in his hand …' Is this going to be about gardening, or playing cards? People with Parkinson's can be particularly prone to tripping up on (mis)expectations (Holtgraves & Giordano, 2017). Listeners may be unaware that the person with a PND wishes to speak (see sociolinguistic complexity below). When the person does speak, there can be uncertainty over what they wish to say due to hesitations with word retrieval, selecting the wrong word and/or over-relying on non-specific vocabulary (e.g., 'this', 'thing'). Motor disability means methods that could compensate for word retrieval difficulties, such as non-verbal strategies (e.g.

facial expressions, gestures) are unavailable (Perez et al., 2020; Saldert & Bauer, 2017).

Conversations are non-verbally and sociolinguistically complex

Part of general linguistic acculturation involves acquiring the knowledge of when and how one can enter an exchange. To signal one wishes to take a turn and retain the floor in a conversation there are key non-verbal postural, facial, eye, and gestural signs that inform other participants of one's intentions. To avoid one's turn being interrupted one must sustain fluent, audible speech without hesitations, or, if one hesitates, be able to exploit non-verbal signals to indicate one's turn is not finished.

Such non-verbal support encompasses body posture, rules of proximity of conversation partners, hand and arm gestures that accompany speech. It covers facial expression and eye contact. For people with Parkinson's, especially, misreading others' facial expressions is common (Jin et al., 2017; Prenger et al., 2020; Ricciardi et al., 2017). Importantly, non-verbal gestural communication does not follow universal rules. There can be marked differences across cultures/languages concerning which body proximity (how close people sit/stand; rules on whom and where one can touch) – postural, gestural, facial, eye-contact – signals are employed and interpreted (e.g., Arapova, 2017). In cross-cultural encounters, such variables add further layers of potential misunderstanding or misconstruing. The same applies to how prosodic features of speech are manipulated in different languages to express emotions, nuances of meaning, politeness, and disinterest.

Non-verbal cues go hand-in-hand with sociolinguistic conventions dictating who can speak to whom in which circumstances, about what topics; who is allowed to initiate and continue an exchange; who must wait to be addressed and be silent once they have responded. Again, these rules vary markedly across (sub)cultures and potentially mislead communication. PNDs may also alter behaviours around social norms, (dis)inhibition, and social and psychological insight (Holtgraves & Giordano, 2017; Prenger et al., 2020).

PNDs affect all the above requisites

Attention and attention switching are impaired. Cognitive–linguistic processing speed and capacity are diminished. Slowness initiating speech, dysfluency, and pauses during conversations mean people with PNDs may lack the precise timing needed to take up turns of talk, and listeners, often inadvertently, exclude people with PNDs from participation. Motor changes impair nonverbal gestural support for turn taking and conveying meaning. Thus, even for someone who sounds intelligible, let alone for more affected individuals, the effort of speaking and maintaining intelligible speech as well as the attentional, cognitive, physical, and cultural challenges all conspire to render conversations highly problematic, with a constant risk of exclusion and misapprehension.

The aim of interlocutors ideally should be to build an auditory–visual space conducive to allowing the person time to comprehend, to see as well as hear others, giving time to prepare and signal their desire to contribute and the opportunity to reformulate and repeat messages without losing their turn. Employing strategies to check the person has said everything they wish, and that others have understood precisely what they intended are key. The interlocutor should be aware of cross-cultural variations in non-verbal signalling in conversations and culturally different ways of expressing emotional/affective tone of voice. Suggestions to help with this appear below in Table 9.2.

Speech as identity

Speech and voice are intimate parts of our anatomy

How we speak provides a potent medium to project our inner self, the kind of person we want people to think we are. We gain information from someone's speech on their gender, age, geographical and social place, even their political and moral views. We build an opinion about their mood, health, desire (or not) to communicate or build a relationship, what their spoken and unspoken intentions are. Listeners can quickly construct a complex picture around a speaker regarding their perceived trustworthiness, calmness, openness, empathy, warmth, level of interest in others, and many other qualities.

For people with communication changes associated with PNDs, adeptness in signalling mood, desires, views, projecting social and psychological persona through speech and accompanying non-verbal communication gradually decreases. The subtleties of voice, pronunciation, rate and loudness, intonation, and the many other shades of speech one employed in this universal drama of human discourse, no longer come out as planned.

Without the verbal and nonverbal dexterity, intended messages can be unnoticed, ignored, misconstrued, or misunderstood. Instead of the politeness one wanted to express, listeners might perceive aggression; instead of conveying calmness speech may sound agitated; instead of expressing a humorous tone speech can sound depressed or unfeeling; instead of certainty listeners hear tentativeness; instead of motivation and keenness to cooperate, listeners pick up disinterest (Bambini et al., 2020; Holtgraves & Giordano, 2017). Some remarks by people with PNDs illustrate these problems e.g., 'I feel like I am showing that I'm sad to say goodbye but people don't see that'. 'My biggest fear, when I speak to her, I don't think it sounds like I love her any more. It comes out wrong.'

In some disorders, there is a mirror image to this. People with PND (Parkinson's provides a prime example), may themselves misperceive the non-verbal or verbal intended content of the talk of others (Jin et al., 2017; Montemurro et al., 2019; Yunusova et al., 2019). They have a receptive dysprosody and/or altered theory of mind (Pell et al., 2014). Hence, someone might miss the irony or concern expressed in 'ah, you've arrived at last' spoken with exasperation versus worried relief; or the differing implications of 'no' spoken with a definite, tentative, or 'no, but' tone.

Receptive dysprosody can affect understanding of different stress patterns in sentences too. Someone may miss the distinction between 'they're HUNTing dogs' and 'they're hunting DOGS'; 'the kids played in the TOY shop vs 'toy SHOP'. Such difficulties often accompany problems comprehending figurative or metaphorical speech. There is a tendency to favour the literal meaning of phrases – e.g., 'don't knock people with disabilities' is taken to refer to poor balance; 'what's your view' can be misunderstood as enquiring what you can see; 'she's a real fighter' is mistaken to imply belligerence.

These difficulties comprehending prosody and figurative meanings or disambiguating multiple meanings may be one factor behind relatives often reporting the person with PND has lost their sense of humour, cannot follow jokes, and gets the wrong end of the stick. They all add another layer of potential communication breakdown.

Psychosocial impact

Given the above challenges, it is unsurprising that speech changes exercise profound influences on the psychological and social well-being of individuals and their families, the roles one performs, and places one communicates. Struggle and failure to communicate can sap confidence and damage self-esteem. Sensing people are avoiding you, talking over, through, or for you can be belittling and lonely. Having people constantly ask 'What did you say?' or pretending they understood when they did not can be demoralising. It can be depressing, exasperating and feel unjust – the final insult – when even family and close friends seem to follow societal trends, stigmatizing one's speech and showing embarrassment in public about how one speaks. Discovering that listeners believe disordered speech is synonymous with being mentally incompetent, or drunk, and that one has nothing of value to express, further demoralises and isolates.

Given language is central in shaping and transmitting one's feelings, identity, cultural values, and norms, multilingual speakers have a heightened risk of feeling these effects in a health and education service that does not acknowledge or validate their other language(s). Cross-cultural factors may also enter the equation. Views on why a person has become speech disordered (not to mention why they have a PND), what implications this has for how they should themselves behave, how one should react to them and treat them, what the solution(s) to their situation might be differ widely across cultures (Andersen et al., 2018; Smith et al., 2020) with direct consequences for psychosocial impact of communication changes.

Faced with these circumstances the danger is that individuals may delegate communication to a partner, withdraw from all but the most pressing social interaction, and/or give up speaking. Friends and workmates who might have offered encouragement can be put off because they struggle to understand or know how best to communicate. Hence the importance in rehabilitation of including significant others in therapy. Communicating is a social, at least two-way affair; treating and educating only the person with PND does only half the job. Feeling one's speech and voice are no longer faithful companions can lead to feelings of grief and loss. Worrying that the situation is only due to get worse tests resolve. The net outcome, if not urgently addressed in preventative intervention, is social and psychological isolation, a lost voice, and increased affective burden.

Summarising, listeners may fail to respond to or understand the wishes and views of someone with altered communication because of speech intelligibility issues. However, equal, and most times greater, breakdown in communication stems from failure to appreciate the prosodic, non-verbal, cognitive-linguistic, psychosocial and cross-cultural dimensions of communication. Compensating for, adjusting to, and avoiding the negative consequences of these variables represents a prime, active responsibility of the listener/interlocutor, not (just) the person with PND.

It is because of this that impaired communication represents a risk factor for not receiving optimum health and social support (Forsgren et al., 2016; Palmer, Newsom, & Rook, 2016; Stransky, Jensen, & Morris, 2018). The affected person is less able to make their needs and wishes known; health and social care workers are more likely to miss or misunderstand needs and wishes; they can find it more difficult to form a constructive therapeutic relationship; and are more likely to perceive the person as less of a 'good patient'. Such antipathy need not arise from any conscious prejudice, but from the ear and brain being unconsciously misled by distorted, unfamiliar verbal/non-verbal signals. Finding time in a busy clinic to adjust to the added time people with PNDs require to communicate can exacerbate the situation.

It can be difficult enough negotiating the hidden conventions of how one accesses health care, presents one's views/concerns/questions to health service workers, how one establishes and understands what the possibilities are for support and intervention, let alone someone with communication changes, who is likely to face additional attitudinal barriers. Hence the need for health professionals to acknowledge (a) the challenges the person may be having in maintaining and conveying their personality, wishes and hopes; (b) the challenges they may be experiencing in reconceptualising themselves as someone with a PND/with communication changes; (c) the potentially negative effects for this that can arise from carers/family/careworkers being unaware of these dimensions. It is important that health professionals develop disability competencies, including an awareness of their own attitudes towards and assumptions about the lived experiences, the needs of those with communication disabilities. This will enable professionals to work alongside those with PNDs to support them in finding and expressing their true selves, and make sure the view of the situation from their side becomes and remains clear and central.

The chapter now turns to how to act upon observations from above to assure optimum care for people with altered communicative ability.

Communication guidelines for working with this population

This section addresses how healthcare professionals can enact personalised care with those who have PNDs, ensuring prioritisation of their views and wishes in their own healthcare interventions. Personalised care and support happen through 'a series of facilitated conversations, in which the person being cared for, or those who know them well, actively participate to explore the management of their health and well-being within the context of their whole life and family situation' (NHS England and NHS Improvement, 2019).

It is important to check whether the person is receiving support for their communication difficulties. Contact local speech and language therapy services and refer people if they are not already receiving support. People in the early stages of PNDs should be referred as soon as possible to a speech and language therapist for assessment, education and advice: see The National Institute for Health and Care Excellence (NICE: UK) guidelines listed in the resource chapter. Important therapy techniques and adaptive strategies started early have more benefit in the long term than support left until difficulties become severe.

Simple strategies have the power to enhance participation and increase the likelihood that people will stay engaged, will not give up on communication, and will be able to contribute to conversations about their own healthcare. The following tables summarise some strategies that can optimise communication, based on both research evidence and clinical experience. Table 9.1 provides advice on setting the right circumstances for successful communications to occur ('setting the scene') and Table 9.2 outlines strategies for managing specific types of communication challenges. Some of these strategies are 'speaker oriented', techniques a speaker with communication difficulties can practise to enhance communication; some are 'listener oriented' where interlocutors adapt how they communicate (Griffiths et al., 2012, 2015). In reality, supporting successful conversations often involves both parties adapting as a collaborative effort. The strategies used depend on personal preference, e.g., what one person finds disabling, another might find enabling, so if it is not obvious, it can be good to check with people about whether they find what you are doing helpful.

Table 9.1 Clinical recommendations: setting the scene for successful communication

Find out about any strategies already being using to enhance interaction

Examples:

For people with Parkinson's, 'attention to effort' techniques can have positive outcomes for improving vocal volume, breath support, articulation and prosody. Ask the person about the therapy they are receiving and whether there is anything you can do to encourage the use of techniques e.g., some people value and benefit from a prompt like *'Can you say that a bit louder please?' 'Can you slow down a bit?'* Or, they may have developed a system at home where a companion uses a 'secret signal' to prompt them e.g., thumbs up means raise volume.

The person may use a high- or low-tech AAC aid (see Chapter 4) - e.g. an alphabet board for pointing to first letter of word as spoken (Cave & Bloch, 2021; Kentner & Miller, 2009; Nobematsu & Takahashi, 2020), combining this strategy with introducing each new topic or pointing to words/pictures in a communication book. Make sure they have their device. Learn how it works and how to interact with someone employing AAC.

Ask about preferences for when there is a problem, e.g., whether and when to step in; whether to offer suggestions for word retrieval problems (see also Table 9.2: 'When the person has difficulties with word retrieval').

The person may find it easier to make themselves understood when reading aloud than during conversational speech. Ask if this applies. If so, suggest that the person write down key points they wish to discuss prior to the meeting, with help from others where needed. Reading these out in the session serves as a basis for conversations.

Some people with upper-limb control can use handwriting to convey a message. As the person is writing, read aloud what they have written to display your understanding and show that you are 'with them' (Bloch & Clarke, 2013). If you can anticipate the full message before completed, verbalise this. It can save the 'author' time and physical effort – although be aware that some people like to write the full message anyway, to demonstrate competence. This applies also to people who use spelling aloud as a strategy to improve intelligibility.

Maximise hearing, vision, and the environment (theirs and yours)

Check that everyone has their glasses and hearing aids. Is orientation, proximity, and lighting conducive to seeing each other's face, maintaining eye contact, and hearing each other? Eliminate glare and intrusive background noises. Listen purposefully and actively work at comprehension. Some people prefer to communicate in a very private setting where others cannot overhear their altered speech and voice.

Allow time

Schedule crucial conversations when the person is less tired, allowing more time for meetings in order to accommodate the longer time and attention to effort required to speak and explain. If discussions are prolonged, plan regular rests. Allowing more time ensures healthcare professionals do not contribute to an often gradual and pervading diminishment of self-esteem if people with PNDs feel others are too much in a rush to hear their views.

Demonstrate a willingness to wait; to try and problem solve difficulties arising (*'I'm sorry I didn't quite get that'* or *'I'm finding it hard to understand, can we try again? Would it help to write it down/say it in a different way?'*) This may seem unrealistic, given time pressures inherent in delivering effective healthcare. The important thing is to convey that the person's thoughts are important, whilst being honest about time constraints.

Involve caregivers/family members to best effect

Carers are often very 'tuned in' to the communication needs of their loved one, skilfully supporting their involvement by simplifying information, using shared knowledge to put things in context, and spotting signs of fatigue. Hence the helpfulness of involving carers as much as possible in healthcare interactions. Simultaneously, be alert to well-intentioned carers unnecessarily speaking for/answering on behalf of the person with the PND. Use strategies such as using the person's name, directing eye gaze/body orientation towards them and verbally signalling who the expected next speaker should be e.g., '*What do you think Jack (the person with the PND)?*'

Don't make assumptions

Just because the person smiles, nods, says 'aha' does not mean they have understood you. Thinking you have heard their words does not necessarily mean you have understood them. Regularly check back. *'So, you're saying xyz. Is that right?' 'So, can you summarise in your words what you think we're going to do?'* Give a written summary of your points and/or explanations. Make sure carers have also understood.

Table 9.2 Strategies for managing specific communication challenges

Dealing with unexpected pauses

The person may produce an incomplete utterance, followed by a long pause; a common feature of communication in PNDs, with multiple causes, e.g. delayed speech initiation, cognitive difficulties, or word retrieval problems (also see 'When the person has difficulties with word retrieval difficulties').

Repeat back the 'turn so far', with flat intonation (i.e., the intonation signals the repetition is intended as a display of understanding rather than a request for verification), which can sometimes help the person complete the utterance and allow conversation to progress. Can also be used when speakers use spelling aloud as a strategy.

Examples:

- Person with PND: *'I went to see my …'* (long pause – listener is not sure if more time is needed or whether to provide help). Listener: *'You went to see your …'*
- You might sometimes (without overdoing it) repeat back complete and understandable utterances, to demonstrate what you have understood and that you are fully engaged in the conversation. *'So you said X and Y and Z. What's the other bit you're wanting to tell me?'*
- Maintain eye gaze during a pause where it is clear that the person is still trying to complete an utterance. This allows you to obtain visual cues from their face/lip movements and demonstrates you are still listening.

When the person is hard to understand and you often find yourself asking them to repeat

Vary the way in which you request a repeat, e.g., '*Sorry? ... Pardon? ... Could you say that again?*' You can also use non-verbal methods, e.g., an enquiring head movement breaks up frequent requests for repeats. This softens the impact of being frequently asked for a repeat

When a person seems to go off topic. You were following OK and suddenly they seem to be talking about something else. You've lost the thread

Try using prompts to return to topic e.g., '*We were talking about …*' or '*Can you tell me the topic we are talking about now? I've got a bit lost.*'

When the person takes long turns in the conversation and you are finding it hard to understand

Break into a turn to resolve a difficulty hearing/understanding, instead of waiting until it is too late and you have completely lost track e.g., '*Sorry can I just stop you for a moment – I want to make sure I understood that last bit.*'

When it is hard for the person to express choices verbally

Use visual methods to provide choices/forced alternatives e.g., ask the person to point to one of a range of written choices.

When a person is being talked over because their voice is quiet or they take a long time to initiate speech

Be alert to this happening, by you or others. Where you find yourself talking over the person, allow an opportunity for the speaker to repeat his/her overlapped turn.

When the person has difficulties with word retrieval

Request clarification/make a suggestion (if you have understood enough) '*Do you mean x?*' (Carlsson, Hartelius, & Saldert, 2014).

Request modification – e.g., '*Can you describe it?*' (a strategy of 'talking around the word or 'circumlocution') '*Can you tell me the first letter?*' '*Can you write it on your communication device?*'

Recap the conversation – say what you have understood so far (and the word may be triggered).

Redirect the conversation if it is proving too difficult. You may want to acknowledge this: '*It's really tricky isn't it? Perhaps we can come back to this another time.*'

As there is some overlap between the language problems experienced by those with PNDs and those with aphasia, some of the strategies outlined in Chapter 11 may also be helpful.

When people with PNDs are used to only being asked questions focused on the business of the healthcare encounter

Include everyday 'rapport building' conversation openers into your encounters. This risks conversational difficulty BUT allows people to pursue topics of interest, demonstrate competence and negotiate identity. In turn, this can help with relationship building and trust and help tune the clinician into their speech.

Because people with PNDs often have a reduced ability to convey emotions and meaning through facial expression and speech tone, leading to healthcare practitioners forming negative judgements about their mood and personality

Where possible, avoid purely relying on problem-focused questions like: '*What have you found difficult in the last week?*' These can exacerbate reduced expressiveness and appearance of apathy and hopelessness. Include adaptive coping questions like '*What did you enjoy in the last week?*'

To counter the negative judgement bias, encourage people to be active, rather than passive participants in the encounter; to tell their stories about what matters most to them and what strategies they currently use to self-manage

Summary

In this chapter, we have outlined typical communication features associated with PNDs and highlighted the challenges they can pose to achieving successful healthcare interactions. We have suggested a range of evidence-based strategies to enable practitioners to achieve optimal circumstances for communication success and develop specific techniques to overcome communication breakdowns. We conclude this chapter by presenting three case vignettes, illustrating the importance of attending to communication needs in each of the PNDs focused on in this chapter.

Case studies

Case study 9.1 Brenda

Brenda has had MND for three years. Controlling breathing for speech had become a major difficulty. It was effortful, tiring, and she managed only a few words per breath. The frequent breaths decreased understandability as their random positioning disrupted the grammar of the phrase. To eke out breath and reduce effort Brenda tended to speak in telegrammatic (i.e. key words only: see her phrases below). Because this altered her tone of voice and grammar, listeners could misunderstand or misconstrue her intentions. An exchange she reported with her husband illustrates this. 'I said "Want coffee". Husband shout at me. "You ask properly!". But can't say long. Can't sound polite'. Three intervention priorities for communication arose from this. We worked on breath control and taking breaths at points that did not obscure meaning. We targeted work on grammatical stress/intonation and emotional tone, especially in her shortened phrases. We increased her husband's appreciation of her limitations and how to interpret her tone. Even though Brenda had not intended an impatient command tone, the incident highlighted her husband's exasperation and strain. He heard just another order to 'jump to it' without any sense of appreciation from others. This triggered more intervention targeting his stress and strategies to 'care for the carer'.

Case study 9.2 Arun

One of the first Parkinson's symptoms Arun experienced was reduced vocal volume. His wife, Roshni, would constantly say 'Pardon?' when he spoke, and getting cross with him for not speaking louder, because she knew he could raise his volume sometimes. Arun did not think his speech was too quiet. He thought the problem was that Roshni was hard of hearing. He found it frustrating to be asked to repeat himself all the time. As the Parkinson's progressed, Arun's facial mobility reduced and his voice became less melodic. Eventually, Arun stopped talking unless absolutely necessary. Roshni felt that Arun was not showing any interest in her or the wider family, and both of them became quite lonely and depressed. Eventually, Roshni spoke to her GP. The couple were referred to a speech and language therapist who raised their awareness of the communication difficulties associated with Parkinson's (e.g., that it can be difficult for people to monitor their own loudness), arranged a hearing test for Roshni, worked with Arun on improving his ability to monitor and increase his volume and suggested strategies like announcing his feelings e.g. '*I'm happy for you*' or checking his volume '*Can you hear me? Shall I speak louder?*'

Case study 9.3 Marie

As a result of having MS, Marie was experiencing language processing difficulties. She had always enjoyed meeting up with friends for a meal and saw herself as 'the life and soul of the party'. However, when in a group, she was feeling increasingly overwhelmed and unable to keep up with the speed of conversation and picking out multiple voices amongst background noise. She wanted to contribute, but it was difficult finding a 'way in' and by the time she had formulated what she wanted to say, the conversation had moved on. When she did speak, she would often struggle to retrieve a specific word she wanted to say and ended up fading into the background. She ended social occasions feeling exhausted and sad, thus compounding the fatigue caused by MS. After discussing her situation with her speech and language therapist, Marie explained to each friend in turn what she was experiencing. She suggested ways they could help, e.g., making space for her to enter the conversation ('*What do you think Marie?*'), and giving her time to contribute. As a group, they decided to try meeting up for a meal in a quiet restaurant, or in one of their homes.

Key clinical recommendations (for details refer to Table 9.1)

- Find out about any strategies already being used to enhance interaction
- Maximise hearing, vision and contextual/environment communication facilitators (theirs and yours).

- Allow time for communication.
- Involve caregivers/family members to best effect.
- Don't make assumptions (e.g., that you have understood each other). Regularly check to see if a shared understanding has been reached.

Recommended resources

1. Yorkston, K., Miller, R., & Strand, E. (2012). *Management of speech and swallowing in degenerative diseases.* 3rd ed. (Austin, TX: PRO-ED).
2. www.Parkinsons.org.uk in particular; www.parkinsons.org.uk/information-and-support/speech-and-communication-problems which includes tips for those communication with people who have Parkinson's.
3. www.mndassociation.org in particular; www.mndassociation.org/support-and-information/living-with-mnd/speech-and-communication/ for information on communication, including voice banking; www.mssociety.org.uk/ includes a link to a booklet on 'Speech Difficulties'.
4. National Institute for Health and Care Excellence (UK). Parkinson's disease in adults: diagnosis and management. London: National Institute for Health and Care Excellence (UK); 2017 Jul. (NICE Guideline, No. 71.). www.ncbi.nlm.nih.gov/books/NBK4471
5. Motor neurone disease: assessment and management. London: National Institute for Health and Care Excellence (UK); 2019 Jul. (NICE Guideline, No. 42.). www.ncbi.nlm.nih.gov/books/NBK554746/

References

Andersen, P. M., Kuzma-Kozakiewicz, M., Keller, J., Aho-Oezhan, H. E. A., Ciecwierska, K., Szejko, N., … Lulé, D. (2018). Therapeutic decisions in ALS patients: cross-cultural differences and clinical implications. *Journal of Neurology, 265*(7), 1600–1606.

Arapova, Maria A. (2017). Cultural differences in Russian and Western smiling. *Russian Journal of Communication*, 9(1), 34–52.

Bambini, V., Bischetti, L., Bonomi, C. G., Arcara, G., Lecce, S., & Ceroni, M. (2020). Beyond the motor account of amyotrophic lateral sclerosis: verbal humour and its relationship with the cognitive and pragmatic profile. *International Journal of Language & Communication Disorders, 55*(5), 751–764.

Bloch, S., & Clarke, M. (2013). Handwriting-in-interaction between people with ALS/MND and their conversation partners. *Augmentative and Alternative Communication, 29*(1), 54–67.

Carlsson, E., Hartelius, L., & Saldert, C. (2014). Communicative strategies used by spouses of individuals with communication disorders related to stroke-induced aphasia and Parkinson's disease. *International Journal of Language & Communication Disorders, 49*(6), 722–735.

Cave, R., & Bloch, S. (2021). Voice banking for people living with motor neurone disease: views and expectations. *International Journal of Language & Communication Disorders, 56*(1), 116–129.

El-Wahsh, S., Ballard, K., Kumfor, F., & Bogaardt, H. (2020). Prevalence of self-reported language impairment in multiple sclerosis and the association with health-related quality of life: an international survey study. *Multiple Sclerosis and Related Disorders, 39*. Retrieved from www.sciencedirect.com/science/article/pii/S2211034819309678?casa_token=J4tiP9hyo_UAAAAA:GWE9-25Ix-yonv-GJ3C-S8aWTvWlariZr8U-HyLFV-aN4UZUmezpEPWP5gbWamd8B

Forsgren, E., Skott, C., Hartelius, L., & Saldert, C. (2016). Communicative barriers and resources in nursing homes from the enrolled nurses' perspective: a qualitative interview study. *International Journal of Nursing Studies, 54*, 112–121.

Griffiths, S., Barnes, R., Britten, N., & Wilkinson, R. (2012). Potential causes and consequences of overlap in talk between speakers with Parkinson's disease and their familiar conversation partners. *Seminars in Speech and Language, 33*(1), 27–43.

Griffiths, S., Barnes, R., Britten, N., & Wilkinson, R. (2015). Multiple repair sequences in everyday conversations involving people with Parkinson's disease. *International Journal of Language and Communication Disorders, 50*(6), 814–829.

Holtgraves, T., & Giordano, M. (2017). Parkinson's disease without dementia. In L. Cummings (Ed.), *Research in Clinical Pragmatics* (pp. 379–407). Cham: Springer International.

Jin, Y. Z., Mao, Z. Q., Ling, Z. P., Xu, X., Zhang, Z. Y., & Yu, X. G. (2017). Altered emotional recognition and expression in patients with Parkinson's disease. *Neuropsychiatric Disease and Treatment, 13*, 2891–2902.

Johansson, K., Schalling, E., & Hartelius, L. (2021). Self-reported changes in cognition, communication and swallowing in multiple sclerosis: data from the Swedish Multiple Sclerosis Registry and from a national survey. *Folia Phoniatrica et Logopaedica, 73*(1), 50–62.

Kentner, J., & Miller, N. (2009). Effects of visible versus concealed alphabet cues on speech intelligibility in dysarthria. *International Journal of Therapy and Rehabilitation, 16*, 272–279.

Miller, N. (2017). Communication changes in Parkinson's disease. *Practical Neurology, 17*(4), 266–274.

Montemurro, S., Mondini, S., Signorini, M., Marchetto, A., Bambini, V., & Arcara, G. (2019). Pragmatic language disorder in Parkinson's disease and the potential effect of cognitive reserve. *Frontiers in Psychology, 10*. Retrieved from www.frontiersin.org/articles/10.3389/fpsyg.2019.01220/full

NHS England & NHS Improvement. (2019). *Personalised care*. Retrieved on 12 March 2021 from www.england.nhs.uk/personalisedcare/

Nobematsu, A., & Takahashi, K. (2020). Timing of communication device introduction defined by ALSFRS-R score in patients with amyotrophic lateral sclerosis. *Progress in Rehabilitation Medicine, 5*, 20200013–20200013.

Noffs, G., Boonstra, F. M. C., Perera, T., Butzkueven, H., Kolbe, S. C., Maldonado, F., … Vogel, A. P. (2021). Speech metrics, general disability, brain imaging and quality of life in multiple sclerosis. *European Journal of Neurology, 28*(1), 259–268.

Palmer, A. D., Newsom, J. T., & Rook, K. S. (2016). How does difficulty communicating affect the social relationships of older adults? An exploration using data from a national survey. *Journal of Communication Disorders, 62*, 131–146.

Pell, M., Monetta, L., Rothermich, K., Kotz, S. A., Cheang, H. S., & McDonald, S. (2014). Social perception in adults with Parkinson's disease. *Neuropsychology, 28*(6), 905–916.

Perez, B. D. D., Luna, E. C., Cloutman, L., Rog, D., Preston, E., & Conroy, P. (2020). Anomia in people with rapidly evolving severe relapsing-remitting multiple sclerosis: both word retrieval inaccuracy and delay are common symptoms. *Aphasiology, 34*(2), 195–213.

Prenger, M. T. M., Madray, R., Van Hedger, K., Anello, M., & MacDonald, P. A. (2020). Social symptoms of Parkinson's disease. *Parkinson's Disease, 2020.* Retrieved from www.hindawi.com/journals/pd/2020/8846544

Ricciardi, L., Visco-Comandini, F., Erro, R., Morgante, F., Bologna, M., Fasano, A., … Kilner, J. (2017). Facial emotion recognition and expression in Parkinson's Disease: An emotional mirror mechanism? *PloS One, 12*(1), e0169110.

Saldert, C., & Bauer, M. (2017). Multifaceted communication problems in everyday conversations involving people with Parkinson's disease. *Brain Sciences, 7*(10), 123.

Schalling, E., Johansson, K., & Hartelius, L. (2017). Speech and communication changes reported by people with Parkinson's disease. *Folia Phoniatrica et Logopaedica, 69*(3), 131–141.

Smith, E. R., Perrin, P. B., Tyler, C. M., Lageman, S. K., & Villaseñor, T. (2020). Cross-cultural differences in Parkinson's disease caregiving and burden between the United States and Mexico. *Brain and Behavior, 10*(9): e01753.

Stransky, M. L., Jensen, K. M., & Morris, M. A. (2018). Adults with communication disabilities experience poorer health and healthcare outcomes compared to persons without communication disabilities. *Journal of General Internal Medicine, 33*(12), 2147–2155. doi:10.1007/s11606-018-4625-1

Yorkston, K., Baylor, C., & Mach, H. (2017). Factors associated with communicative participation in amyotrophic lateral sclerosis. *Journal of Speech Language Hearing Research, 60*(6), 1791–1797.

Yunusova, Y., Ansari, J., Ramirez, J., Shellikeri, S., Stanisz, G. J., Black, S. E., … Zinman, L. (2019). Frontal anatomical correlates of cognitive and speech motor deficits in smyotrophic lateral sclerosis. *Behavioural Neurology.* Retrieved from www.hindawi.com/journals/bn/2019/9518309/

10

Dementia and conversation patterns helpful to practitioners

Trini Stickle and Jean Neils-Strunjas

Chapter contents:

Introduction

This chapter explores how several common dementia symptoms can create challenges for doctor–patient communication, just as these symptoms may impede any interaction. During the clinical visit, common linguistic symptoms of neurocognitive disorders such as word- or concept-finding difficulties and loss of memory of recent events (Bäckman et al., 2001; Blair et al., 2007), perseveration (Bayles et al., 1985; Fuld et al., 1982), or severe syntactic disfluency (Fraser et al., 2016) erode rapport and trust and impede efficacy of care and treatment (Karnieli-Miller et al., 2007). At the same time, cognitive deficits do not impede conversation in a vacuum, rather conversational partners have the potential to facilitate interactions that serve a social purpose, which goes beyond exchanging information (Kindell et al., 2017).

DOI: 10.4324/9781003142522-14

In this chapter, we present interactional strategies that work toward ameliorating potentially negative patient–doctor conversations. The strategies and practices we present arise from close analyses of conversations between persons with Alzheimer's dementia (AD) diagnoses and their non-impaired co-participants. Use of such heuristic approaches are shown to demonstrate interactional choices that progress conversation and preserve the well-being and identity of the person with AD (Kindell et al., 2017). Additionally, we highlight strategies best to avoid, those that yield little progression and are evidenced by participant stress and/or withdrawal from the conversation. Finally, we illustrate ways to move an unproductive conversation toward a more productive engagement for all participants. To better facilitate this goal, this chapter presents two clinical case studies that serve as instructional models of better interactional practices and then culminates with a summary of five strategies for better clinical (or any) interactions with persons diagnosed with AD or any number of neurological conditions that result in similar linguistic and interactional impairments.

Aims and goals: toward application

Our aims and objectives for this chapter are to identify conversation patterns common to persons experiencing dementia, particularly those with an AD diagnosis, alongside patterns of talk employed by their co-participants that yield productive interactions despite challenges that arise from the linguistic difficulties such neurological conditions create. Additionally, we present conversational patterns that impede the progress of such interactions. From our analyses, we distil communication patterns expected to better facilitate clinical interactions.

Clinical relevance

The purpose of our chapter is to inform clinicians and provide them with helpful conversational strategies for the medical history interview. Engel and Morgan describe the medical history interview as the most powerful, sensitive, and versatile instrument available to the physician (1973, see update in Nichol et al., 2020). Key to the medical history's power are clinicians' interview skills, as these skills allow for diagnostic accuracy, sufficient treatment plans, patient adherence to therapy, and patient health outcomes (Hatem et al., 2007). During these intake moments when dementia patients' interactional competencies are compromised, clinician interview skills are placed under exceptional stress, stress that without additional preparation may, indeed, fail. Obtaining a thorough history is important, but the questioning should reflect understanding of the patient and their condition. Persons with dementia may experience increased anxiety if they are questioned in a way that causes the conversation to turn in a negative direction or if they feel rushed (Nichol et al., 2020).

Using our data in accord with the guidance from the National Institute on Aging (2021), the primary goal of this chapter is to hone clinician interviewing skills for persons with dementia. Because dementia affects episodic memory or memories for specific events particularly recent events, the clinician should verify all information obtained directly from the patient. At the same time, the physician needs to care for the patient with dignity and respect that is grounded in productive communication strategies that promote an emotional connection with the patient.

Brief review of conversational difficulties per dementia

Figure 10.1 summarizes the four most prevalent forms of dementia and their respective conversational, linguistic, or interactional difficulties (as compiled from the following sources: Alzheimer's Association, 2021; Banovic et al., 2018; Reilly et al., 2010; The World Health Organization, 2021).

Method

We employ a social–interactional analytical approach that focuses on discourse, or language in use, as the social phenomenon in which meanings are collaboratively made and actions are achieved (see Edwards & Potter, 1992).

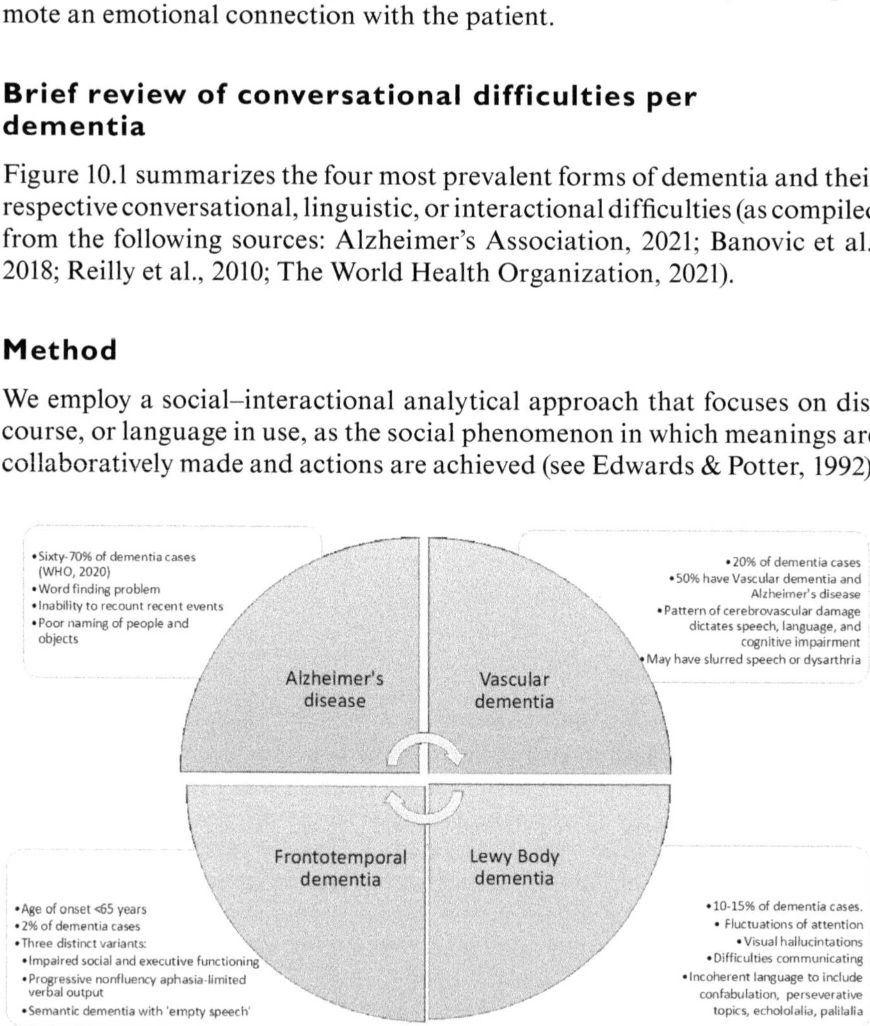

Figure 10.1 Four most prevalent forms of dementia and their respective conversational, linguistic, or interactional difficulties

For our purposes, "language in use" refers to spoken language used in the real world, on a day-to-day basis. This stands in contrast to elicited responses employed in experimental data collection methods. In essence, we are using strategies employed in actual conversations to arrive at our understandings of how persons with dementia and their co-participants derive meaning as they more or less successfully engage in social activities. Terms used in conversation may reflect the social aspect of language rather than provide accurate information. For example, Müller and Mok (2012) used a language analysis of discourse between two nursing home residents and two students. The analysis revealed that one of the women with AD used a term of endearment, "maman" (Grandma) for the other older women because of a constructed but incorrect remembrance about how the other resident took care of her when she first entered the nursing home. It was noted that the remembrance could be labelled *confabulation* in clinical terms, yet the function of the term and related memory served to positively impact the social connectiveness of the participants. Similarly, we study language used in the following conversations to draw conclusions about the mechanics of language, to understand how linguistic structures are employed within actual interactions, and to identify how patterns of language use help the participants achieve social actions (e.g., acknowledge a new idea or situation, agree on a course of action, arrange for a next meeting).

Conversation analysis (CA) is employed here to examine the ways in which one "turn" of talk, with its construction from lexical, syntactic, and prosodic features, engenders another participant's turn—and its unfolding linguistic construction—in the emerging collaborative process of sense making and action completion. Such conversation analytic methods have been employed profitably in studying interaction between clinicians and patients (e.g., Goodwin, 2003; Maynard, 2003).

Using discourse analysis (DA), we turn our attention to the ways that language use may function within a conversation beyond its traditional grammatical classifications. DA looks at how persons with dementia can use *grammatical structures* in ways beyond what traditional grammatical descriptions predict (see Davis & Maclagan, 2009; 2020). This approach lets us demonstrate the often-needed flexibility placed upon co-participants' in both their expectations and interpretations of the talk produced by persons with dementia.

CA and DA analytical approaches bring into relief both beneficial and problematic practices employed to elicit and convey information, especially considering the challenges of any patient population affected by communicative difficulties.

Participants

Our data are of audio and/or video clips and corresponding transcripts of 36 persons with AD diagnoses and their numerous, 65 non-impaired co-participants engaged in 104 clinical and mundane conversations collected as part of the Carolina Conversation Collections (CCC) (http://carolinaconversations.musc.edu) Each person with dementia is identified with a pseudonym that includes their title (Ms. or Mr.) plus a family name that is abbreviated to three letters (e.g., Ms. Smith > Ms. SMT) while the co-participant volunteers are simply given a given-name pseudonym (e.g., Jim). One shortfall of the CCC database is its inability to track the progression of each participant's disease or the stage of disease at the time each conversation took place as the consenting processes for the original data did not request accesses to that information. When possible, information provided on a subject's age, data collection period, and/or other contextual information is included to help provide a window to subjects' stage of disease. The audio and/or video data are transcribed using the symbols associated of Jeffersonian CA practices (2004) (see Appendix A for a key to the symbols).

Analysis

Analyses of these conversations provide verbal practices likely to increase responses, such as eliciting patient histories or fulfilling task requests (e.g., complying with exam protocols). Also of import, we illustrate practices that result in negative effects in particular circumstances that are likely to shut down needed conversations. While we caution the over-generalizability of either of these positive or negative practices, they are meant to offer some guidance for, primarily, clinical application but also daily conversations with persons diagnosed with AD. The following conversations demonstrate how the physician can look beyond patients' cognitive deficits, build rapport with patients, and elicit patients' concerns. What follows, then, is a close examination of four interactions. We start with two conversations that demonstrate positive progression despite interactional difficulties, followed by two in which the negative trajectories cause the person with dementia to retract, but we then show how one of the negative interactions turns toward a positive trajectory that allows the conversation to progress.

Overall findings

From minimal to complex linguistic production

Importantly, most of the participants with a dementia diagnosis were able to converse with little trouble. Nine of the 36 participants displayed communicative difficulties within various conversations that impaired meaningful communication, at least initially. From a close analysis of those conversations, the fundamental productive strategy for eliciting relevant and understandable information is the duration and tenor provided by the conversation partner.

Fluctuations in the complexity of syntactic production in the talk of persons diagnosed with AD during conversations followed similar patterns. During the initial stages of talk, single words or phrases with minimal syntax were often the patterns produced by the participants with dementia, often without sufficient syntax or lexical cohesion. These utterances, consequently, created clarity and comprehension problems for the co-participant. As expected, within the first few minutes of talk, co-participants often responded in ways that demonstrated their assessment of the linguistic abilities of the person with dementia to be severely impaired and, many, as expected, attempted to fill in the gaps or solve the disfluency through their own turns at talk. This often led to signs of distress and a propensity to withdraw from the conversation.

Still, productive strategies employed by many of the co-participants proved to be incredibly helpful in progressing the talk. We present a preview of those strategies here and then explicit details along with explanation following.

One key observation is that when the non-impaired co-participant yields control of the conversation to persons with AD, without attempting to talk for them or correct them, most often, the participants with dementia would begin to produce greater syntactic complexity, alternating with simplistic ones. We noticed that after about seven to 12 minutes of talk, minimal utterances and/or less complex syntactic patterns re-emerged. This finding concurs with the warm-up period noted by Stickle and Wanner (2016). It should be noted that the average time in a medical appointment is very short and that the short time of the visit could limit the quality of the interaction.

Tai-Seale, McQuire, and Zhang (2007) observe the median visit length was 15.7 minutes covering a median of six topics. About 5 minutes were spent on the longest topic whereas the remaining topics each received 1.1 minutes. Therefore, we suggest that information is obtained when possible prior to the appointment and that all the office staff are coached in conversational techniques. To illustrate the movement from minimal to complex linguistic production, we present two sets of co-participant interactions in which the persons with dementia begin their respective conversations with great communication challenges: however, within a short duration, their talk transforms, incredibly, to robust conversations.

Palilalia

In the first example (Extract 1), we see in the transcript a residential patient engaged in a palilalia loop,[1] the involuntary repetition of one's own speech utterances (Larner, 2015).[2] Berthier et al. (2017) report that infractions within the bilateral executive-control network[3] that acts as a "brake" preventing inappropriate repetition in healthy brains cannot exert such control and palilalia (or echolalia) may result. This ongoing situation would appear to impede any productive conversation.

Extract (1) BGG 002a (The Kathy): Palilalia looping

```
Ms. B: the Kathy, the Kathy, was Kathy, was Kathy,
       that was Kathy,
       and that was Kathy, so, have we, and Kathy,
       and the Kathy
       and the Kathy and the Kathy, and the Kathy.
       But, that
       was the Kathy, the Kathy, the Kathy, the
       Kathy, the Kathy,
```

What occurs is the co-participant Tom treats the palilalia loop as a question (Extract 2):

Extract (2) BGG 002b (I hadn't seen Kathy): Breaking the palilalia loop

```
Ms. B:  [The Kathy, the Kathy, ]
Tom:    [I hadn't seen Kathy.]
```

This leads to the resident producing several coherent turns of talk, approximately three minutes, in which the two Ms. BGG and Tom hold a coherent conversation that Ms. BGG controls.[4]

Extract (3) BGG 002b (I hadn't seen Kathy): Breaking the palilalia loop

```
MS B:   is there anything else, anything else
        there is?
        (0.4)
Tom:    ha(ah)-I, I think we're all set.
```

After the several minutes of competent talk, Ms. BGG, upon closing the conversation, turns and walks away from Tom and the recorder. As she does so, the palilalia loop begins again with "the Kathy, the Kathy."

We find this interaction to be a potential model within clinical interactions as it demonstrates the power of treating incoherent talk as meaningful rather than dismissing it. As Tom treats the palilalia loop as accomplishing social, linguistic, and interactional actions—namely an inquiry as to the location of Kathy—the palilalia loop is interrupted and Ms. BGG can participate in a coherent conversation. In fact, Ms. BGG becomes the "host," if you will, of her environment and takes control of the conversation floor for a few minutes. Within the clinical environment, such an exchange may allow for a brief duration in which the patient is able to discuss their concerns, pain, or needs. While our inferences remain conjectures, we offer them to be proofed in the hope that the medical needs of persons with dementia can be better addressed through even a brief meaningful exchange during the medical interview.

Severe Impairment

A resident between the ages of 79 and 84[5] is displaying severe linguistic and interactional impairment for nearly 15 minutes of talk and appears unable to produce a coherent utterance (see Extract 4):

Extract (4) THW 001a (They give you a diamond): Impaired syntax

```
Mr. T:       I but no waste but waste to him.
             (0.8)
             Yeah.
             (12.7)
             I'd-

             (4.0)
             I don't know.
```

The non-impaired co-participant displays active listening responses (e.g., uh huh, yeah, it must be hard). Our suppositions are that with the aid of these cues and by granting the person with dementia a sufficient warm-up time and yielding control of the conversation without trying to speak for the participant, the person with dementia commandeers the role of interviewer allowing him to access coherent syntax (see Extract 5).

Extract (5) THW001b (Being heard): Interactional competency

```
Mr. T:       Where bouts are you?

             (2.1)
Jim:         (ahh)Me?
             (0.4)
Mr. T:       yeah.
Jim:         I'm in, uh,
             (0.7)
Jim:         Charlotte.
```

The co-participant Jim's respond “Me?” is initiated with a near gasp “(ahh)” as it appears he is taken aback by the transformation of Mr. THW's communicative ability. Mr. THW continues this coherent production of language as he interviews Jim, the non-impaired co-participant, for another fifteen minutes.[6]

We find these two examples helpful reminders that a moment of incoherent talk can be transcended. That within the clinical visit, time should be allotted for the patient to warm up, if need be, prior to a history, intake, or update being taken, as demonstrated by Clinical Case 1 (later in this chapter).

Moving from these cases of severe expressive communication impairment, we continue this chapter, demonstrating a series of conversation, each with their own, but lesser, challenges. For many, a particular problematic situation is resolved through various emergent strategies; these include strategies of active listening, yielding control, asking questions about overlearned, remote autobiographical memories, or allowing sufficient time without overt corrections. Practices leading to negative outcomes of focus here include overcorrection and/or speaking for the co-participant with dementia, diminishing the concerns of the co-participant with dementia, and/or overtly controlling the conversation through questions.

Perseveration

Perseveration is a well-documented feature of AD (Bayles et al., 1985; Fuld et al., 1982) in which a neurocognitive loop puts in motion an action that is difficult to alter or stop. One type of loop occurs with a repetition of speech, which consequently interferes with interaction. For persons diagnosed with AD, perseveration has been noted to manifest early in the disease, to increase in severity with the progression and with a stuck-in-set of perseverations emerging in the later stages (Pekkala et al., 2008; 2013). Recommended mediation of such perseverating incidents includes redirecting attention and/or engaging the person in a different task (Gillen & Brockmann Rubion, 2016). We present an example of verbal perseveration with analysis of the co-participant strategies used to redirect the conversation and facilitate interaction. We then build upon these strategies within case study 10.2 for clinical education and practice.

In Extract (6), Ms. WAL, age 83,[7] has been perseverating on the notion that someone stole one of her slippers. Despite the non-impaired co-participant's attempts to interject doubt over someone stealing one slipper and not both slippers, Ms. WAL continues her complaint for over five minutes.

Extract (6) WAL001 (Stolen slipper): Perseveration

```
Ms. WAL:    I went to bed last night and somebody
            took my bedroom
            slipper.

            ...
Ms. WAL:    People steal, you know.
```

At one point, the co-participant Jen continues to express doubt that someone would steal just one slipper and attempts to alter Ms. WAL's narrative. Ms. WAL becomes so agitated, she expressed the desire to physically injure the person that she believes has stolen the slipper: "I said if I saw one of those people that took my bedroom shoe, I would knock the hell out of 'em." Without any resolution, Jen attempts a different strategy. Jen interjects a new focus, something physical within the environment (see Extract 7).

Extract (7) WAL 001 (Bird): Perseveration

```
Ms. WAL:    And the one, the other girl had it on.
            She had it on.
            (3.7)
Jen:        Aren't those just beautiful colors on
            this bird?

            ((looking outside through a window))
Ms. WAL:    M'hm. They are. They are.
```

Jen's strategy appears to interrupt the perseverative talk of the slipper narrative, aiding Ms. WAL's move to a new topic. Additional interactions within the data in which perseverative talk is impeding progression, non-impaired co-participants interject noticings of physical attributes (e.g., shoes, a recent haircut, holiday décor). It would have also been possible for the conversational partner to move the topic to a related but different one. I like the shoes that you have on. Are they comfortable?

We find redirection to be potentially helpful in the clinical setting when persons with dementia may perseverate on a particular health or social issue. While it may be unusual and/or interpreted as impolite to interject a non sequitur in a typical conversation, a turn such as this may be one way to move the intake process to a relevant point.

Case study 10.1

Mrs. James attends her medical examination with her daughter.

The receptionist (R) greets them and engages Mrs. James in conversation.

R: "Mrs. James, I see you came with your daughter."

(Provides ample response time).

MRS. JAMES: "Um, traffic."
R: "So you hit a lot of traffic on some days."

(Expands)

MRS. JAMES: "Yes, over on Green."
R: "Oh, Green street, yes, that's not far."

(Expands)

MRS. JAMES: "Doctor, doctor."
R: "Yes, the doctor will be here soon."

Of note, the receptionist is engaging Mrs. James in conversation to better allow for a sufficient warm-up time before she enters the exam room to interact with her physician. The receptionist also expands on Mrs. James' talk to ensure she treats it as completing coherent social actions (i.e., a complaint, an inquiry). Additionally, she provides ample time for Mrs. James to respond. Providing for a staff—administrative or clinical—the time, resources, and opportunity to engage with patients with dementia or geriatric patients, in general, could facilitate the clinical interaction as this priming time could lead to more productive clinical interviews, particularly when these patients may lack the daily social interactions of younger patients. Studies have reported social interaction for many geriatric persons residing in nursing homes to be six to eleven minutes per day (Thorsell et al., 2010). For older persons remaining in their homes, the Pew Research Center reported in a 2019 study that "Americans ages 60 and older are alone for more than half of their daily measured time. All told, this amounts to about seven hours a day; and among those who live by themselves, alone time rises to over 10 hours a day" (Livingston, 2020). This increased isolation may exacerbate the interactional decline, and clinical visits may, indeed, be one of the few places older persons can experience social interactions and human engagement.

Extremely negative trajectories

We now look closely at interactions that are stymied by the interactional choices that create difficulties due to the heuristic nature of typical conversations.

Assuaging difficulties

One common interactional strategy that we observe used by non-impaired participants that has the effect of temporarily or completely shutting down the progression of talk is the diminishing or assuaging of life's difficulties expressed by a co-participant with dementia. We present several of the exchanges that have interrupted the progression of talk.

One participant, Ms. Yarrow, a person with dementia, expresses difficulty remembering the number of grandchildren she has. In response, her co-participant attempts to dismiss her inability to remember such a detail: "Oh, okay, well, it's okay." The effect on Ms. Yarrow is anything but reassuring: "I don't think it's okay. I think that's *bad*." The co-participant quickly changes her strategy, allowing Ms. Yarrow to talk about this difficulty and her inability to accept this kind of forgetting. This type of active listening and its positive effects are what we saw with the second interaction presented with Mr. T and Jim, where allowing for difficulties to be expressed maintained the flow of conversation.

Other co-participants with dementia have produced similar outrage at their inability to remember personal or family details: "Well, this is ridiculous!" (WEA_001, line 74); "I've lost it" (WEA_001, line 75). The progression of the interaction is often incumbent upon the non-impaired co-participant response. Yielding the floor to such talk along with making eye contact and using an empathetic tone of voice often work to encourage progression while dismissals or diminishing the importance of those experiences more often than not causes a retreat from and refusal to continue the interaction.

In one difficult interaction, Mr. WHE, the co-participant with dementia (age 84–89),[8] is discussing a list of new physical difficulties—loss of mobility, increased pain—and ultimately expresses that the end of life may be near: "I think I'll getta close to da(h) enda(h) the road I think." Research indicates that these types of remarks may be end of life initiators (Travers & Taylor, 2016). In a typical conversation pattern, the non-impaired co-participant attempts to dismiss Mr. WHE's complaints and fears: "Oh, *no*: don't say that you've got plenty of years left on you." Rather than working to ease Mr. Wheiten's concerns, Mr. WHE, instead, expresses anger and moves to end the interaction: "I tell ya this livin' to a ripe old age is a bunch of CRAP."

While our findings call for simple modifications in interactional patterns, namely empathetic and active listening cues, additional clinical training may be the necessary course of action, one borrowed from recommendations currently discussed in medical education literature. Similar findings are noted within hospice settings in which clinicians are reluctant to engage in end of life discussions initiated by the patient (Travers & Taylor, 2016). As a result, a variety of interactional clinical training interventions have been suggested (Chua & Shorey, 2021; Kerr et al., 2018), to include theatrical or scripted responses. Our suggestion is more tempered in that we recommend a natural but conscious employment of common active listening cues:

- Simple displays of backchanneling and space to tell: "yes," "uh huh," "I hear that."
- Offers of support: "What can I do to help?"
- Demonstrated empathy: "You are going through a challenging time."
- Displays of affirmation and understanding: "I understand. It must be difficult."

Questions and correction

The last observation we present is the consequence of an overuse of the interrogative structure, or questions. Warning on the negative effects of yes/no and open-ended question formats to elicit conversations with persons diagnosed with dementia has been presented (e.g., De Vries, 2013); however, much of the advice is contradictory. Some research advises the use of discrete information-seeking questions (Hopper et al., 2001; Small et al., 2003; Small & Perry, 2005) while others advise open-ended questions (Davis et al., 2011). Consequently, the following exchange is of no surprise in the co-participant's retraction from the interaction. Still, we present the exchange and its resolution as offering possible ways to accomplish the medical interview.

In the first two minutes and 48 seconds, the non-impaired co-participant asks the co-participant with dementia 15 yes/no questions, two discrete information-seeking questions, and two open-ended questions. Upon receipt of continued questioning, the co-participant with dementia shuts down the interaction in a most disturbing way, particularly considering the interaction is occurring in a residential center.

Extract (8) TDD 001 (Help): Interrogative overload

```
Lisa:       It will be nice to see your daughter,
            right?
Ms. TDD:    Tsk. YES. Don't ASK (0.9) those questions.
Lisa:       Why not?
            (1.7)
Ms. TDD:    HE:LP.
```

A negative interaction turns positive

After an undesignated time (the recording device is turned off and then back on), Lisa finds a way to interact with Ms. TDD, age 80 to 85.[9] Lisa begins talking about her own likes and dislikes of the coming holiday, Thanksgiving.

Finding common ground

Extract (9) TDD 001 (Thanksgiving): Common ground

```
Lisa:       I hafta agree with you, turkey is my
            favorite part.
            (1.3)
Lisa:       It makes you tired though.
            (0.5)
Ms. TDD:    It does?
            (0.5)
Lisa:       It makes me tired any time I eat it.
            It makes me wanna take a nap.
Ms. TDD:    Ha-
```

By turning to the holiday and offering up personal experiences, Lisa re-engages Ms. TDD in the conversation, and they can proceed in a congenial manner.

While this interaction may seem significant to interpersonal relationships, we posit that geriatric care and, particularly, care of persons with dementia may require time designated within the interaction in which history inventory questions can be paced in order that the person with dementia is not overtasked. Additionally, it is important to recognize that the breakdown in the conversation does not just limit information shared, it also has the potential to expose a lack of competence on the part of the person with dementia and this, in turn, has social consequences, including placing the individual's positive identity at stake at that point in the interaction. Yet, at the same time minimizing challenges may also not be helpful or appear to be disingenuous.

Case study 10.2

Returning to Mrs. James's appointment, she is taken to the exam room.

The doctor sits down in front of her at eye level. "Tell me what is bothering you."

MRS. JAMES: "Difficult, really hard. To talk."
DR.: "Yes, it must be incredibly difficult."
MRS. JAMES: "To remember."
DR.: "Yes, that, too. Tell me about your days."
MRS. JAMES: "She shouldn't, have to."
DR.: "You mean your daughter?"
MRS. JAMES: "Yes, too hard."
DR.: "Maybe we need to look for help."

As illustrated in case study 10.2, before any physical exam or traditional medical interview questions, the physician begins with acknowledging the patient and allowing space for her to begin the conversation with concerns and with the language she can produce. *The physician's initial inquiry is formulated as a declarative and, importantly, it is syntactically simpler than the language recommended by the NIA website* (National Institute on Aging, 2021). As the physician displays active listening strategies, they[10] fill in the gaps with clarification statements and address the patient's concerns before moving to the clinical exam.

Clinical relevance revisited

From our analysis, we recommend the following five strategies to better ensure positive clinical interactions with persons with dementia.

Clinical practice recommendations

1. Allow for sufficient warm-up time before assessing competency or seeking information. The warm up may begin in the waiting room by a receptionist or by a nurse who begins with taking vitals.

Employ active listening strategies (see also *Assuaging Difficulties section*). In essence, allow sufficient time for conversation.

2. If possible, allow the person with the dementia diagnosis to exert control over the trajectory of the conversation, guided by clinician responses.
3. Limit inquiries that employ interrogatory/question structures; questions asked should focus on autobiographical memory rather than recent memories (questions like who brought you to your last appointment should be avoided.
4. Avoid explicit corrections and, instead, seek clarification or employ redirection.
5. Do not diminish quality of life difficulties.

Summary

Our findings align with the key principles of person-centered practice. Making the most of every minute of an appointment is partly a matter of giving clinical and non-clinical staff the tools, resources, and latitude they need (Gray, 2007), and we recommend adding clinical training on common interactional strategies that progress along with those that could stymie or prematurely stop interactions. Modest changes in physicians' actions and demeanor can help immensely, says Helen Riess, MD, director of the Empath and Relational Science at Massachusetts General Hospital and an associate professor of psychiatry at Harvard Medical School.

"It begins with creating a space where your patients feel like they're being listened to," Riess says (2021). To that end, she recommends that doctors sit down and make eye contact when they talk with their patients, reminding doctors that they should not try to type data into an EHR at the same time they are talking with a patient. We find providing patients with dementia the extended courtesy of conversational practices to be effective, particularly when a patient is unable, initially, to form syntactically or interactionally coherent talk. As noted in our data, making that extra effort to display cues of actively listening and treating the talk as completing social actions often lead to more coherent, productive conversation. While every physician's time is precious, we concur with Riess: Give each patient your full attention, "and it won't feel like a waste of time for them—and you'll make the best of your time as well."

Recommended readings

Alsawy, S., Tai, S., McEvoy, P., & Mansell, W. (2020). "It's nice to think somebody's listening to me instead of saying 'oh shut up'." People with dementia reflect on what makes communication good and meaningful. *Journal of Psychiatric and Mental Health Nursing, 27*(2), 151–161.

Kindell, J., Keady, J., Sage, K., & Wilkinson, R. (2017). Everyday conversation in dementia: A review of the literature to inform research and practice. *International Journal of Language & Communication Disorders, 52*(4), 392–406.

Morris, L., Horne, M., McEvoy, P., & Williamson, T. (2018). Communication training interventions for family and professional carers of people living with dementia: A systematic review of effectiveness, acceptability, and conceptual basis. *Aging & Mental Health, 22*(7), 863–880.

Swan, K., Hopper, M., Wenke, R., Jackson, C., Till, T., & Conway, E. (2018). Speech-language pathologist interventions for communication in moderate–severe dementia: A systematic review. *American Journal of Speech-language Pathology, 27*(2), 836–852.

Appendix A

Understanding the transcription system

Transcriptions of talk employ an agreed-upon set of symbols that represent or encode how the speakers actually say utterances. These general transcription practices are set forth by Jefferson (2004) and provided below in Table 10.1.

Table 10.1 Jefferson transcription symbols (2004)

Symbol	*Explanation*
(.)	When a full stop symbol is surrounded by round brackets, it shows that a micro pause happened in the conversation.
(0.2)	A number inside brackets denotes a timed pause. This is a pause long enough to time and subsequently show in transcription.
[ ]	Square brackets denote a point where overlapping speech occurs. This shows the exact point in the turn where the overlap or interruption happened.
> <	Arrows surrounding talk like these show that the pace of the speech has speeded up.
< >	Arrows in this direction show that the pace of the speech has slowed down.
()	When rounded brackets are shown with nothing between them, it shows that the words could not be heard by the analyst.
((note here))	Double brackets are used to present a note to the reader; for example, it may show that the speaker nods their head, or shakes their hand, or other non-verbal behavior.
Under	If the word or part of a word is underlined, it denotes a raise in volume or emphasis.
↑	An upward arrow means there is a rise in intonation.
↓	A downward arrow means there is a drop in intonation.
→	An arrow like this denotes a particular sentence of interest to the analyst.
CAPS	Where capital letters appear, it denotes that something was said loudly.
=	The equal sign represents latched speech, a continuation of talk.
:::	Colons appear to represent elongated speech, a stretched sound.

Notes

1 The CCC provides no age, medical, or admittance information on this resident. Pąchalska and Łukaszewska (2011) report that the presence of palilalia and/or echolalia often occur in late state dementia, often seen in Frontotemporal dementia.
2 Also referred to as *recurrent perseveration*, e.g., Bayles et al. (1985).
3 This area is composed of premotor, posterior parietal and frontal-parietal opercula cortices, right inferior frontal, superior temporal cortices, and basal ganglia.
4 For a complete analysis of the data, see Stickle and Wanner, 2020.
5 Resident's date of birth is 1927. Multiple data collection conversations occurred between 2006 and 2011.
6 See Stickle and Wanner (2020) for a complete analysis of this full thirty-three-minute conversation.
7 Resident was born in 1924 and data collection occurred in 2007.
8 Resident was born in 1919. Multiple data collection conversations occurred between 2003 and 2008.
9 Resident was born in 1926. Multiple data collection conversations occurred between 2006 and 2011.
10 Singular 'they' is used in accordance with APA 7th edition (https://apastyle.apa.org/blog/singular-they).

References

Alzheimer's Association. (2021). *Alzheimer's disease facts and figures.* [Ebook]. Chicago. Retrieved from www.alz.org/alzheimers-dementia/facts-figures

Bäckman, L., Small, B., & Fratiglioni, L. (2001). Stability of the preclinical episodic memory deficit in Alzheimer's disease. *Brain, 124*(1), 96–102. https://doi.org/10.1093/brain/124.1.96

Banovic, S., Zunic, L., & Sinanovic, O. (2018). Communication difficulties as a result of dementia. *Materia Socio-medica, 30*(3), 221–224.

Bayles, K., Tomoeda, C., Kaszniak, A., Stern, L., & Eagans, K. (1985). Verbal perseveration of dementia patients. *Brain and Language, 25*(1), 102–116.

Berthier, M. L., Dávila, G., & Torres-Prioris, M. J. (2017). Echophenomena in aphasia: Causal mechanisms and clues for intervention. In P. Coppens and J. Patterson (Eds.), *Aphasia Rehabilitation: Clinical Challenges* (pp. 143–172). Burlington, MA: Jones & Bartlett Learning.

Blair, M., Marczinski, C., Davis-Faroque, N. & Kertesz, A. (2007). A longitudinal study of language decline in Alzheimer's disease and frontotemporal dementia. *Journal of the International Neuropsychological Society, 13*, 237–245.

Chua, J., & Shorey, S. (2021). Effectiveness of end-of-life educational interventions at improving nurses and nursing students' attitude toward death and care of dying patients: a systematic review and meta-analysis. *Nurse Education Today, 101*, 104892.

Davis, B., & Maclagan, M. (2020). Signposts, guideposts, and stalls: Pragmatic and discourse markers in dementia discourse. In T. Stickle (Ed.) *Learning from the Talk of Persons with Dementia* (pp. 63–83). Berlin: Springer Nature.

Davis, B., & Maclagan, M. (2009). Examining pauses in Alzheimer's discourse. *American Journal of Alzheimer's Disease & Other Dementias, 24*(2), 141–154.

Davis, B., Maclagan, M., Karakostas, T., Hsiang, S., & Shenk, D. (2011). Watching what you say: Walking and conversing in dementia preliminary studies. *Topics in Geriatric Rehabilitation, 27*(4), 268–277.
De Vries, K. (2013). Communicating with older people with dementia. *Nursing Older People, 25*(4), 30–37.
Edwards, D., & Potter, J. (1992). *Discursive psychology*. London: Sage.
Engel, G. & Morgan, W. L. (1973). *Interviewing and patient care*. Philadelphia, PA: Saunders.
Fraser, K., Meltzer, J., & Rudzicz, F. (2016). Linguistic features identify Alzheimer's disease in narrative speech. *Journal of Alzheimer's Disease, 49*(2), 407–422.
Fuld, P., Katzman, R., Davies, P., & Terry, R. (1982). Intrusions as a sign of Alzheimer dementia chemical and pathological verification. *Annals of Neurology: Official Journal of the American Neurological Association and the Child Neurology Society, 11*(2), 155–159.
Gillen, G., & Brockmann Rubion, K. (2016). Treatment of cognitive-perceptual deficits: A function-based approach. In G. Gillen (Ed.) *Stroke rehabilitation* (4th ed., pp. 612–646). Maryland Heights, MI: Mosby.
Goodwin, C. (Ed.). (2003). *Conversation and brain damage*. New York: Oxford University Press.
Gray, J. (2017). *Giving physicians what they need to thrive*. Athena Health. www.athenahealth.com/knowledge-hub/practice-management/physician-capability-tools-needed-thrive-burnout
Hatem, D., Barrett, S., Hewson, M., Steele, D., Purwono, U., & Smith, R. (2007). Teaching the medical interview: Methods and key learning issues in a faculty development course. *Journal of General Intern Medicine, 22*(12), 1718–1724.
Hopper, T., Bayles, K., & Kim, E. (2001). Retained neuropsychological abilities of individuals with Alzheimer's disease. In *Seminars in Speech and Language, 22*(4), 261–274.
Jefferson, G. (2004). Glossary of transcript symbols with an introduction. *Pragmatics and Beyond New Series, 125*, 13–34.
Kerr, A. M., Biechler, M., Kachmar, U., Palocko, B., & Shaub, T. (2018). Confessions of a reluctant caregiver palliative educational program: using readers' theater to teach end-of-life communication in undergraduate medical education. *Health Communication, 35*(2), 192–200.
Karnieli-Miller, O., Werner, P., Aharon-Peretz, J., & Eidelman, S. (2007). Dilemmas in the (un) veiling of the diagnosis of Alzheimer's disease: walking an ethical and professional tight rope. *Patient Education and Counseling, 67*(3), 307–314.
Kindell, J., Keady, J., Sage, K., & Wilkinson, R. (2017). Everyday conversation in dementia: A review of the literature to inform research and practice. *International Journal of Language & Communication Disorders, 52*(4), 392–406.
Livingston, G. (2020). On average, older adults spend over half their waking hours alone. Pew Research Center. Retrieved from www.pewresearch.org/fact-tank/2019/07/03/on-average-older-adults-spend-over-half-their-waking-hours-alone/
Maynard, D. (2003). *Bad news, good news: Conversational order in everyday talk and clinical settings*. Chicago, IL: University of Chicago Press.
Müller, N., & Mok, Z. (2012). Applying systemic functional linguistics to conversations with dementia: The linguistic construction of relationships between participants. In *Seminars in Speech and Language* (vol. 33, no. 01, pp. 05–15). Thieme Medical Publishers.

National Institute on Aging. (2021, May). *Alzheimer's and Dementia Resources for Professionals.* U.S. Department of Health and Human Services, National Institute on Aging,

National Institutes of Health. Retrieved from www.nia.nih.gov/health/alzheimers-dementia-resources-for-professionals.

Nichol, J., Sundjaja, J., & Nelson, G. (2020). Medical history. StatPearls Treasure Island (FL): StatPearls Publishing. Retrieved from www.ncbi.nlm.nih.gov/books/NBK534249/

Pąchalska, M., & Łukaszewska, B. (2011). Progressive language and speech disturbances in two different types of dementia. *Acta Neuropsychologica*, *9*(2), 193–208. http://1035.indexcopernicus.com/fulltxt.php?ICID=969744.

Pekkala, S., Wiener, D., Himali, J., Beiser, A., Obler, L., Liu, Y., McKee, A., Stanford, A., Seshadri, S., Wolf, P., & Au, R. (2013). Lexical retrieval in discourse: An early indicator of Alzheimer's dementia. *Clinical Linguistics & Phonetics*, *27*(12), 905–921.

Pekkala, S., Albert, M., Spiro, A., & Erkinjuntti, T. (2008). Perseveration in Alzheimer's disease. *Dementia Geriatric Cognitive Disorders*, *25*(2), 109–14.

Riess, H. (2021). Empathy and Relational Science Program. Massachusetts General Hospital. Retrieved from www.massgeneral.org/psychiatry/research/empathy-and-relational-science-program.

Reilly, J., Rodriguez, A., Lamy, M., Wilson, J., & Neils-Strunjas, J. (2010). Cognition, language, and clinical pathological course of non-Alzheimer's dementias: An overview. *Journal of Communication Disorders*, *43*, 438–452.

Small, J., Gutman, G., Makela, S., & Hillhouse, B. (2003). Effectiveness of communication strategies used by caregivers of persons with Alzheimer's disease during activities of daily living. *Journal of Speech, Language, and Hearing Research*, *46*, 353–367.

Small, J., & Perry, J. (2005). Do you remember? How caregivers question their spouses who have Alzheimer's disease and the impact on communication. *Journal of Speech, Language, and Hearing Research*, *48*(1), 125–136.

Stickle, T., & Wanner, A. (2020). Making sense of syntactic error in conversations between persons with dementia and their non-impaired co-participants. In T. Stickle, (Ed.). *Learning from the talk of persons with dementia: A practical guide to interaction and interactional research* (pp. 85–109). Berlin: Springer Nature.

Stickle, T., & Wanner, A. (2016). Transitivity patterns exhibited by persons with dementia in conversation. *Applied Linguistics*, *40*(1), 43–63.

Thorsell, K., Nordström, B., Fagerström, L., & Sivberg, B. (2010). Time in care for older people living in nursing homes, *Nursing Research and Practice*, www.ncbi.nlm.nih.gov/pmc/articles/PMC3169199/

Tai-Seale, M., McGuire, T., & Zhang, W. (2007). Time allocation in primary care office visits. *Health Services Research*, *42*(5), 1871–1894.

Travers, A., & Taylor, V. (2016). What are the barriers to initiating end-of-life conversations with patients in the last year of life? *International Journal of Palliative Nursing*, *22*(9), 454–462.

World Health Organization. (2021, March 22). "Dementia." Retrieved from www.who.int/health-topics/dementia#tab=tab_1

Part IV

Practical guidance on specific conditions resulting in atypical communication

11

Supporting meaningful conversations in stroke-induced aphasia

Elizabeth Hoover and Anne Carney

Chapter contents:

Introduction

The experience of aphasia following a stroke often begins with the individual waking suddenly in a hospital bed unaware of what has happened to bring them there. The individual with aphasia (IWA) recognizes family and caregivers but doesn't understand what is being said to them. The individual becomes upset and frightened because they know what they want to say, but each time they try to speak the words come out wrong (Simmons-Mackie, 2018).

Aphasia is defined as a language disorder resulting from damage to areas of the brain which subserve the formulation and understanding of language (Helm-Estabrooks, Albert, & Nicholas, 2013). Importantly, aphasia does not impact intelligence, but rather impacts an individual's ability to *communicate* and thus participate fully in social and daily activities.

Primary symptoms of aphasia include difficulty producing and understanding spoken language (speaking and listening) and difficulty with reading and writing. In general, the type and severity of the aphasia profile varies depending on the location and extent of damaged brain tissue; the larger the

DOI: 10.4324/9781003142522-16

area of brain damaged, the more severe the symptoms. Aphasia can be mild, affecting only a single aspect of communication, or it can be so severe that typical communication is almost impossible. While many people with aphasia will make significant improvements, residual language and communication problems often persist, yielding a high frequency of long-term aphasia (Flowers et al., 2016). This means that aphasia is often a chronic condition.

This chapter will provide a brief overview of aphasia and its subtypes, as well as the impact of aphasia on the individuals, families, and the broader society. We will introduce strategies for using communication supports with this population and illustrate the advantages of using the strategies in clinical case scenarios. Supportive communication techniques can assist with all aspects of clinical care for this population, including more effective case history intakes, clinical evaluations, assessments of pain and complaints, and goal setting to name a few. We hope this chapter will help healthcare and social providers feel more comfortable in their understanding of the different manifestations of aphasia, feel equipped to engage in everyday healthcare interactions as well as have meaningful conversations and create opportunities for people with aphasia to share their concerns, in order to provide the best levels of care.

Prevalence of stroke and aphasia

Stroke is a leading cause of chronic disability in adults (Berthier, 2005). Recent statistics estimate that the global prevalence of stroke in 2019 was 101.5 million people, of which 94.9 million survived (AHA, 2021). Studies show that approximately one-third of stroke survivors, an estimated 31.63 million people worldwide, develop aphasia (Berthier, 2005).

Aphasia, when compared to other acquired conditions, is more than double the *combined* estimated global prevalence of Huntington's disease, Parkinson's disease, multiple sclerosis and amyotrophic lateral sclerosis. Despite this relatively high prevalence, aphasia remains one of the least-known conditions (Code et al., 2021). Indeed, the general public seem "woefully" uninformed when asked to describe or define the term aphasia (Simmons-Mackie, 2018). A series of international public surveys were conducted in Argentina, Canada, Croatia, Greece, Norway, and Slovenia (Code et al., 2016). In total, 3483 members of the public responded to the survey and indicated whether they had heard of aphasia, where they had heard of it and what they knew about it. Overall, 37.1% of respondents said they had heard of aphasia, but only 9.2% demonstrated a basic knowledge of the condition. This proportion is similar to the findings from a public survey completed by the National Aphasia Association (NAA) in the United States which revealed that only 8.8% of respondents had heard of the term and correctly described it as a language disorder (NAA, 2016).

A low level of public awareness directly contributes to the fear, stigma, and isolation that people experience when living with aphasia, because when individuals suddenly experience an unknown and confusing condition, the individual and their loved ones have no frame of reference for understanding the sequelae.

Unfortunately, it is not just the general public who have poor levels of understanding of aphasia, many healthcare providers and physicians are also under-informed (Simmons-Mackie, 2018). Patients with post-stroke aphasia and their families report feeling excluded from healthcare discussions, receiving inadequate information to make decisions, and reduced involvement in decision making particularly surrounding hospital discharge (Tomkins, Siyambalapitiya, & Worrall, 2013; Helmsley, Werninck & Worrall, 2013). People with aphasia report that physicians did not discuss their medical condition with them; did not explain the condition of aphasia with them or their care-partners while in the hospital; and did not receive information about resources, services and potential outcomes (Welsh et al., 2009). Additionally, physicians seem to overestimate the communication abilities of their patients with aphasia which leads to conversations that are not understood by their patients (McClenahan et al., 1990). Many healthcare professionals appear to have outdated or limited knowledge of the long-term impact of aphasia as they continue to repeat the *now disproved* opinion that prognosis for meaningful improvement ends around 12 months post-onset of the stroke. The compound effect of the reported and observed concerns is that people with aphasia are left feeling confused about the condition of aphasia and their future, many believing that they are experiencing mental health issues or are suffering from a type of dementia (Simmons-Mackie, 2018).

Studies observing interactions between people with aphasia and healthcare providers support the perspectives reported above. Observations revealed unbalanced conversations, with clinicians directing the topic, timing, and flow of the conversation. Conversational responses for people with aphasia were largely limited to closed or forced-choice questions and focused on physical care tasks, with no evidence of conversations about the patient's goals or individual concerns (Gordon, Ellis-Hill, & Ashburn, 2009).

A recent study interviewed healthcare providers from a diverse range of discipline backgrounds and work settings about their experiences working with IWAs (Carragher et al., 2020). Participants engaged in focus groups and responses were analyzed using an inductive thematic approach. Table 8.1 details the five major themes named from the data. Themes reveal a lack of comfort and training within the focus group participants; the good news, however, is that the healthcare professionals indicated a strong desire to get more training and communicate successfully with people with aphasia.

Table 11.1 Major themes relating to health professionals working with people with aphasia (adapted from Carragher et al., 2020)

Theme	*Subthemes*
Health professionals find communicating with patients with aphasia to be a negative experience	Communication is time consuming Communication is really hard Negative perceptions
Health professionals do not know how to help	Inadequate skills Speech pathologist cannot always help Strategies are not always effective
Health professionals limit their conversations with patients with aphasia	
Health professionals want to know how best to help patients with aphasia	Want to help and to do a good job Know there are things that can help The speech pathologist/therapist plays an important role.
Staff feel good after successful communication with patients with aphasia	

Clinical relevance

Based on the evidence reviewed above, it is clear that stroke-induced aphasia is a relatively common condition that remains poorly understood by the general public. It is also apparent that many healthcare providers have a cursory or outdated understanding of the complexities of the condition and feel both unprepared and uncomfortable engaging in natural conversations with their patients who have aphasia. As members of the healthcare community, we have an opportunity to mitigate feelings of fear, frustration, and depression by educating about aphasia and demonstrating how to communicate effectively.

Overview of aphasia

The study of aphasia has shown us that specific aspects of language may be damaged in aphasia. The focus of this chapter is aphasia related to stroke; however, a sudden onset of aphasia may also result from a focal head injury or infection, or develop slowly as a result of a brain tumor or a progressive neurological disease (primary progressive aphasia). Aphasia may also co-occur with a motor speech disorder such as dysarthria or apraxia of speech.

Over the past few decades, several different aphasia taxonomies have been developed to describe the symptoms of aphasia. The simplest classification divides profiles into Expressive or Receptive subtypes to indicate whether the primary deficit is experienced in the production or understanding of speech. This categorization is under-refined because there are cases where *both* understanding and production are significantly affected; this classification also does not account for overall severity and significant variability within each category. Aphasia profiles can also be described using models of psycholinguistics; wherein linguistic components such as semantics (the meaning of words), phonology (the sound system of words), and syntax are individually analyzed across language contexts to provide a *detailed* profile of an individual's strengths and challenges (Caplan & Bub, 1990).

The most common classification system is based on neurological sites of damage and associated descriptions of behavioral deficits. This syndrome classification was initially described by Goodglass and Kaplan (1972) and is still considered to be the most widely used classification taxonomy for aphasia (Gordon, 1998; LaPointe, 2005; Spreen & Risser, 2003). Currently, eight types of aphasia are described within this taxonomy, two of which are named for the scientist who first discovered the location of damage and correlated deficits (i.e., Broca's and Wernicke's). The remaining six types may occur from varied locations of damage and are therefore described on the bases of the linguistic deficits (Baker et al., 2008). The diagnosis of the profile of aphasia is made based on relative strengths in the following *spoken language* tasks: (1) naming or word retrieval, (2) fluency and informational content of the individual's speech, (3) auditory comprehension, and (4) repetition of sentences. A rating of relatively good or relatively poor performance across these linguistic areas will manifest a differential diagnosis. Figure 11.1 illustrates the pathway by which the subtypes of aphasia are designated.

Broadly speaking, aphasia profiles within the syndrome classification can be considered along a continuum of severity with global aphasia presenting as the most severe non-fluent subtype and anomic aphasia as the mildest fluent subtype. All subtypes of aphasia include the core symptom of *anomia*, or word-retrieval problems. Word-retrieval difficulties can range from mild difficulty coming up with words in conversation to an extreme difficulty producing any meaningful words in any environment (Helm-Estabrooks, Albert, & Nicholas, 2013). Diagnosis of aphasia begins with demonstrating the presence of word-finding difficulties that cannot be explained by memory problems, thought disorders, or confusional states. The second factor is the "fluency" of verbal expression, that is the ease of production, length of utterance, and presence of melodic line. Strength of auditory comprehension and ability to repeat spoken sentences are also considered in the "syndrome diagnosis." Figure 11.1 provides brief descriptions and the pathway to diagnosis within the profiles of the syndrome classification.

A comprehensive clinical evaluation should be completed by a qualified speech therapist with expertise in neurologic communication disorders.

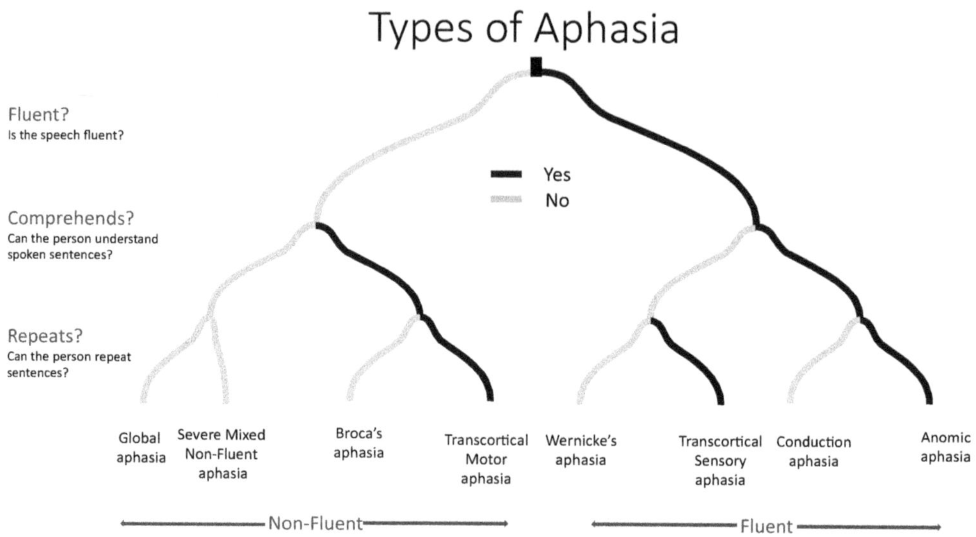

Figure 11.1 Syndrome Classification of Aphasia profiles (adapted from www.aphasia.org/aphasia-definitions/)

Although the classification of the profile depends on the client's performance on the language tasks described above, the therapist will ideally also investigate performance across many other language and communicative contexts, including a measure of reading, writing, functional communication, and a patient-reported outcome measure to understand the impact of the aphasia on the individual's quality of life. While these classifications of aphasia profiles are helpful in broadly understanding the condition, it is important to remember that the characteristics of aphasia tend to vary. Some researchers note that as many as 40% of aphasia profiles do not fit neatly into the syndrome classification.

Importantly, these profiles are not static and may evolve as areas of language improve throughout the recovery process, for example, an individual with a Broca's profile of aphasia immediate post-stroke, may evolve to an anomic subtype by 12-months post-stroke (Kertesz, 1984). Regardless of the location and degree of brain damage from the stroke, we are all *individuals*, each with different personalities, education, and vocational experiences, and as such, will have different goals and communication needs.

Understanding the unique communication profile of the person with aphasia is a *critical* first step to having a successful exchange of information and a meaningful conversation. It is important for all communication partners (whether family members, care partners, or healthcare providers) to know how this individual best understands, how they can best communicate their wants and ideas and, which conversational supports are helpful.

Boston Classification: Non-Fluent Aphasias

Broca's Aphasia

Characterized by word retrieval difficulties (anomia), short phrase length (1–5 words per utterance), good understanding of simple sentences, and difficulty repeating simple sentences. People with this profile of aphasia show signs of agrammatism (syntactic difficulties) in their speech – their utterances consist primarily of substantive words (nouns and main verbs) with fewer supportive words (prepositions, pronouns, etc.).

Word production errors (paraphasias) are common and may include substitution of sounds within the word known as a phonemic parahasias (e.g., shable for *table)* or substitution of related or unrelated whole words (chair for *table* [semantic paraphasia], car for *table* [verbal paraphasia]).

> Tell me why you are here today?
>
> **"Umm ... ah ... well, January ... thirty ... um ... um ... Germany, no ... um ... France ... um ... I can stay it but I can't say it ... Umm I ... holiday ... I ... um ... hotel ... um ... I fall ... um ... hospital ... um ... here ... um ... can't shpek, um ... no ... speak."**

Transcortical Motor Aphasia (TCM)

Like Broca's aphasia, TCM is characterised by reduced initiation of speech, anomia, short phrase length and relatively good auditory comprehension, ***but*** shows relatively preserved ability to repeat sentences.

Global Aphasia

Characterised by severe anomia with very little speech under any conditions accompanied by poor auditory comprehension. Sometimes, stereotypic utterances are present and produced during all attempts to speak. These stereotypic utterances may be well articulated and spoken with natural intonation and include nonsense words or neologistic paraphasias, (e.g. tono, shpay) or real words (e.g., same time, a party).

> Tell me why you are here today?
>
> **"*Grunts* ... shpay, ah ... sphpay ... um ... shpay"**

Severe Mixed Non-Fluent Aphasia

This profile presents somewhere between a global and Broca's aphasia with performance being neither as poor as a global nor as strong as a Broca's profile in any of the language areas.

> Tell me why you are here today?
>
> **"Um ... no ... and uh ... uh ... went ... and the oh my ... oh my! ... Hackers ... she ... the boy ... no ... sorry"**

Boston Classification: Fluent Aphasias

Wernicke's Aphasia

Characterized by severe anomia, poor auditory comprehension and difficulty repeating words and sentences. Language is often empty of meaning due to the prevalence of paraphasias (phonemic, semantic and neologistic). In some cases, the paraphasias may be so frequent that the speech sounds like jargon. The speech is often rapidly produced and excessive – a phenomenon known as "press of speech." Individuals with this profile often do not understand simple questions or instructions, they have little awareness of their communication difficulties and often persist with the conversation unaware of the communication breakdown.

> Tell me why you are here today?
>
> **"Well to tell you the truth it's all a ditty on the filly and the who's-a-call it happened so sudden and boom and a boom on waycycle and fall and the ditty filly. I have the stuff here and he said he would but the boom on the filly."**

Transcortical Sensory Aphasia (TCS)

This profile presents similarly to the Wernicke's aphasia profile (described above), but like the TCM profile, has a relative strength in the ability to repeat sentences.

Conduction Aphasia

Characterized by anomia with normal phrase length. Flow of speech may be interrupted by pauses to retrieve word or self-correction or errors. This profile is unique for the prevalence of phonemic paraphasias and the attempts by the individual to self-correct those errors. Auditory comprehension is good. Errors are also seen in ability to repeat spoken words and phrases.

> Tell me why you are here today?
>
> **"I had one of these over here (points to heart)...you know tac an tack a heart attack and then the thing I know they tell me I had toke, a coat a stroke...and here we are."**

Anomic Aphasia

Characterized by word-finding difficulties across all tasks requiring retrieval of specific substantive words. Auditory comprehension and repetition are relatively intact. Paraphasias are rare, but when they occur they are likely to be closely related semantically.

> Tell me why you are here today?
>
> **"To tell the truth, I am still not right. I see the words, but they um...just don't come quickly enough. I know, it but I just can't find the right word...or I have one word, but I really want a different word. It is very frustrating"**

Figure 11.2 Descriptions of the Syndrome Classification of Aphasia subtypes

The impact of aphasia

The consequences of aphasia are far reaching and often severe. Aphasia disrupts language processing, which in turn disrupts communication. Communication is essential for most aspects of daily life, and thus, its disruption results in a cascade of other social corollaries including social isolation, reduced participation in work and hobbies, and a loss of friendships (Brown et al., 2013; Code, 2003; Cruice, Worrall, & Hickson, 2006; Parr et al., 1997). Not surprisingly, aphasia has been shown to have a significant negative affect on quality of life at a higher level than those stroke survivors without aphasia (Simmons-Mackie, 2018; Hilari, 2011). In fact, when compared to 60 diseases and 15 health conditions, aphasia was reported as the largest negative impact on health-related quality of life in a large cohort of individuals living in long-term care (Lam & Wodchis, 2010). People living with aphasia report negative impacts on relationships between family and friends, which is associated with a high prevalence of loneliness and social isolation (Simmons-Mackie, 2018). Loneliness and degrees of social isolation matter because studies have shown social isolation is associated with "increased rates of premature death, lower general well-being, more depression and a higher level of disability from chronic disease" (World Health Organization, 2003, p. 16). There are several studies that detail the risk of adverse health consequences associated with loneliness or social isolation; social isolation caused by aphasia can result in higher risk of recurrent strokes, infection, and falls. Researchers even suggested that reduced social relationships should be viewed similarly to other risk factors such as obesity or alcohol abuse and that reduced social contact is "equivalent to smoking up to 15 cigarettes a day" (Holt-Lundstat & Smith, 2012).

Aphasia is also associated with a high risk of depression, low mood, or emotional problems that often persist over time. Hilari and colleagues (2012) found that people with aphasia were more likely to experience significantly higher levels of emotional distress three months after stroke than stroke survivors without aphasia. This is important because levels of mood have been shown to be the highest predictors of living well with aphasia in the first year after onset (Worrall et al., 2017) and that depression is associated with a plethora of negative consequences such as poor quality of life; lower functional outcomes from rehabilitation; poorer recovery of physical and cognitive functions; higher healthcare costs; longer hospitalizations and increased mortality (Simmons-Mackie, 2018). Depression is detrimental to health and quality of life, in addition to elevating healthcare costs; therefore prevention and treatment of emotional problems should be prioritized for people with aphasia.

Aphasia also impacts an individual's sense of self and identity. Early in the course of recovery, interactions can be challenging and people with aphasia may experience breakdowns in their communication. Changes in abilities, roles, relationships, and community-life may diminish one's sense of identity. Shadden (2005) describes this process as having a potentially devastating impact on self-esteem and identity and that the onset of aphasia therefore may be likened to "identity theft." Debra Meyerson (Meyerson & Zuckerman, 2019) chronicles her recovery along with the stories of other stroke survivors and their care partners in her book *Identity Theft: Rediscovering Ourselves After Stroke*. Meyerson describes how recovery programs, focused primarily on rehabilitation, often leave survivors with a sense of "failure" if they don't regain all their capabilities. She proposes the need to reconstruct positive identities in the face of whatever disabilities remain, to rebuild rewarding lives.

Communication access: a basic human right

According to the International Communication Project (2014), "The opportunity to communicate is a basic human right … everybody has the potential to communicate." This is certainly the case for people with aphasia. Even in the case of the most severe forms of aphasia, communication is possible. Below we review some guidelines for communicating successfully with people with aphasia.

Communication guidelines

Communication supports encompass a variety of strategies and techniques that seek to improve access to communication for people with aphasia. These include any strategies or techniques used by either the person with aphasia or their communication partner to maximize the success of the communication exchange, such as the use of facial expressions, gestures, writing, drawing, photos, pictographs, other visual aids (e.g., rating scales, calendars, maps), and technology. Given the various presentations of aphasia discussed earlier, communication supports both help people who have aphasia with understanding what is being communicated to them and also provides people with alternative ways to communicate their message, e.g. pointing, writing, drawing, answering a yes/no question, choosing from a field of options, etc. Underlying the usage of communication supports is a respect for the inherent competence of the person with aphasia and a desire to support their participation in meaningful communication exchanges.

The concept of communication supports is widely employed by speech–language pathologists and is reflected in approaches such as multimodality or total communication, augmentative and alternative communication (AAC), and compensatory strategy training, as well as specific programs for training communication partners, such as Supported Communication for Adults with Aphasia (SCA™; Kagan, 1998). Rather than conceiving of communication supports as a specific type of treatment or approach, there is a growing movement among the aphasia community to ensure that the usage of communication supports is integrated across communication partners, across settings, and across the continuum of care in support of maximizing communication participation for people with aphasia (Simmons-Mackie, King, & Beukelman, 2013).

In 2014, Aphasia United, an international organization of aphasia researchers, clinicians, and consumers, published a set of Best Practice Recommendations for Aphasia (www.aphasiaunited.org). Several of the ten recommendations speak to the use of communication supports and training communication partners to support the communication of people with aphasia. One recommendation specifies the training of healthcare and social care providers who work with people who have aphasia across the continuum of care – "acute care to end of life." Given that healthcare professionals are often among the first individuals that a person with aphasia may encounter after their stroke or brain injury, ensuring that they are equipped to effectively communicate with this population is paramount. In a study by Worrall and colleagues (2011) entitled "What People with Aphasia Want," people with aphasia reported wanting *control and independence*, noting specifically that they were frustrated by not being involved in decisions about their care. Excluding people with aphasia from decisions about their care is reflected in comments from a stroke team's perceptions of delivering healthcare to people with aphasia (Carragher et al., 2020). In order to save time, healthcare professionals reported that they speak to family members rather than directly to the person with aphasia. Beyond reasons of basic dignity, respect and the right to communication access, healthcare professionals oftentimes must communicate critical information, further necessitating an understanding of how to use communication supports with their patients who have aphasia.

SCA™ Kagan, 1998) is a training program that was developed by the Aphasia Institute in Toronto. SCA™ is a method that employs a range of communication supports, underlying which are the fundamental goals of *acknowledging competence* and *revealing competence* of the person with aphasia. The method uses spoken and written keywords, body language and gestures, drawing, and detailed pictographs to address the communication barriers that can result from aphasia (www.aphasia.ca).

Acknowledging competence involves both the way in which one communicates with the person who has aphasia (e.g., natural tone and volume of voice) as well as making specific statements such as "I know that you know" during appropriate times. To *reveal competence*, the SCA™ method employs techniques to: (1) support the person who has aphasia with understanding the information or message that is being communicated to them (getting the message "IN"); (2) support the person who has aphasia with expressing themselves (getting the message "OUT"); and (3) confirm that the person with aphasia's message has been understood (verifying the person with aphasia's message "VERIFY"). Figure 11.3 details strategies for acknowledging and revealing competence in conversation.

Getting the message ...

IN:
Techniques that can assist with ensuring the message is being understood by the person with aphasia include:

- using short, simple sentences;
- using gestures while speaking;
- writing down keywords or topics of conversation;
- using pictures or other visual supports;
- eliminating distractions (e.g., noise or visual distractions);
- observing the person with aphasia (e.g., facial expression, body language, etc.) to assess level of comprehension

OUT:
Techniques that can support the person with aphasia to communicate their message include:

- asking yes/no questions; asking forced choice questions (Was your stroke in May or June?);
- asking the person with aphasia to gesture, point or write;
- giving the person with aphasia "wait time" or an adequate time to respond.

VERIFIED:
Techniques that can support verification of the person with aphasia's message include:

- restating the person with aphasia's message;
- recapping the conversation.

Figure 11.3 Strategies for acknowledging and revealing competence (SCA™) (adapted from www.aphasia.ca/communication-tools-commmunicative-access-sca)

The extensive pictographic library developed by the Aphasia Institute has been employed by innumerable speech therapists to support the communication of their patients with aphasia across topics ranging from educating the patient about aphasia and its different presentations to goal setting, discharge planning, COVID-19, and countless other topics. At the time of this book's publication, the Aphasia's Institute's pictographic library was available for free search and download at www.participics.ca/. Figures 11.4 and 11.5 illustrate how pictographs can be used to support the discussion of complex and critical topics such as dealing with depression and medical decision making.

When sharing written information with patients who have aphasia, healthcare professionals and institutions can also adapt their written materials to ensure that they are more accessible or "aphasia-friendly." When faced with an unfamiliar and life-altering condition such as aphasia, people with aphasia reported *wanting more information* about stroke and aphasia for themselves and their loved ones (Worrall et al., 2011). They also reported wanting information about their prognosis and the potential course of recovery through the stages of rehabilitation. While IWAs

You may feel **frustrated** or **helpless** because of

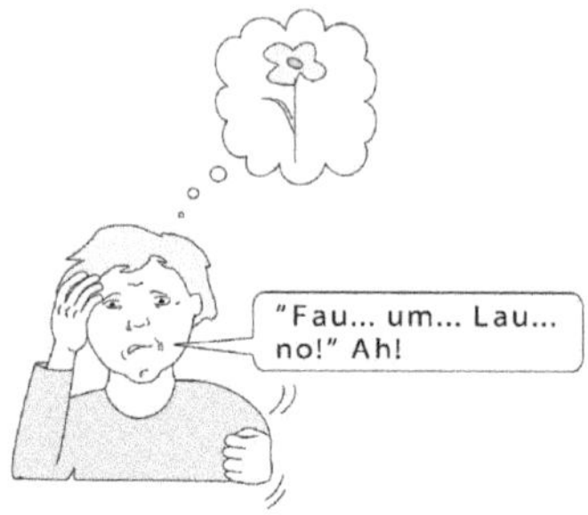

Difficulty **expressing** yourself.

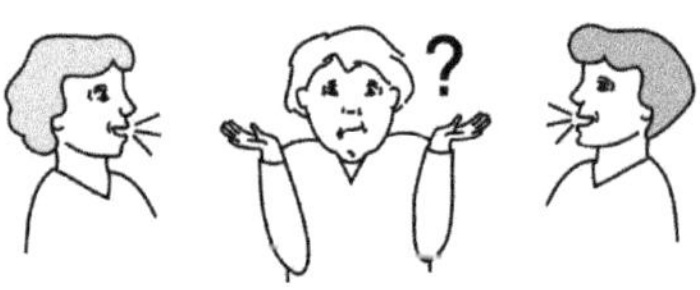

Difficulty **understanding** others.

You may feel **frustrated** or **helpless**

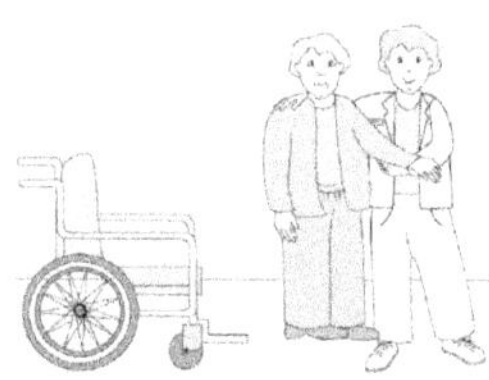

because you must **rely** on **others**.

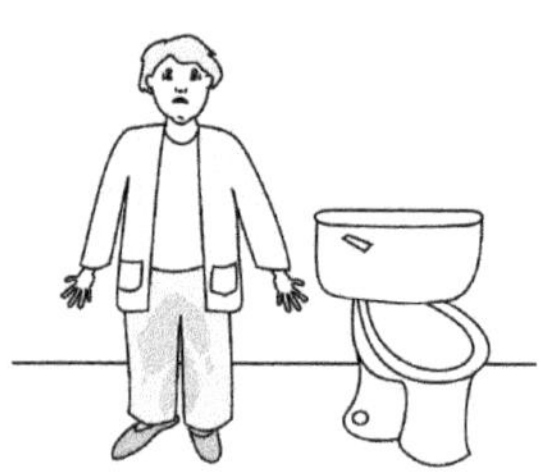

because of **changes** in your **body**.

Feeling frustrated and helpless could lead to **depression**.

Figure 11.4 Communication supports for a conversation about depression in aphasia

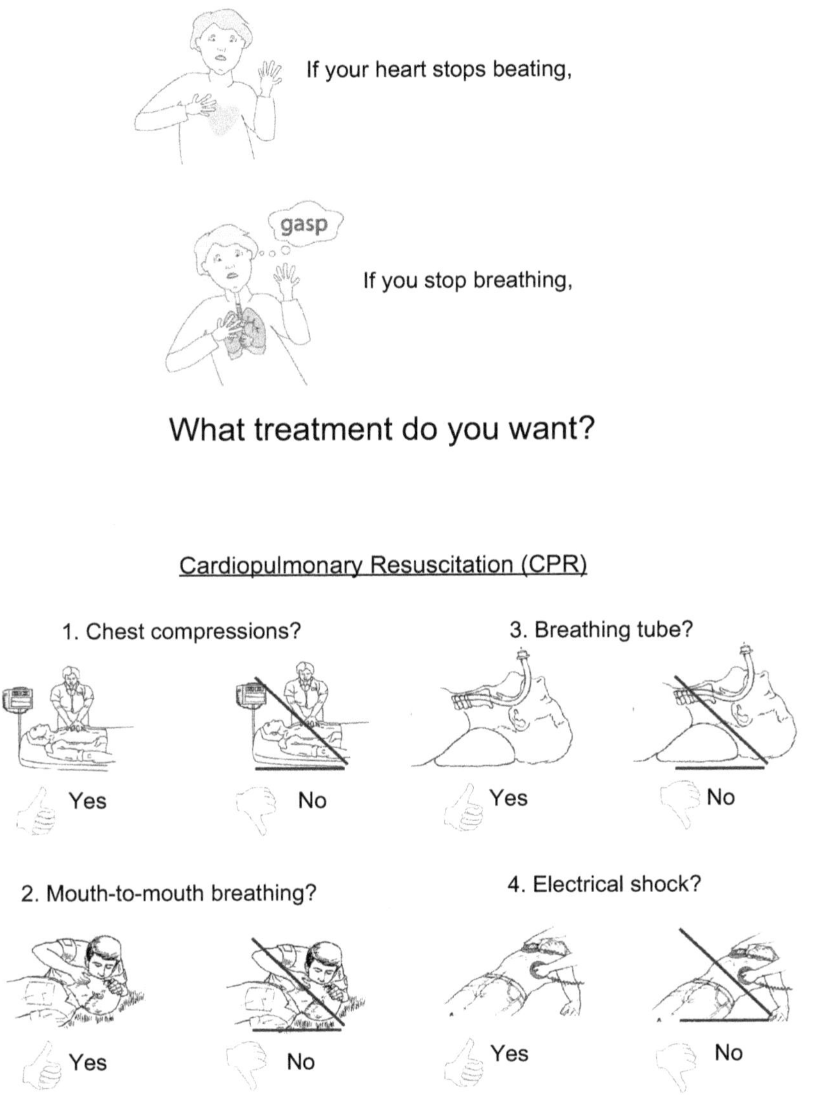

Figure 11.5 Communication supports for a conversation about medical decision making

and their loved ones are undoubtedly receiving some information from healthcare professionals about aphasia, their prognosis and what to expect during rehabilitation, it is likely that the information could be provided in a more accessible way and repeated or reviewed at different intervals to allow for the IWA and their loved ones to process the information. Figure 11.6 lists "suggested guidelines" for use when creating

Adult Speech-Language Intake Form

NEED HELP FILLING OUT THIS FORM? ☐**YES** ☐ **NO**

Today's date: ______________________________

Last Name:	First Name:
Address:	City: Postal Code:
Telephone #: ( )___-________	Email Address:
Date of Birth:	Gender: ☐Female ☐Male ☐Non-Binary
Emergency Contact Person:	Contact Person's Phone #: ( )___-________
Present/ Past **Occupation**:	Highest Level of **Education**:
First Language:	**Other** Languages Spoken:

PHYSICIAN INFORMATION.

Family Physician name: ______________ **Phone:** ( )___-_____

Other physicians involved in your care:

MEDICAL DIFFICULTY (related to communication difficulty)

Date of occurrence of difficulty/ illness/injury

____

Cause of difficulty/ illness/injury:

Accident	Brain Injury	Stroke	Disease	Other:
			Type:	________ ________

Please list any **medications** that you are currently taking:

Allergies:

Do you have any allergies? Yes No

If **yes** please list them: ______________________________

Do you use an Epipen? Yes No

Figure 11.6 Guidelines for aphasia-friendly written information

aphasia-friendly written information, adapted from a study conducted by Rose et al. (2010) in addition to guidelines published by Simmons-Mackie and King (2013). In summary, text should be large and easy to read. Sentences should be clear, short, and simple in syntax. Word choice should be accessible with an emphasis on everyday terminology versus medical or technical jargon. Photos, pictographs, maps, icons, and other graphics should be used to supplement text as relevant. Ample amounts of white space and few distractions are also recommended.

Using technology to support communication

In addition to the growth of high technology AAC tools discussed in Chapter 4, the proliferation of mobile technology has increased the accessibility of technologically based communication

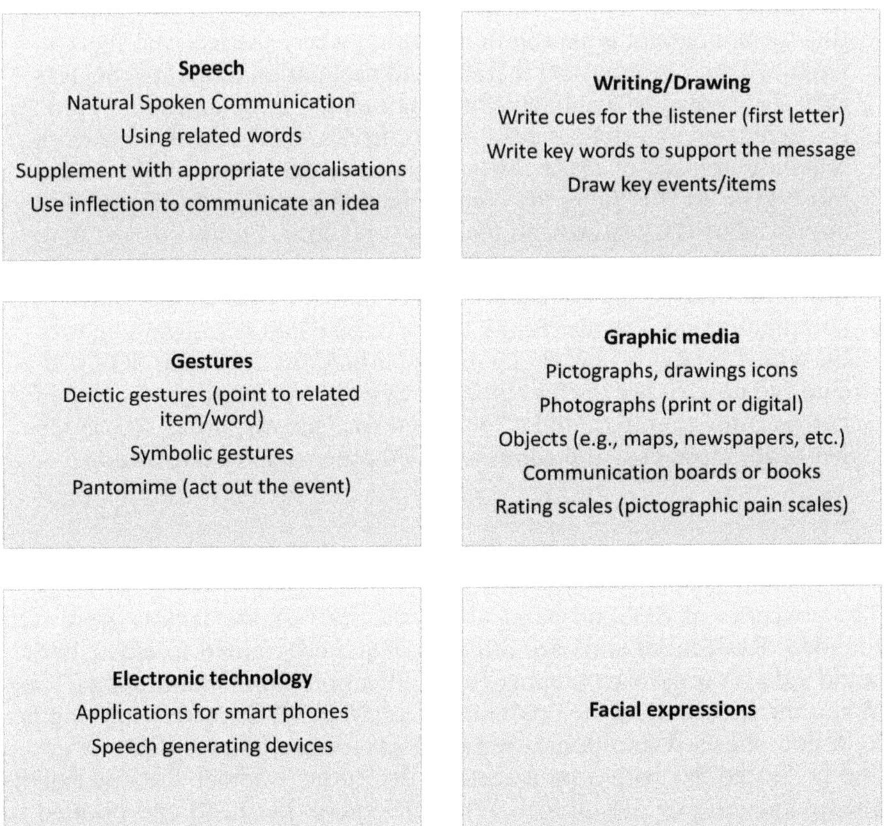

Figure 11.7 Communication supports (adapted from Simmons-Mackie & King., 2013)

supports. Given that the sequelae of post-stroke aphasia may involve vision, dexterity, and cognitive issues, people with aphasia may benefit from accessibility features (e.g. enlarged font, text to speech, assistive touch, etc.) to support their usage of mobile devices. They may also benefit from step-by-step introduction for how to use specific apps in support of their communication as well as opportunities to practice these skills in a supportive environment.

Clinical case examples

Case study 11.1 Subacute/nursing facility

SG sustained a left hemisphere haemorrhagic stroke that resulted in a severe mixed non-fluent aphasia and apraxia of speech. She also had a right hemiplegia that necessitated the use of a wheelchair. Once medically stable, SG was discharged from her acute care hospital setting to an inpatient rehabilitation hospital where she received speech–language therapy, physical therapy, and occupational therapy. SG was then discharged to a subacute/nursing facility. SG's husband, Frank, is a dedicated and tireless advocate for her care. He adjusted his work schedule in favor of night shifts so that he could be with SG during most days. At this time, SG communicated primarily in single word approximations, gestures, and facial expressions. Frank worried that, due to the severity of her aphasia and co-occurring motor speech disorder, the staff at the facility would not take the time to support SG's communication. Despite Frank's efforts, he could not always be with his wife. One day, a speech–language pathologist arrived at SG's bedside and noticed her visible agitation. SG had refused to participate in her morning therapies and when asked why she was upset, SG shook her head, grimaced, and communicated other signs of frustration.

Discussion

The concerns of SG's husband about the staff at the facility were well founded. Residential staff are often inadequately trained to either understand aphasia or how to support communication (Simmons-Mackie, 2018). When the speech–language pathologist arrived at SG's bedside seeing her agitation, she used communication supports to ascertain why SG was upset. She presented SG with a pain scale to determine whether she was experiencing any pain or discomfort. When SG shook her head and pointed to "0" on the pain scale, the speech-language pathologist then verified with SG that pain was not the issue at hand. She then employed other supportive communication strategies to support SG in getting her message "OUT," such as asking SG if she could point to what was wrong and asking yes/no questions. SG then pointed to her shirt and placed her hand on her chest. Through these supported communication techniques, the speech–language pathologist ultimately learned that the nursing staff was not dressing SG in her undergarments, leaving her vulnerable and uncomfortable and as a result unwilling to participate in therapies. This example illustrates that when healthcare professionals and staff have little understanding of aphasia or how to support communication, IWAs often struggle to have their basic needs and dignity met. It also shows how employing a few simple communication supports and techniques, e.g. a pain scale, verifying the patient's message, encouraging the use of gesturing/pointing, and asking yes/no questions can result in a successful communication exchange.

Case study 11.2 Inpatient rehabilitation

MB sustained a left hemisphere stroke because of a ruptured arteriovenous malformation. After three weeks in the ICU, she was discharged to an inpatient rehabilitation hospital. MB recalls not being able to speak at all when she arrived and learning from her speech–language pathologist that she had aphasia. MB had never heard of aphasia, which is consistent with both anecdotal and public awareness data. MB progressed from communicating yes/no via head nodding to verbally saying yes/no and vividly remembers saying "more work – speech only" as soon as she could. As a self-described "talker," MB was desperate to get her speech back. While still at the inpatient rehabilitation hospital, MB describes an appointment she had with a neuropsychologist who she thought would somehow miraculously cure her aphasia. The neuropsychologist began administering reading and writing tests, which MB could not complete. In those moments, MB became overwhelmed with emotion, devastated by the realization that she may not make a full recovery from her aphasia. Despite her tears, the neuropsychologist persisted with testing until MB finally told him that she wanted to go back to her room.

Discussion

MB is now more than ten years post-onset from her stroke and has a mild anomic profile of aphasia. She returned to work in a different capacity than prior to her stroke and regularly volunteers as a sample patient to help train physical therapy students. When MB was asked about why she thought the neuropsychologist wanted to proceed with testing despite seeing her so visibly upset, MB speculated that "maybe it was going to disrupt his schedule." MB's retelling of this exchange, over ten years after it took place, and speculation regarding the neuropsychologist is consistent with the findings of

Carragher and colleagues (2020) described above: healthcare professionals find communicating with patients who have aphasia to be time consuming and challenging and they limit their conversations with those patients. In this scenario, MB could have benefited from any number of communication supports. People with aphasia report that they are offered few rationales before beginning therapeutic activities and that when provided with oral and written information it is often inaccessible due to jargon and complexity (Parr, 2007). To begin the testing, the neuropsychologist could have explained the rationale for the measures in a more accessible way. When it was clear that MB was upset, the neuropsychologist should have discontinued testing. At this point, he should have engaged MB in a conversation about why she was upset. Using the "IN," "OUT," and "VERIFY" techniques, he could have acknowledged her distress, asked whether her performance on the testing was upsetting her and verified her response. From there, it may have been appropriate to make a referral to a social worker or other mental health professional so that MB could be screened for depression. The speech language pathologist on MB's team could have also been brought in to discuss the implications of MB's performance and provide accessible patient education about how aphasia can affect reading and writing and to also share that evidence-based treatment approaches exist for addressing acquired reading and writing impairments related to aphasia.

Case study 11.3 University-based aphasia center

When RM began participating in group treatment at a university-based aphasia center, he was two years post-onset from a left hemisphere stroke that resulted in Wernicke's aphasia. RM's verbal expression was "fluent but empty" due to his frequent phonemic and semantic paraphasias and he had poor auditory comprehension. During his intake interview, the speech–language pathologist and occupational therapist both used communication supports to account for RM's auditory comprehension difficulties (e.g. increased visuals, simplified syntax, highlighting keywords and topic changes in writing, etc.) as well as to clarify and confirm his verbal responses. Given RM's background and affinity for IT, he enrolled in the center's technology group, which sought to explore ways in which accessibility features (e.g. text to speech, reader) and apps (e.g. maps, calendar, camera/photos, video calling, etc.) could support speech and language comprehension and production for people with aphasia. One day, RM arrived at the center looking distraught. When asked why he was upset, RM began speaking and gesturing but his language was vague and nonspecific and due to paraphasias and neologisms (non-words), he was not initially understood.

Discussion

The occupational therapist who was facilitating the group began using communication supports to clarify RM's message. She confirmed that something was wrong and that it involved a family member. The technology group had recently reviewed ways in which the maps app could be used to support discussions about locations (e.g. where the group members live, locations they frequent in their community, places they have traveled, as parts of discussions related to current events, etc.). The occupational therapist asked if RM could show her where the problem was taking place using the maps app on his iPad. Using the maps app, RM zoomed into another region of the country and pointed to a city where it was confirmed that his wife had traveled due to a death in the family, which he communicated using a gesture. Through the use of a generic family tree that was retrieved in an online search, RM pointed to "brother-in-law." The occupational therapist and other group members shared their condolences with RM. In this scenario, RM effectively used technology to support his communication. As discussed above, the proliferation of mobile technology allows for a wealth of communication supports at our finger tips. To support the effective usage of technology, however, people with aphasia may benefit from specific instruction and practice for using apps and accessibility features to support their communication.

Summary

Aphasia is a complex disorder characterized by difficulties in language processing that include speaking and understanding, most obviously, but may also extend to reading and writing. These language difficulties can vary significantly by individual, but nonetheless directly impact the ability to communicate. Because communication is critical in most aspects of daily life, aphasia typically has a negative impact on social relationships, participation, and well-being. Aphasia does not impact intelligence; however, intelligence can be masked by difficulty communicating. People with aphasia are mentally competent and able to make decisions about their well-being and participate in activities that are made communicatively accessible. Healthcare services for people with aphasia should be person-centered and collaborative. Best practice recommendations for healthcare or community services involving people with aphasia include: (1) receiving information regarding aphasia and options for treatment regardless of point in recovery continuum, and providing an effective means of communicating the individual's needs and wishes; (2) involving families or care partners of people with aphasia in the rehabilitation process; and (3) providing education and training to healthcare and social care providers on communication supports for people with aphasia (www.aphasiaunited.org/).

Attention to meaningful conversation and life participation should begin soon post-onset of aphasia. All healthcare partners should attempt to share information and resources about aphasia and invite questions and opinions from people with aphasia about their care in an accessible manner. Sadly, research shows that healthcare providers are uncomfortable having conversations with people with aphasia. Conversations lack an equal amount of turn-taking, with healthcare partners directing the topic, timing, and flow of the conversation. Conversational responses for people with aphasia were largely limited to closed- or forced-choice questions and did not include discussion about goals or individual concerns.

People with aphasia can communicate their wants and needs when given enough time and support. Use of communication supports should be integrated across communication partners, settings, and the continuum of care to maximize communication participation for people with aphasia. In this chapter, we have provided an overview of aphasia-friendly resources and shared access to adaptable communicative supports in a variety of health-related and participation-based topics. We have also illustrated how the course of care can be positively impacted when time is taken to use these communicate strategies with clinical case examples. Healthcare partners should strive to support and verify the IWA's *understanding of a conversation message* and provide multimodal supports to enable the individual to *create their own message* (SCA™). These central tenants foster equity in the conversation and help to cultivate a more inclusive environment. The consequences of aphasia can be wide reaching and severe. Taking the time to have meaningful conversations throughout the course of recovery can have a positive impact on outcomes and mitigate adverse health consequences.

Recommended reading

1. Aphasia Access website for State of Aphasia in North America White Paper (Simmons-Mackie, 2018) and Aphasia survival guides: www.aphasiaaccess.org
2. Aphasia Institute – Life's a conversation: www.aphasia.ca
3. Holland, A. L. & Elman, R. J. (2021). *Neurogenic Communication Disorders and the Life Participation Approach: The social imperative in supporting individuals and families.* Plural Publishing
4. Meyerson, D., & Zuckerman, D. (2019). *Identity theft: rediscovering ourselves after stroke.* Andrews McMeel Publishing
5. Simmons-Mackie, N., King, J. M., & Beukelman, D. R. (2013). *Supporting communication for adults with acute and chronic aphasia.* Brookes Publishing.

References

American Heart Association (2021). *Heart Disease & Stroke Statistical Update Fact Sheet Global Burden of Disease.* Retrieved on 4 December 2021 from: www.heart.org

Baker, J. C., Leblanc, L. A., & Raetz, P. B. (2008). A behavioral conceptualization of aphasia. *The Analysis of Verbal Behavior, 24*(1), 147–158.

Berthier, M. L. (2005). Poststroke aphasia: epidemiology, pathophysiology and treatment. *Drugs and Aging, 22*, 163–182.

Brown, K., Davidson, B., Worrall, L., Howe, T. (2013). "Making a good time": the role of friendship in living successfully with aphasia. *International Journal of Speech–Language Pathology, 15*(2), 165–175.

Caplan, D., & Bub, D. (1990). *Psycholinguistic assessment of aphasia.* Mini-seminar presented at the annual convention of the American Speech–Language–Hearing Association, Seattle, WA.

Carragher, M., Steel, G., O'Halloran, R., Torabi, T. Johnson, H. Taylor, N., & Rose, M. (2020). Aphasia disrupts usual care: the stroke team's perceptions of delivering healthcare to patients with aphasia. *Disability and Rehabilitation, 41*(2)1, 3003–3014.

Code, C. (2003). The quantity of life for people with chronic aphasia. *Neuropsychological Rehabilitation, 13*(3), 379–390.

Code, C., Papathanasiou, I., Rubio-Bruno, S., de la Paz Cabana, M., Villanueva, M. M., Halland-Johansen, L., Prizl-Jakovac, T., Leko, A., Zemva, N., Patterson, R., Verry, R., Rochon, E., Leonard, C., & Robert, A. (2016). International patterns of the public awareness of aphasia. *International Journal of Language and Communication Disorders, 51*(3), 276–284.

Code, C., Simmons-Mackie, N., Armstrong, E., Stiegler, L., Armstrong, J., Bushby, E., Carew-Price, P., Curtis, H., Haynes, P., McLeod, E., Muhleisen, V., Neate, J., Nikolas, A., Rolfe, D., Rubly, Simpson, R., & Webber, A. (2001). The public awareness of aphasia: an international Survey. *International Journal of Language and Communication Disorders, 36*, 1–6.

Cruice, M., Worrall, L., & Hickson, L. (2006). Quantifying aphasic people's social lives in the context of non-aphasic peers. *Aphasiology, 20*(12), 1210–1225.

Flowers, H., Skoretz, A., Silver, F., Rochon, E., Fang, J., Flamand-Roze, C., & Marinto, R. (2016). Poststroke aphasia frequency, recovery and outcomes: a systematic review and meta-analysis. *Archives of Physical Medicine and Rehabilitation, 97*(12), 2188–2201.

Goodglass, H., & Kaplan, E. (1972). *The assessment of aphasia and related disorders.* 1st ed. Philadelphia, PA: Lea & Febiger.

Gordon, J. K. (1998). The fluency dimension in aphasia. *Aphasiology.* 12:673–688.

Gordon, C., Ellis-Hill, C., & Ashburn, A. (2009). The use of conversational analysis: nurse–patient interaction in communication dis-ability after stroke. *Journal of Advanced Nursing, 65*(3), 544–553.

Helm-Estabrooks, N., Albert, M. L., & Nicholas, M. (2013). Manual of aphasia and aphasia therapy, 3rd ed. Austin, TX: Pro-Ed Publishers.

Hilari, K. (2011). The impact of stroke: are people with aphasia different to those without? *Disability and Rehabilitation, 33*(3), 211–218.

Hilari, K, Needle, J., & Harrison, K. (2012). What are the important factors in health-related quality of life for people with aphasia? A systematic review. *Archives of Physical Medicine and Rehabilitation, 93*, 586–595.

Hemsley, B., Werninck, M., & Worrall, L. (2013). "That really shouldn't have happened": people with aphasia and their spouses narrate adverse events in hospital. *Aphasiology, 27*(6), 706–722.

Holt-Lundstat, J. & Smith, T. (2012). Social relationships and mortality. *Social and Personality Psychology Compass, 6*, 41–53.

International Communication Project. (2014). The Universal Declaration of Communication Rights. Retrieved 14 December 2016 from www.internationalcommunicationproject.com/wp-content/uploads/2014/09/English-Declaration.pdf

Kagan, A. (1998) Supported conversation for adults with aphasia: methods and resources for training conversation partners. *Aphasiology, 12*(9), 816–830.

Lam, J., & Wodchis, W. (2010). The relationship of 60 disease diagnoses and 15 conditions to preference-based health-related quality of life in Ontario hospital-based long-term care residents. *Medical Care, 48*, 380–387.

LaPointe, L. (2005). *Aphasia and related neurogenic language disorders.* New York, NY: Thieme Publishers.

McClenahan, R., Johnston, M., & Densham, Y. (1990). Misperceptions of comprehension difficulties of stroke patients by doctors, nurses and relatives. *Journal of Neurology, Neurosurgery, and Psychiatry, 53*, 700–701.

Meyerson, D., & Zuckerman, D. (2019). *Identity theft: rediscovering ourselves after stroke.* Kansas City, MO: Andrews McMeel Publishing.

National Aphasia Association (2016). Aphasia Definitions. Retrieved from www.aphasia.org/aphasia-definitions/

Parr, S., Byng, S., Gilpin, S., & Ireland, C. (1997). *Talking about aphasia: Living with loss of language after stroke.* Maidenhead, UK: Open University Press.

Parr, S. (2007) Living with severe aphasia: Tracking social exclusion. *Aphasiology, 21*(1), 98–123.

Rose, T., Worrall, L., Hickson, L., & Hoffmann, T. (2010). Do people with aphasia want written stroke and aphasia information? A verbal survey exploring preferences for when and how to provide stroke and aphasia information. *Topics in Stroke Rehabilitation, 17*(2), 79–98.

Rose, T., Worrall, L., Hickson L., & Hoffmann, T. (2011). Exploring the use of graphics in written health information for people with aphasia. *Aphasiology, 25*(12), 1579–1599.

Shadden, B. (2005). Aphasia as identity theft: Theory and practice. *Aphasiology, 19*(3/4/5), 211–223.

Simmons-Mackie, N. (2018). *The state of aphasia in North America: A white paper.* Aphasia Access. Retrieved from www.aphasiaaccess.org/white-papers/

Simmons-Mackie, N., & King, J. (2013). Communication support for everyday situations. In N. Simmons-Mackie, J. King, & D. Beukelman (Eds.), *Supporting communication for adults with acute and chronic aphasia.* Baltimore, MD: Paul Brookes publishing

Simmons-Mackie, N., King, J., & Beukelman, D. (2013). *Supporting communication for adults with acute and chronic aphasia.* Baltimore, MD: Brookes Publishing.

Spreen, O., & Risser, A. (2003). *Assessment of aphasia.* New York: Oxford University Press.

Tomkins, B., Siyambalapitiya, S., & Worrall, L. (2013). What do people with aphasia think about their health care? Factors influencing satisfaction and dissatisfaction. *Aphasiology, 27*(8), 972–991.

Welsh, J., Abbanat, G., & Szabo, G. (2009). Development of an aphasia training program for medical residents. Presentation at the Clinical Aphasiology Conference, Keystone CO.

World Health Organization (2003). *The social determinants of health: the solid facts*. 2nd ed. Geneva: WHO.

Worrall, L., Sherratt, S., Rogers, P., Howe, T., Hersh, D., Ferguson, A., et al. (2011). What people with aphasia want: their goals according to the ICF. *Aphasiology*, *25*(3), 309–322.

Worrall, L., Hudson, K., Khan, A., Ryan, B., & Simmons-Mackie, N. (2017). Determinants of living well with aphasia in the first year post stroke: a prospective cohort study. *Archives of Physical Medicine and Rehabilitation*, *98*, 235–240.

Communication and people with learning disabilities

Jonathan Beebee

Chapter contents:

- Clinical relevance
- Communication guidelines
- Mental capacity
- General communication advice for people with learning disabilities
- Cultural implications
- Recommended reading
- References

Introduction

People with learning disabilities are an integral part of our communities. Gone are the days where those with learning disabilities are secluded from the general population and cared for in large institutional settings. This will mean that you will be very likely to support people with learning disabilities whatever setting you work in.

A learning disability is defined as a significant impairment of intelligence, requiring significant support to meet daily living skills, and onset before the age of 18. Intelligence is generally measured with IQ scores, with an IQ score of 70 or below being generally accepted as diagnostic criteria, this being those in the 2nd centile of standard distribution of IQ. However, services are relying less on arbitrary IQ scores in contemporary practice and referring more to the support that people need in their lives. A learning disability is a lifelong need and a global condition, not to be confused with specific learning difficulties such as dyslexia, or mental health needs that are treatable. Learning disability has been used as the term to describe this client group in the United Kingdom since the 1990s. Internationally, the term 'intellectual disabilities' is used.

DOI: 10.4324/9781003142522-17

It is believed that up to 90% of people with learning disabilities have some form of communication difficulties, with around 50% of people having difficulty with both expressing themselves and understanding what other people say (RCSLT, 2010). This is why communication is an essential consideration for this client group.

People with learning disabilities are a non-homogenous group with an incredibly wide range of diversity in how their learning disabilities present. Some conditions associated with learning disabilities have clear physical characteristics that are easily identifiable, such as for people with Down Syndrome, whilst others may have no clear identifying characteristics at all. The range of communication needs is equally diverse.

For healthcare professionals, working with a patient with learning disabilities can be an intimidating experience, particularly if you are not familiar with supporting people with these needs. If a person is largely communicating through behaviours and you are not familiar with them they may appear unpredictable. They may be frightened and distressed in the healthcare setting which may lead to behaviours that cause disruption to the environment and other patients, and make meeting their healthcare needs more challenging. If you are intimidated then this will likely add to their anxiety, instead of providing them with the reassurances they need to feel safe.

Knowing whether the patient is giving full informed consent to your intervention can also be challenging, and knowing what to do if people are unable to consent can be complicated. This chapter aims to explore these challenges and provide recommendations on how to address these issues.

Clinical relevance

Some people with learning disabilities will not use conventional methods for their expressive communication. They may use Makaton (a simplified form of sign language), picture exchange methods of communication, or other forms of augmentative and alternative communication (see Chapter 13 on autism for more on AAC). Some may have no identified method of expressive communication and rely on their behaviours and actions in order to make their needs and wishes known. Others may have very fluent expressive communication.

Those skilled in expressive communication can often mask difficulties in receptive communication needs. Some may have learnt specific 'cocktail conversational speech' in order to mask a lack of understanding. Not wanting to draw attention to our shortcomings is a feeling we can all probably relate to. Yet this can create challenges in healthcare when it can be hard to ascertain if a patient has understood the information they have been provided with or are simply providing the answers they believe we want to hear.

Additionally, many people with learning disabilities have lifelong impairments around social communication, social interaction, and social imagination (Department of Health, 2010). This can mean that social interactions may appear unusual, and conventional social rules may not be understood or followed. People with learning disabilities may therefore not have an understanding of things like social space, what is public and private, or when others are showing social disapproval. This can make their actions seem strange and occasionally frightening for people who do not know them.

People with learning disabilities experience significant disadvantages in getting their health needs met. The Confidential Enquiry into Premature Deaths in People with Learning Disability (Heslop et al., 2013) found that 38% of deaths of people with learning disability were avoidable. Communication barriers clearly contribute to this where people are unable to understand or express their symptoms or access the health services they need. The Learning Disability Mortality Review (University of Bristol, 2019) also found that people with learning disabilities die 20–30 years younger than the general population. These figures highlight the grave inequalities people with learning disabilities face in having their health needs met.

The Equality Act (2010) places a duty on all public services to make reasonable adjustments for diversity, which includes learning disabilities. Health services must consider access issues for all of their patients, which should include considering for each patient what their access needs are. An example of reasonable adjustments could include producing 'easy read' versions of documents where documents are re-written to be in shorter, plain English language, with pictures to accompany the text. Easy read documents are now more often being referred to as 'easier read' to acknowledge that they will still not be easy for everyone to read and that providing easy read versions of documentation alone may be seen as a tokenistic method of trying to meet accessibility without considering each patient's individual access needs. Reasonable adjustments must be considered on an individual basis.

The Mental Capacity Act (2005, Amended 2019) has been one of the most influential pieces of legislation in England and Wales for contemporary learning disability practice. Scotland similarly has the Adults with Incapacity Act (2000). Northern Ireland also has a Mental Capacity Act (MCA NI, 2016). The focus on this chapter will be on the Mental Capacity Act for England and Wales, although it is believed the underpinning principles are the same.

This act has brought together case law to form legislation detailing the duties we all must follow with regard to obtaining consent from patients. It also lays out duties in assessing someone's ability to consent when there is reason to question this, and steps to take to make decisions in people's best interest when they cannot consent whilst protecting their human rights. It further describes the actions required when people may be deprived of their liberties and rights, to safeguard them from harm and abuse.

This legislation makes it mandatory to present information to people in their preferred method of communication, and to ensure time and effort is given to support people to understand complex decisions so as they can make informed choices.

The term 'diagnostic overshadowing' is used in learning disability support to describe when people's health needs may be overshadowed by their presenting characteristics. For example, if a patient with learning disabilities and autism is repeatedly hitting himself on the cheek with his fist, it may be that this behaviour is accounted to his learning disability or autism and not investigated any further. It may be that the diagnosis of learning disability or autism here is overshadowing an underlying health need, such as dental pain. As health professionals we are often encouraged to be parsimonious in our approach and the simplest answer is usually the right answer. However, we need to acknowledge for many people with learning disabilities that, if they are not able to express what they are feeling, we will not be working with as full a picture as we may be with other patients. Therefore it is important that healthcare practitioners are encouraged to show additional diligence when investigating the health needs of people with learning disabilities to avoid missing significant health needs that their presenting needs may mask.

Communication guidelines

Due to the individuality of need for this client group, it is difficult to provide guidelines that will be universally applicable for all. It should be noted that any guidance given here is advisory and thought will need to be given as to how this relates to each individual you support.

Five Good Communication Standards

The Royal College of speech and language therapists developed Five Good Communication Standards (RCSLT, 2013) for services supporting people with learning disabilities. Although these are primarily aimed at learning disability services they are still worthy of consideration for all services, as they may support people with learning disabilities at some time. The standards are:

- Standard 1: There is a detailed description of how best to communicate with individuals.
- Standard 2: Services demonstrate how they support individuals with communication needs to be involved with decisions about their care and their services.
- Standard 3: Staff value and use competently the best approaches to communication with each individual they support.

- Standard 4: Services create opportunities, relationships, and environments that make individuals want to communicate.
- Standard 5: Individuals are supported to understand and express their needs in relation to their health and well-being.

It is worth considering how these standards apply to your workplace and whether any improvements can be made.

Mental capacity

Everyone should be assumed to have the capacity to consent to a decision, unless there is good reason to question this. Having a learning disability does give healthcare practitioners a reason to question capacity to consent, but diagnosis alone does not prove lack of capacity to consent. We must demonstrate that all practical steps have been attempted to give someone capacity to consent to a decision before it is deemed that they do not have capacity. An unwise decision is not evidence of lacking capacity and people can make what we consider unwise decisions if they wish. It is also important to remember that capacity is decision specific and time specific. A person may have the capacity to make some decisions and not others, and their capacity may change over time.

When making decisions that are in a person's best interest we must ensure that those decisions are firmly in the person's best interest and not being made to serve the interests of others. We must also consider what is the least restrictive and least aversive way we can provide this intervention and be person centred in our approach.

The person who is responsible for deciding whether someone has capacity is the person undertaking the procedure. When considering capacity and best interest decisions it is important to involve people who know the person well, such as their family and those who support them regularly. It may also be beneficial to consult experts in learning disabilities, such as Learning Disability Nurses.

In order to determine capacity you will need to consider four questions:

- Can the person understand the information given to them about the decision, when given all practical steps to do so?
- Are they able to retain that information long enough to make a decision?
- Are they able to weigh up the pros and cons of deciding for or against the decision as part of the decision making process?
- Are they able to communicate their decision, utilising their preferred method of communication?

Some people with learning disabilities may have a family member that has applied for deputyship through the Court of Protection. This can give them powers to consent on behalf of their loved one. Evidence of these court orders needs to be seen as without the court order no one can consent on behalf of another adult.

Case study 12.1

'Charles' is 26 and has severe learning disabilities and autism. He communicates with behaviours rather than words, and has made up some of his own Makaton signs that those who support him understand.

Charles' support team had noticed that he had begun banging his head against the wall more than usual recently. Self-injurious behaviours like this were common for Charles, but his support knew there was something different about how he was doing it this time. They began giving Charles pain relief and called the Community Learning Disability Team for support. With pain relief the behaviours immediately reduced.

The Learning Disability Nurse visited and thought it might be something to do with his teeth. A dentist from the hospital Maxillofacial Unit agreed to visit him at his home, as it was explained to her that due to his learning disabilities he would find the hospital frightening.

The dentist confirmed that Charles had cavities and needed to have dentistry that would involve drilling and filling these cavities, and possibly may need an extraction. The dentist found that Charles could not consent, so held a best interest meeting with his parents and his support team. It was agreed that the work was essential and in his best interest. It was also acknowledged that he will find the experience distressing so it would need to be done under sedation. The remaining challenge was planning how to help Charles go to hospital without being distressed.

Charles was given the first appointment of the day. His team had two weeks to prepare. The team gradually changed the time Charles got out of bed in the morning, so getting up early for this appointment would not be a surprise. They took him for daily visits to the hospital where they would go up to the ward, have a seat where he would be waiting before his appointment, and then had a cup of coffee in the hospital cafe. This all helped Charles be familiar with the hospital environment and routine. He was also prescribed diazepam to take on the morning of his procedure as a pre-med to reduce his anxieties on the day and support the general anaesthetic to be effective.

On the day of the procedure Charles was up ready to go for the procedure, went to the hospital in a relaxed state, and went straight into the treatment room with no concerns. He was sedated for his procedure and discharged back to the care of his support team the same day.

General communication advice for people with learning disabilities

Address anxieties

Attending a healthcare appointment can cause anxieties for most of us. This can be heightened if you have a learning disability. People may have limited understanding about what the appointment is for. The environment may be confusing and frightening for them. They may lack social skills related to waiting. Increased anxiety will result in reduced communication.

Plan beforehand what can be done to reduce these anxieties. Discuss what will help with the person, their family, or those who support them. There may be some simple practical things that can be done, such as making their appointment first thing so as there isn't any waiting, or ensuring they have a safe place to go to if they are feeling overwhelmed.

Review how communicative your environment is

The best kind of environments are those that speak for themselves. Visual prompts, structure, predictability, and routine can help environments tell you where you are and what you need to do without the need for human interaction. Consider the layout of your environment, how easy it is to find the area you will be seeing the person in, how engaging and welcoming the environment is, and how predictable it is to understand what is happening before your interaction and whether there is anything more that can be done to meet the needs of this person.

Can you reduce distractions in the environment?

People with learning disabilities may struggle to process lots of different information at the same time. If you are trying to communicate with them and there is a radio on in the background, children playing loudly in the room next door, flickering lights, activity going on outside the window, air conditioning humming, then all of these things will reduce the person's ability to focus on what you are saying and effectively communicate with you.

Avoid assuming that people cannot understand

Having a learning disability and/or a lack of expressive communication does not automatically mean that someone does not understand you. Direct your communication directly to the person wherever possible and avoid asking questions to those supporting them on their behalf, unless this has been agreed in advance.

Use plain English

Ensure that your communication is as simple as possible. Try avoiding jargon, metaphors, or phrases that they may not understand. Phrases like 'pull yourself together' could be taken literally, and sarcasm or subtleties may be missed.

Support communication visually

Understanding spoken language is a highly complex skill we develop and many people with learning disabilities struggle with the reception and interpretation of the spoken word. Where possible, support spoken communication with visual prompts. This can include gestures, objects, pictures, or drawings, or anything else that you have that visually gives context to what you are saying.

Remember to also give people time to process information before they answer you. If someone has to interpret each word you say and connect the words together to figure out what you are saying it may take them longer to reply. Interrupting and rephrasing the question may mean that the person then has to begin the interpretation process again from the start, further delaying their response.

Case study 12.2

Charlotte is a young woman with moderate learning disabilities. She has verbal speech, but she is aware that she has difficulties and desperately doesn't want to show others that she finds understanding things difficult. she will therefore try and give you answers that she thinks you want to hear. Charlotte often uses strategies like choosing the last option you give to her, saying 'yes' if she has not understood, and picking up cues from others for what she thinks you want her to say.

Charlotte has been living in residential care for the last four years and it was felt that her needs would be better met and she would be more independent if she lived in her own tenancy. It was felt that Charlotte could have capacity to make some decisions about moving on, but it was acknowledged that discussing this verbally would not work for her.

A speech and language therapist from the Community Learning Disability Team became involved and introduced to the team a 'Talking Mat'. This is a mat like you would have in a doorway. Three pictures were put at the top of the mat that indicated 'yes', 'no', and 'maybe'. Charlotte was then presented a variety of pictures to sort under these headings to find out what was important to her.

Within the pictures there were also some that tested for 'double negatives'. For example there was a picture for 'living by myself' and a picture for 'living with others'. If Charlotte put both of these pictures under 'yes' it would indicate she is not understanding the process and is giving answers based on what she thinks we want to hear.

Listen to people who know the person well

Those who spend most time with the person build up a tacit knowledge of them, where they are able to pick up on the smallest changes to their presentation or slightest signs that something isn't right. Being told by a health professional that there is nothing wrong could go two ways: either you will allay fears and concerns they have; or you will make them feel like they aren't being heard.

Remember to be mindful of diagnostic overshadowing, and if those who know the person well think that something is not right then there is probably something not right so ensure you have taken the time to fully listen to concerns and ensure all assessments have been conducted diligently to give you full confidence that you have not missed something.

Those who know the person well can often act as a communication partner for people with learning disabilities, so use their knowledge and expertise of the person to identify how you should best communicate with the person or how they can facilitate you to effectively communicate with them.

Pause regularly to check understanding

Regular pauses help to chunk the information the person is receiving so helps with their processing. When checking understanding avoid closed questions. Asking 'do you understand?' will undoubtedly result in the answer being 'yes' regardless of whether they have understood or not. We also need to be aware of acquiescent responses where people may try to give us the answer they think will make us happy.

Avoid closed questions. Try instead asking 'can you repeat back to me what I have said?' Or ask questions to provoke more of a conversational response to gauge understanding, like 'what do you think about that?'. If you present an option of two it is worth repeating the question and switching the order of the options to ensure the person isn't simply repeating the last word you said.

Consider having a communication champion on your team

A communication champion could have additional training in communication methods, like Makaton. They could audit how communicative the environment is. The role could also be responsible for ensuring anyone with communication needs that you encounter has a communication passport and that this is clearly alerted to when they have an appointment.

Liaise with local learning disability services for support

Each area will have a community learning disability team, and some hospitals have learning disability liaison nurses. Familiarise yourself with what NHS learning disability services there are in your area, and approach them if you need support.

Top 5 Clinical Practice Recommendations

1. Check how communicative the environment is
2. Consider what reasonable adjustments each person needs, such as time or accessible information
3. Always speak directly to the person, unless it has been agreed otherwise
4. Ask the person to tell you what you have said to check their understanding

Cultural implications

Learning disabilities can affect people of different cultures the same. Some conditions are more prevalent in certain cultures, for example Tay-Sachs disease generally affects people of Jewish descent. It is important to be mindful of peoples diversity needs when working with diverse cultures, as this can often lead to people with learning disabilities facing double discrimination (Fulton & Richardson, 2010).

Some cultures may see a learning disability as a spiritual punishment for something wrong they have done, or may see it as something to be ashamed of. It is not unusual for non-British cultures to have beliefs that they should care for each other internally, and this may lead to reluctance to let in professionals.

If the person with learning disabilities you are supporting is from another culture then English may not be their first language and this may make their learning disabilities appear more significant than they are. It may be that they need a translator, and it is not uncommon for family members to act in a translator role, although this may be unethical at times and there may be issues to consider with this whether the person's voice is being truly independently given.

Summary

People with learning disabilities are an integral part of all of our communities, and it is very likely that at some point a person with learning disabilities will use your healthcare setting.

Communication needs for people with learning disabilities can be complex. However, by taking time to prepare and involving the person and those who know them well, plans can be made to overcome communication challenges and involve people in meeting their healthcare needs. There are also learning disability services that can support you if needed.

As people with learning disabilities face significant health inequalities it is important to make reasonable adjustments to ensure people with learning disabilities can access your services. This will also ensure your services are compliant with the Equality Act.

Recommended reading

1. CHANGE (2010) How to make information accessible: a guide to producing easy read documents. Leeds, CHANGE.
2. Coakes, L. (2004) *It's My Book: Creating ownership of a communication passport* (first published in *Communication Matters Journal*, 18, number 1 (2004)). Available from: www.communicationpassports.org.uk/Resources/Passport-Articles/
3. Grove, N. (2000) See what I mean (SWIM) Guidelines to aid understanding of communication by people with severe and profound learning disabilities. BILD Publications. Kidderminster
4. Matthews, A. *Communication Dictionaries and Communication Passports.* Available from: www.communicationpassports.org.uk/Resources/Passport-Articles/
5. Millar, S., & Caldwell, M. (1997) *Personal Communication Passports.* Paper presented at the SENSE Conference, Westpark Centre, University of Dundee, 13 September 1997. Available from: www.communicationpassports.org.uk/Resources/Passport-Articles/
6. Millar, S. (2006) *Auditing passports.* Available from: www.communicationpassports.org.uk/Resources/Good-Practice/
7. NHS Leicestershire Health Informatics Service (2013) *If You listen you will hear us, Guidelines on involving people with profound and multiple learning disabilities.* Available from: www.leicspart.nhs.uk/InformationLibrary-Easyreadinformation.aspx
8. The experience of aphasia following a stroke often begins with the individual waking suddenly in a hospital bed unaware of what has happened to bring them there. The individual with aphasia recognises family and caregivers, but doesn't understand what is being said to them. The individual becomes upset and frightened because they know what they want to say, but each time to they try to speak the words come out wrong (Simmons-Mackie, 2018).

References

Department of Health (2010). *Fulfilling and rewarding lives: the strategy for adults with autism in England.* London: Department of Health.

Equality Act (2010). London: HMSO.

Fulton, R., & Richardson, K. (2010). *Towards race equality in advocacy services: people with learning disabilities from black and minority ethnic communities.* London: Race Equality Foundation.

Heslop, P., et al. (2013). *CIPOLD The Confidential Inquiry into premature deaths of people with learning disabilities.* Bristol: Norah Fry Research Centre, University of Bristol.

Mental Capacity Act (2005, amended 2019). London: HMSO.

RCSLT. (2010). *Adults with learning disabilities: position paper.* London: Royal College of Speech and Language Therapists.

RCSLT (2013) *Five Good Communication Standards: Reasonable adjustments to communication that individuals with learning disability and/or autism should expect in specialist hospital and residential settings.* London: Royal College of Speech and Language Therapists.

University of Bristol (2019). *Learning disability mortality review programme: annual report 2019.* Bristol: University of Bristol.

13

Communication with autistic adults

Alison Drewett and Samuel Tromans

Chapter contents:

- Clinical relevance
- The Unite study: autistic inpatients and staff interaction in mental health
- An investigation of autism prevalence in adults admitted to acute mental health wards: a cross-sectional study
- Communication guidelines
- Clinical practice recommendations
- Key resources
- References

Introduction

This chapter will discuss principles to facilitate effective communication with autistic adults, with reference to two research studies involving this patient group, both conducted within adult mental health settings. The purpose of presenting the two research studies, each from a different research paradigm, one qualitative and one quantitative, is to offer principles grounded in research findings and researcher reflections. Each study takes a distinct methodological approach, reflecting the diversity of autism research, but both nonetheless present recommendations relevant to clinical practice. Following a general introduction to autism and communication, the studies are discussed in turn with subsequent presentation of communication guidelines.

Clinical relevance

Communication difficulties are central to both how autism is conceptualised, and how autistic people are perceived by healthcare professionals.

DOI: 10.4324/9781003142522-18

Communication challenges are traditionally understood to be the result of difficulties residing in the individual. However, more recently, the role of communication partners is understood to be key to effective communication, and rather than problems being perceived to be living within the autistic person, they are viewed as located within the interaction itself. It is important for staff to be aware of this and to be able to reflect on their role in facilitating effective communication in clinical care.

Autism is defined as a neurodevelopmental condition, characterised by persistent difficulties in social communication and interaction, as well as a repertoire of restricted, repetitive patterns of behaviour, interests, or activities. Symptoms should be present during the early developmental period and have a substantial impact on functioning (American Psychiatric Association, 2013).

Autistic people[1] represent a highly heterogeneous group, with the manner in which their autistic features manifest, and the severity of functional impairment varying widely. For example, social communication covers a broad range of potential difficulties, including pragmatics or language use, emotional understanding, and non-verbal expression. As such, autism encompasses diverse communication features, ranging from individuals who are completely non-verbal to verbal, reticent to talk or overly formal to verbose, and socially isolated with no or few friends to engaging in frequent social interactions (Brugha, 2018).

Others view autistic communication as a reflection of diversity rather than representing a disorder or abnormality (Woods et al., 2018). Such authors regard the categorisation of these differences as evidence of atypicality rather than impairment or deficit although significantly this also evokes binary ways of viewing autistic and non-autistic persons. The theory underlying this perspective is that firstly autistic individuals have sometimes been inappropriately measured against neurotypical norms, and secondly that some scholars have failed to recognise communication as an interactional achievement rather than a reflection of a specific individual's competencies (Wilkinson, 2019).

On the first point, Milton (2017) argues that there is a double-empathy problem, whereby neurotypical persons are equally unable to empathise or understand autism and autistic communication, rather than lack of empathy solely being the preserve of autistic persons. Crompton et al (2020) provide evidence for this phenomenon in their empirical research, showing that autistic matched pairs are able to create rapport and exchange information as effectively as their neurotypical matched pair peers, with the poorest performing pair being the mixed neurotypical and autistic pairs.

On the latter point, Wilkinson (2019) argues that interactions between typical and atypical communicators are not 'normal', not just because of deficits in the impaired individual alone but also because staff make adaptations to their communication to address the perceived impairment of the atypical communicator. For healthcare staff, this raises the need for them to recognise the part they play in challenges pertaining to social communication. As neurotypical communication partners in the main, staff play a central role in how meaningful or natural interactions are with autistic patients (Cummins, Pellicano, & Crane, 2020). It is not competent communicator (staff) meets incompetent communicator (patient), but rather a mix of differences in communication approaches and resultant adaptations that lead to challenges with communication.

The Unite study: autistic inpatients and staff interaction in mental health

The Unite research study is a video-reflexive ethnography (VRE) study of staff and autistic inpatient communication in mental health (Iedema, 2018; Drewett, 2021).[2] In particular, it examines interaction between staff and autistic individuals during routine ward rounds to investigate talk as it happens during the real-world scenario of meetings set up to discuss the care management of patients.

By profession, author one is a speech and language therapist with previous experience of working in an inpatient mental health setting. As a practitioner on the wards, she noticed the additional communicative and psychological demands being placed on autistic people by being present in their ward rounds. There appeared to be a tension between the laudable principles of shared or supported decision making, patient involvement and person-centredness, and the challenges felt by autistic people of participation in such events. The Unite study enabled the thorny problem to be explored by shining a light on hitherto tacit practices that constitute the machinery of the ward round, and to hear from autistic people themselves as well as staff their perceptions of what is good and bad about communication in these environments.

The research took a VRE approach to exploit its theoretical underpinnings as well as its advances in methods (Iedema et al., 2018). As a methodology, it combines a view of practices as inherently embodying, and being embodied by, the tacit understandings of participants. These hidden or unconscious expectations, ways of doing and meaning-making can be revealed to the participants and the researcher–clinician by videoing everyday events, and then allowing reflective spaces to collaboratively look at and talk about what is going on either in interviews or focus groups. In short, the VRE approach places a central value on starting with work-as-done, for example via the video-recordings of naturalistic occasions, rather than work-as-imagined, such as the perceptions of how people do things that are remembered or reported in interviews. However, in VRE, interviews are key to *subsequently* explore the video-data in order to facilitate reflective practice and foster quality improvement in clinical practices among staff.

This sequencing in the research design (video and then interviews) is also underpinned by a foundational principle in VRE called exnovation. Exnovation refers to the competencies of participants themselves to identify and find solutions to challenges, rather than a reliance on more external measures. This epistemological position underpins the value placed on the interview as reflexive and collaborative, fully exploiting the skills of both the researcher–clinician, and the participants as experts. In this case, both staff and autistic individuals are valued as equally able to recognise and unravel how to address communication barriers. Furthermore, they are also able to highlight good practices and ascertain the reasons why these are either positive or negative.

The sequencing of the different stages of the research is also important. The research sits broadly within a qualitative paradigm but there are also key VRE considerations with regard to the sequencing of the methods. In the Unite study, there are three key phases: video-recordings of the ward rounds, interview with the patient concerned, and finally an interview with two of the individual's corresponding staff members. Briefly, the reasons for this sequencing were to maintain an emphasis on the work-as-done (the video of the actual ward round communication), and to keep the focus on patient-identified communication barriers/facilitators for the purposes of later discussion in the staff interview. In this way, the events of the specific ward round (as well as more generic experiences) are the focus of patient interview so that the autistic person has the opportunity to discuss communication in a concrete way. Thus, the event and the patient's perceptions of the event detailed via the interview are paramount; they are the focus of the staff interview and provide staff with an opportunity to reflect with the clinical-researcher about their perspectives on their patients views and experiences of ward rounds and hospital generally.

There are notable benefits of this methodological approach in relation to autistic people's involvement in research and the topic of communication challenges. Firstly, it means that real-talk is at the heart of the research rather than people's perceptions about how autistic people communicate. Secondly, it means that the spotlight is on how autistic people talk in interactions with (in this case) healthcare professionals rather than viewing communication in an individualist way as a set of competencies or deficiencies that a person has or does not have. Thirdly, autistic people have a more equal voice to establish for themselves what works or does not work in the communication, rather than having a pre-prescribed set of clinician-identified criteria for what constitutes an example of successful communication. In the past, there have been many studies that have imposed this kind of external criteria on communication events to determine their merit. In Unite, not only do autistic people determine for themselves what is important, they also rate what they experience in a way that is meaningful for them. Finally, there are specific ways in which the methodology can mitigate some of the perceived difficulties of autistic communication, which will now be examined.

The video-recordings are in one sense a concrete representation of the ward round. Autistic people are often viewed as visual leaners and indeed this has been accepted as widespread by autistic people themselves

(Grandin & Johnson, 2005). It can be a challenge to talk about communication in a meta-theoretical way for anyone, not just autistic participants, as communication is such an ingrained/unconscious way of behaving, and language-wise can be seen as involving abstract ideas like understanding, processing, expressing ideas, and so on. Again, autistic people are viewed as finding concrete concepts easier to express and understand. Clinically, ideas about how difficult autistic people find non-literal language is viewed as related to fixed thinking, problems in generalisation and even theory of mind; all of which it is important to say have been critiqued as too reductionist and neuro-biologically oriented. However, without reference to aetiological arguments about this presentation, for the purposes of research, having a concrete reference point for the research, that is, being able to show excerpts of the video-recordings gave a very clear focus for the interview discussions. It transformed often vague and theoretical notions about communication into more tangible and material phenomena of interest.

Furthermore, video-recordings of routine events are examples of naturalistic data that place no additional demands on the autistic person (Kiyimba, Lester, & O'Reilly, 2018). In contrast to interviews, naturalistic data collection does not require the person to do anything more than they would have done anyway because the ward rounds take place regardless of the research (other than giving consent). In this sense, there are no additional burdens that may cause harm. In order to mitigate the potential harms of the subsequent interviews and to ensure that they generated maximum opportunity for involvement, a participatory approach was adopted by the researcher. For example, participants were able to do the interviews in two shorter half-hour time-periods. They could also opt (as two participants did) to use an augmentative and alternative communication aid called Talking Mats as a visual support (Murphy et al., 2004). These adaptations to the way the interview was conducted allowed autistic people to be involved in research that otherwise may have seemed overwhelming and inaccessible due to their communication difficulties. These adaptations are also critical reminders for healthcare staff generally of the importance of making reasonable adjustments to support someone's ability to focus for longer periods of time, to be able to discuss more abstract topics, to help retention of information in the here and now, and to help evidence a patient's thinking. Total communication approaches that value a variety of means of communication systems, such as signing, picture, photographs, symbols, and easy-read are a key environmental way to embrace diversity in the speech, language, and communication needs of individuals (Royal College of speech and language therapists, 2016).

Trouble in ward rounds

Six autistic adults with additional mental health needs have thus far participated in the UNITE study. This includes video-recordings of six ward rounds, follow-up interviews with all of the autistic participants (n = 6) and two members of their staff (n = 12). Two of the interviews with autistic individuals were facilitated by Talking Mats, and two also opted for 2x30 minute interviews. I shall demonstrate some reflections on communication guidance with reference to a single case study from this research. This is mainly interview data analysis rather than the video-data at this stage.

Case study 13.1 Sue

Sue, a pseudonym, is an autistic woman with an additional hearing impairment, who has achieved highly in education. She has had several inpatient admissions due to depressive episodes, which led to self-neglect and suicidal ideation. In the interview following the ward round, I asked her about (what I called) 'critical communication events' in the ward round; examples of communication that she found difficult. Excerpt one from the video-recording of the ward round is the event she referenced as a communication problem. Excerpt two is taken from Sue's interview where she talks about the doctor's opener.

Excerpt 1 from the ward round: How are we doing?
11: Psychiatrist: How are **we** doing?
12: Sue: Okay
13: Psychiatrist: What would you like **us** to discuss today?
14: Sue: Don't really know

Excerpt 2 from the interview: It drives me barmy

'He always says what do you want us to talk about. Like the fricking weather. I want to talk about my dogs ... and my animals ... *It drives me barmy* because one of the things I struggle with is to initiate conversation. If you ask me questions, I'll happily rabble on ... but to be the person that leads that communication ... it is well tricky. I'd like him to lead and just go from there. (Lines 16–23)

Sue told me that she disliked the psychiatrist's opener; not because she did not recognise the phrases as orienting her to talk about her (mental) health but because she does not like open-ended questions at the start of the interview because it means that she has to take the lead and she finds initiating very hard. The outcome is negative for her mental health (as the phrase in bold indicates). This difficulty in starting off talk or initiating is very common for autistic people. Significantly, even though it looks like the staff member is initiating the interaction, in reality because the onus is being placed on the patient to decide the topic direction, this is *felt by the patient to involve* patient initiation. Sue was also irked by the use of first person plural pronouns (we and us) because he did not really mean that is was a shared view but that he really wanted her to talk about her issues. This pronoun usage can be used by the speaker to soften the communicative demand on the recipient to talk, and it can also be used as a way of the speaker signalling that they are sharing in the responsibility for the talk. In this way, healthcare staff may use *we* instead of *you* to indicate that they are involving the person and being person-centred by asking the person to set the agenda for the ward round talk. However, for the autistic listener, in this case Sue, who by her own account has a tendency towards being literal, the question does not make sense. Sue would prefer to answer direct questions that are aimed at her.

In Sue's interview she also spoke about how her autism and hearing impairment interact to cause communication difficulties that are actually additionally interactionally produced because of organisational and staff practices. These aspects are important to raise here because although they relate to the setting or the context of the talk, they do highlight how communication difficulties are interactionally produced; rather than seeing autistic communication as impaired within the individual it is clear from these example how staff and patient are together (re)producing communication barriers. For example, Sue reports that she relies on watching people's faces to lip read and that this is hard for her because she finds eye contact difficult; on the face of it a demonstration of individual deficit. However, staff do not take these needs into consideration; they cover their mouths when they speak, look away, and look down at computer screens for electronic patient information during ward rounds even when they are talking to her. She also reported that she had never had a deaf interpreter made available to her despite this being identified as a need when she was admitted.

Excerpt 3: I have to be able to look at people

I find it very hard to look at people and to make eye contact and stuff …

It's quite difficult.

But I have to do it because I have to be able to lip read. So that's always uncomfortable.

Excerpt 4: I can't read their faces at all

It can feel a bit them and us and I get stressed by it...they all sit behind computers. I think it's more helpful to talk and listen than to tap away on a computer … I can't read their faces at all … We did ask for sign language support for meeting each week … but they never turned up … which is why I have to ask people to repeat stuff … that then makes my mum and dad think I've got short-term memory loss.

Sue, like many (autistic) people, enjoys to spend time on her own, and as an inpatient this means time in her own room. Sue did have a sign on her bedroom door indicating that she was hearing impaired but this had been lost during one of her four ward transitions. She has missed mealtimes because although she needs prompts to know these things are happening, staff just knock on the door which she cannot hear. The impact of this communication error is critical, because she has diabetes and needs regular meals to maintain her blood sugar levels. She has also missed activities because of this reliance on door knocking too. It is quite usual for autistic people to dislike being touched and have a sensitivity to this but Sue depends on touch for communication. She states that despite informing staff that they should give her a physical prompt (touch) rather than an audible one (knocking) so that she knows what is happening, this is not done by staff. She believes that staff assume that she does not like to be touched because she is autistic.

More generally, Sue also spoke about her communication experiences with healthcare staff. First, she expressed the view that staff expressed mixed messages to her. For example, some staff said to her that she was ready for discharge and others said that she was not ready, and she found this upsetting as she does not manage uncertainty well. Secondly, she reported that important decisions about her care were not relayed to her appropriately, for example, she was given information via ad hoc conversations rather than formally recorded situations (which she prefers). Finally, she stated that because of her deafness and her social communication difficulties, she often needed to ask for verbal information, jokes, sarcasm, and inferential language to be repeated. She felt that staff made the incorrect assumption that she is simple because of this, and this acted as a barrier to her asking for information to be clarified, ultimately leading to her reduced participation in conversations.

This chapter will now discuss a second study, to examine communication principles arising out of an example of quantitative research into autism.

An investigation of autism prevalence in adults admitted to acute mental health wards: a cross-sectional study

Details of study

This study was designed to investigate autism prevalence among adults admitted to acute psychiatric hospital wards, as very little is known about autism prevalence within this vulnerable patient group with complex healthcare needs (Tromans, et al, 2018). Furthermore, previously validated instruments were used to measure rates of co-occurring physical and mental health conditions in the study population (McManus et al., 2016), to compare the prevalence of such conditions among persons meeting diagnostic criteria for autism relative to their non-autistic peers. Study recruitment commenced on 6th March 2019, with the study end date on 30th June 2021.[3]

The study consisted of two phases for adults without intellectual disability. In the first phase, adult participants completed several autism questionnaires, including the 50-item version of the Autism Quotient (AQ-50) (Baron-Cohen et al., 2001), with their corresponding informant[4] also completing autism questionnaires relating to the participant. The AQ-50 score determined the probability of participants being invited into the Phase 2 of the study, which consisted of an autism diagnostic assessment. All participants with intellectual disability[5] bypassed the first phase of the study, progressing directly to the second phase. This is because of the lack of validated autism questionnaires for this patient group, as well as the heightened autism prevalence relative to their peers without intellectual disability.

Phase 2 participant assessment involved both version 2 of the Autism Diagnostic Observation Schedule (Lord et al., 2012) and the autism interview section of version 3 of the Schedules for Clinical Assessment in Neuropsychiatry (World Health Organization, 2023). Informant assessment included a participant neurodevelopmental history, involving the Diagnostic Interview for Social and Communication Disorders (Wing et al., 2002). Autistic cases were determined according to ICD-10-DCR (World Health Organization, 1993) and/or DSM-5 (American Psychiatric Association, 2013) diagnostic criteria for autism.

Figure 13.1 shows a flow chart, summarising the study design (Tromans, 2021). A more detailed protocol for the study is available online (Tromans et al., 2019).

ID denotes intellectual disability, whereas non-ID denotes participants without intellectual disability.

The Phase 2 study population comprised of adults without intellectual disability, selected based on their AQ-50 score (participants with higher scores having an increased probability of selection), as well as all adult participants with intellectual disability. The corresponding informants for all participants were additionally invited back to participate in Phase 2, primarily to provide an in-depth neurodevelopmental history for the participant.

At the time of writing, data collection for the study has recently completed, with the prevalence findings set to be submitted for publication in a peer-reviewed journal. However, based on the experience of undertaking the study, related communication guidelines are discussed in the following section.

Communication issues relevant to the study

While the majority of the study population did not have a pre-existing diagnosis of autism, it was nevertheless important to work on the basis that any participant *could* be autistic. Thus, it was essential that in every stage of the

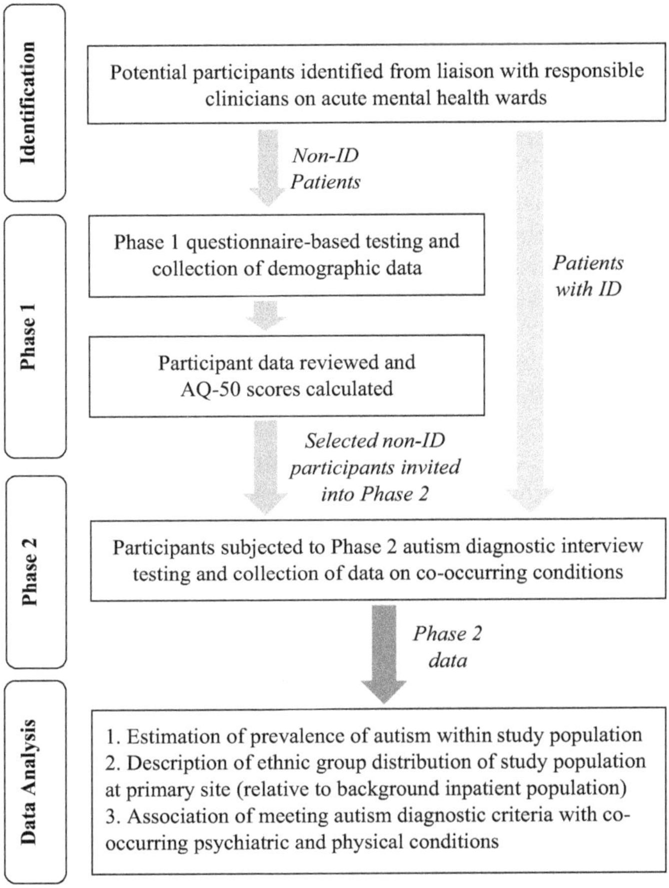

Figure 13.1 Flow chart summary design for study (Tromans, 2021)

study, including the development of study information forms, the consenting process, and all of the resulting study assessments, that the language used was clear, unambiguous, and accessible, avoiding idioms, proverbs, and vague terminology, which are open to misinterpretation, particularly by autistic persons. Involvement of autistic persons at the design stage of the study, including asking them to review study materials in patient and public involvement sessions, was invaluable in identifying issues to be corrected prior to study recruitment. It is also important to check the participant's understanding at regular intervals in the study process, and giving them time to process pertinent information. Such an approach is equally relevant when communicating with autistic persons in other contexts, for example as a healthcare professional, or as a friend or acquaintance of an autistic person.

When working with adults who have been admitted to acute psychiatric hospital wards, it is important to recognise that almost all individuals within this group will have significant psychiatric morbidity. For both autistic and non-autistic individuals, many are likely to have mental health conditions that also affect their communication with others, such as psychotic, mood, and anxiety disorders. Such conditions can also affect observations/ratings on autism diagnostic assessment. For example, a depressed person may demonstrate poor eye contact related to their depression, but there is a risk of this being attributed to autism. Taking a detailed neurodevelopmental history from the study participant as well as their informant can help in determining whether such features are longstanding, and thus potentially a manifestation of autism, or more likely attributable to a deterioration in mental health. In clinical practice, a thorough neurodevelopmental history takes time, but is invaluable in gaining a longitudinal understanding of a persons functioning, development, and symptomatology.

Liaison with healthcare professionals supporting the patient can provide insight as to whether it is appropriate to approach them regarding study participation at a particular time. In some instances, for example where a patient has florid psychotic symptoms, it may be inappropriate for them to take part in the study at that time, though it may be reasonable to approach them at a later point, where such symptoms have partially or fully remitted following treatment. Timing is similarly important with respect to clinical interactions, but particularly so with autistic persons, who may be very routine-based, where an unexpected interruption of their daily routine may cause significant distress.

Furthermore, one should recognise that the tools use to assess for presence of autistic features, such as the AQ-50, can yield different findings depending on the participant's cultural background (Carruthers et al., 2018). Indeed, cultural biases existing both within diagnostic tools as well as among healthcare professionals, may have contributed to a trend of reduced autism identification rates in minority ethnic groups (Tromans et al., 2020). Equally, as healthcare professionals, cultural biases can affect judgements as to whether an individual is autistic (Begeer et al., 2009); this can be reduced by engaging with persons from other cultures and enhancing one's understanding of the cultural norms.

It is important to verbally check during the study participation process that the participant is happy to continue taking part. The facial expression of autistic people are more likely to be atypical in appearance relative to their non-autistic peers (Trevisan, Hoskyn, & Birmingham, 2018), and thus it may be less clear when they are feeling uncomfortable or anxious based on visual observation alone.

When the study was resumed in late September 2020, in the midst of the COVID-19 pandemic, changes to the study procedures were made in order to comply with COVID-19 guidance. The change most likely to have impacted on communication was the wearing of personal protective equipment, including face masks. This would have made it more challenging for the participant to read the emotional expression of the interviewer, in addition to potentially muffling the speech of the wearer, impacting on the intelligibility of verbal communication.

Flexibility with the assessment venue is important, as autistic participants may find certain settings, such as acute psychiatric wards, stressful and over-stimulating from a sensory perspective. It is important to discuss with the participant what setting they would feel most comfortable in, and accommodate such requests wherever possible. When the study resumed in September 2020, COVID-19 related restrictions meant that interviews could not take place in clinical settings, unless the participant was still an inpatient at the time of their interview.[6] This placed limitations on where interviews could take place (prior to the pandemic, all participants were given the option of their interviews taking place in a clinical, university, or home setting). However, wherever possible the research interviews, should take place at a time and place where the autistic person feels comfortable and relaxed, as this is likely to be most conducive to effective communication and a positive participant/patient experience.

Communication guidelines

Research has long documented problematic staff and patient interactions, especially involving people with intellectual disabilities and autism (two groups that are still commonly categorised together). For example, in comparisons of video recordings of real-life interactions against staff reports of the same events, Bradshaw (2001) found that staff underestimate how much they use verbal communication and overestimate their own use of non-verbal communication in their communication with this group. She also found that there was a mismatch between clients' self-reported level of understanding and the complexity of language employed by staff: 45% of expressed language was beyond the client's receptive communication competency. Thus, staff reports of clients' speech, language and communication skills disguise difficulties and overstate competencies.

Currently, there are practical books available providing advice about how people can best communicate with autistic individuals, such as that by Gaynor, Alevizos, and Butler (2020). Milton et al. (2016) and Milton and Mills (2018) have also written and spoken on this subject with specific reference to mental health settings and behaviour that challenges services. The authors underline the importance of an individual approach that recognises autistic heterogeneity, and calls for non-autistic persons to reflect and recognise that their own ideas about best practice are not necessarily ideal for the autistic communication partner, and the need for staff to engage in conscious planning of ways to address differences. Such strategies range from considerations about language use, the timing, pace and place of conversations, and minimising difficult sensory stimuli, such as unpredictable noises and bright lights.

Thus, a key recommendation for any staff member is to develop communication care plans for individuals that are person-centred, acknowledging the individuality of autistic persons. The key to ensuring good communication is consistency of approach, and this is more achievable with a written plan in operation that is shared with staff and reviewed regularly. While one person may be able to manage a small group consultation with people they are familiar with if there is enough notice and the appointment is punctual, another may need the appointment to be one to one, in a certain place and with a key worker that they know very well. Some may manage verbal communication whilst others may require visual supports and longer appointment times.

Nicolaidis et al. (2015) refer to these kinds of recommendations as provider-level changes, as they are able to be implemented by front-line staff in their everyday clinical interactions. However, system-level changes are also needed, including tackling stigma and accessibility of clinical services. In this respect, the language we use to conceptualise autism outside of our direct interactions also needs to be both respectful and empathic.

Clinical practice recommendations

Based on the two studies discussed within this chapter, several recommendations relevant to communicating with autistic adults in the context of clinical practice can be made.

1. Be aware of total communication approaches that recognise the value of using a range of different means of communication to enhance understanding and facilitate expression (e.g., signing systems, easy-read information, visual methods such as photos, drawings, symbols, objects of reference, and writing).
2. It may be hard for staff to give sensitive information without using hedges and softening filler-talk. However, this lengthens utterances and makes them harder to understand as key information is lost within complex construction. Keep language simple: clarity in explanation is not received by the autistic listener as speaker rudeness.
3. Consider carefully how information is collected and especially how questions are asked. Open questions may be stressful for autistic people to answer. Use more direct questions that build on knowledge already known about the person.
4. Be mindful that autistic adults are a very heterogeneous group, and be sensitive to individual differences within this group rather than applying a single approach to communication with all autistic people.

5. Involve autistic persons in the development of any research study involving them, including its design, constituent assessments, and any participant-facing documentation. This can help ensure the study is accessible to autistic persons, as well as participant-facing documents effectively communicating the details pertaining to the study.

Summary

This chapter has provided guidance for how to effectively communicate with autistic adults, with reference to two related research studies conducted within adult mental healthcare settings. Principles of effective communication with autistic adults often transcend context, and thus there is a great deal that can be learnt from a clinical research setting that is similarly relevant to clinical practice.

However, whilst some principles outlined in this chapter will facilitate more effective communication with the majority of autistic adults, it is important to recognise that autistic people represent a heterogeneous group, who frequently have co-occurring mental health conditions, as well as sensory differences. Recognising such individual differences is essential, along with developing approaches tailored to the specific needs of the patient concerned, rather than adopting a 'one-size-fits-all' philosophy.

Key resources

1. Brugha, T. S. (2018). *The psychiatry of adult autism and Asperger syndrome: A practical guide.* Oxford: Oxford University Press.
2. Lord, C., Brugha, T. S., Charman, T., Cusack, J., Dumas, G., Frazier, T et al. (2020). Autism spectrum disorder. *Nature Reviews Disease Primers, 6*(1), 1–23.
3. Nicolaidis, C., Raymaker, D., Kapp, S. K., Baggs, A., Ashkenazy, E., McDonald, K., et al. (2019). The AASPIRE practice-based guidelines for the inclusion of autistic adults in research as co-researchers and study participants. *Autism, 23*(8), 2007–2019.
4. Gaynor, Z., Alevizos, K., & Butler, J. (2020). *Is that clear? Effective communication in a neuro-diverse world: autism inspired tips for allistic (non-autistic) people.* Oxford: Prepare to Publish Ltd.
5. Milton, D. (2017). *A mismatch of salience: Explorations of the nature of autism from theory to practice.* Hove: Pavilion Publishing.

Notes

1 The chapter uses identity-first language to reflect the preferences of autistic people (Kenny et al., 2016).

2 UNITE (Staff and Autistic Communication in Mental Health Hospital Ward Rounds) was given full approval by the Health Research Authority in March 2019. It is funded by a PhD studentship by the NIHR, ARC-EM.
3 Recruitment was extended for 6 months following recruitment being suspended from March to September 2020 due to the COVID-19 pandemic.
4 An individual who knows the adult participant well and also ideally knew them during their developmental period (first 18 years of life).
5 Defined as significant deficits in intellectual functioning (intelligence quotient <70) and adaptive functioning, with onset during the developmental period (American Psychiatric Association, 2013)
6 Prior to COVID-19, most participants had been discharged from their psychiatric hospital stay at the time of their Phase 2 interview.

References

American Psychiatric Association. (2013). *Diagnostic and statistical manual of mental disorders: DSM-5*. Arlington, VA: American Psychiatric Publishing,

Baron-Cohen, S., Wheelwright, S., Skinner, R., Martin, J., & Clubley, E. (2001). The autism-spectrum quotient (AQ): evidence from Asperger syndrome/high-functioning autism, males and females, scientists and mathematicians. *Journal of Autism and Developmental Disorders*, *31*(1), 5–17.

Begeer, S., El Bouk, S., Boussaid, W., Terwogt, M. M., & Koot, H. M. (2009). Underdiagnosis and referral bias of autism in ethnic minorities. *Journal of Autism and Developmental Disorders*, *39*(1), 142.

Bradshaw, J. (2001). Complexity of staff communication and reported level of understanding skills in adults with intellectual disability. *Journal of Intellectual Disability Research*, *45*(3), 233–243.

Brugha, T. S. (2018). *The psychiatry of adult autism and Asperger syndrome: A practical guide*. Oxford: Oxford University Press.

Carruthers, S., Kinnaird, E., Rudra, A., Smith, P., Allison, C., Auyeung, B., … Bakolis, I. (2018). A cross-cultural study of autistic traits across India, Japan and the UK. *Molecular Autism*, *9*(1), 52.

Crompton, C. J., Sharp, M., Axbey, H., Fletcher-Watson, S., Flynn, E. G., & Ropar, D. (2020). Neurotype-matching, but not being autistic, influences self and observer ratings of interpersonal rapport. *Frontiers in Psychology*, *11*, 2961.

Cummins, C., Pellicano, E., & Crane, L. (2020). Autistic adults' views of their communication skills and needs. *International Journal of Language & Communication Disorders*, *55*(5), 678–689.

Drewett, A. (2021). A PhD learning journey: the value of conversational analysis and discourse approaches for speech and language clinical practice. In M. O'Reilly, & J. N. Lester (Eds.), *Improving communication in mental health settings: Evidence-based recommendations from practitioner-led research*. Abingdon, UK: Routledge.

Gaynor, Z., Alevizos, K., & Butler, J. (2020). *Is that clear? Effective communication in a neuro-diverse world. autism inspired tips for allistic (non-autistic) people*. Oxford: Prepare to Publish.

Grandin, T., & Johnson, C. (2005). *Animals in translation: the woman who thinks like a cow*. London: Bloomsbury.

Iedema, R., Carroll, K., Collier, A., Hor, S., Mesman, J., & Wyer, M. (2018). *Video-reflexive ethnography in health research and healthcare improvement: theory and application*. Florida: CRC Press.

Kenny L., Hattersley C., Molins B., Buckley C., Povey C., Pellicano E. (2016). Which terms should be used to describe autism? Perspectives from the UK autism community. *Autism*. *20*(4), 442–462.

Kiyimba, N., Lester, J. N., & O'Reilly, M. (2018). *Using naturally occurring data in qualitative health research: A practical guide*. Cham: Springer.

Lord, C., Rutter, M., DiLavore, P., Risi, S., Gotham, K., & Bishop, S. (2012). *Autism diagnostic observation schedule–2nd edition (ADOS-2)*. Los Angeles, CA: Western Psychological Corporation.

McManus, S., Bebbington, P., Jenkins, R., & Brugha, T. (2016). *Mental health and wellbeing in England: Adult psychiatric morbidity survey 2014*. Leeds: NHS Digital. Retrieved from https://openaccess.city.ac.uk/id/eprint/23646/1/mental_health_and_wellbeing_in_england_full_report.pdf

Milton, D. (2017). *A mismatch of salience: Explorations of the nature of autism from theory to practice*. Hove, UK: Pavilion Press.

Milton, D., & Mills, R. (2018). *10 rules to ensure autistic people obtain poor mental health support … and maybe what to do about it*. Retrieved from https://kar.kent.ac.uk/74104/1/10%20rules%20mental%20health%20-%20RM%20DM-%20final%20presentation%20conference%20%20version.pdf

Milton, D., Mills, R., & Jones, S. (2016). *10 rules for ensuring people with learning disabilities and those on the autism spectrum develop challenging behaviour … and maybe what to do about it*. Hove, UK: Pavilion Press.

Murphy, J., Cameron, L., Watson, J., & Markova, I. (2004). *Evaluating the effectiveness of talking mats as a communication resource to enable people with an intellectual disability to express their views on life planning*. Stirling, UK: University of Stirling,

Nicolaidis, C., Raymaker, D. M., Ashkenazy, E., McDonald, K. E., Dern, S., Baggs, A. E., … Boisclair, W. C. (2015). 'Respect the way I need to communicate with you': healthcare experiences of adults on the autism spectrum. *Autism*, *19*(7), 824–831.

Royal College of Speech and Language Therapists. (2016). *Position paper: Inclusive communication and the role of speech and language therapy*. Retrieved from www.rcslt.org/wp-content/uploads/2021/02/20162209_InclusiveComms_final.pdf

Trevisan, D. A., Hoskyn, M., & Birmingham, E. (2018). Facial expression production in autism: a meta-analysis. *Autism Research*, *11*(12), 1586–1601.

Tromans, S., Chester, V., Kiani, R., Alexander, R., & Brugha, T. (2018). The prevalence of autism spectrum disorders in adult psychiatric inpatients: a systematic review . *Clinical Practice and Epidemiology in Mental Health*, *14*, 177–187.

Tromans, S., Chester, V., Gemegah, E., Roberts, K., Morgan, Z., Yao, G. L., & Brugha, T. (2020). Autism identification across ethnic groups: a narrative review. *Advances in Autism*, *7*(3). https://doi.org/10.1108/AIA-03-2020-0017

Tromans, S. (2021). *An investigation of autism prevalence in adults admitted to acute mental health wards: a cross-sectional multi-site pilot study*. Unpublished Doctoral Dissertation. Leicester, UK: University of Leicester.

Tromans, S., Yao, G. L., Kiani, R., Alexander, R., Al-Uzri, M., & Brugha, T. (2019). Study protocol: an investigation of the prevalence of autism among adults admitted to acute mental health wards: A cross-sectional pilot study. *British Medical Journal Open*, *9*(12), e033169.

Wilkinson, R. (2019). Atypical interaction: conversation analysis and communicative impairments. *Research on Language and Social Interaction*, *52*(3), 281–299.

Wing, L., Leekam, S. R., Libby, S. J., Gould, J., & Larcombe, M. (2002). The diagnostic interview for social and communication disorders: background, inter-rater reliability and clinical use. *Journal of Child Psychology and Psychiatry*, *43*(3), 307–325.

Woods, R., Milton, D., Arnold, L., & Graby, S. (2018). Redefining critical autism studies: a more inclusive interpretation. *Disability & Society*, *33*(6), 974–979.

World Health Organization. (2023). *Section 1: Neurodevelopmental disorders. Schedules for clinical assessment in neuropsychiatry 3.0.* (3rd ed.). Geneva: World Health Organization.

World Health Organization. (1993). *The ICD-10 classification of mental and behavioural disorders: Diagnostic criteria for research.* Geneva: World Health Organization.

Improving engagement with people who stammer

Philip Robinson

Chapter contents:

- Clinical relevance
- Clinical practice recommendations
- Clinical case examples
- Communication guidelines
- Recommended reading
- References

Introduction

Stammering, also known as stuttering (the terms are interchangeable) is a neurological condition affecting between 1 and 3% of the population. Stammering is not caused by low intelligence, anxiety, or any underlying language disorder. Whilst it is known that stammering affects males more than females and has a strong genetic link, its neurological underpinnings are still not fully understood. It is however widely accepted that stammering is a multifactorial condition, with linguistic, environmental, and emotional factors interacting with the neurophysiological predisposition to stammer (Smith and Weber, 2017; Starkweather, 2002).

On the surface, stammering typically takes the form of *repetitions* and *prolongations* of sounds, and the cessation of airflow (*blocks*). People who stammer may also display *secondary behaviours* such as facial grimacing, involuntary movements, and avoidance of certain sounds, words, or speaking situations. Many children – about 8% – will experience a stammer as a natural phase of their language development. The majority of these will go on to develop fully fluent speech, but for between 1 and 3% of the overall population stammering will be a lifelong condition. Many people who stammer can become accustomed to concealing their difficulty, or to dismissing

DOI: 10.4324/9781003142522-19

it as unproblematic, whereas it can in fact have a profound effect on one's self-esteem. It can, for some, be a very isolating and frustrating experience.

There are certain well-observed triggers that typically increase stammering, such as fear, anxiety, frustration, unfamiliar speaking situations, and unfamiliar speaking partners. All of these may, to varying degrees, be relevant in the context of attending a medical appointment, and therefore this communication difficulty is examined in the present chapter. The multifactorial nature of the causes of stammering also mean that it is a highly variable condition, and an individual's experience is likely to be very different between situational contexts. It should also not be assumed that one person's experiences or needs would be the same as another's. This chapter proposes, through reference to the author's experience with a dysfluency caseload, a set of tangible guidelines to help healthcare professionals interact successfully and fruitfully with this population, and to help treat them with the dignity and parity they can often find to be lacking in interactions with health service providers.

Clinical relevance

People who stammer (who will be referred to for the remainder of this chapter by the acronym PWS) comprise a significant proportion of the population. For many children it can represent a typical stage of their language development, and so incidence of stammering in children is high, varying from 5% (Andrews & Harris, 1964) to 8.5% (Yairi & Ambrose, 2013). The present chapter focuses on the experience of adult healthcare service users, and so our attention is drawn to the incidence of stammering in the adult population. This figure has traditionally stood at around 1% (see Canter, 2013), though a recent Omnibus poll undertaken in November 2018 and again in December 2019 by the British Stammering Association and Action for Stammering Children revealed that 3% of adults identify as having a stammer (Stamma, 2020). This poll involved asking participants whether they stammered, with the stipulation

> by 'stammering or stuttering', we mean when someone struggles to get words out, often repeats or prolongs sounds or words, or gets stuck without any sound. Sometimes this includes putting in extra sounds or words. This is different from the problems most people will commonly experience, the occasional hesitation or stumbling around words.

1,975 adults took part in the first poll, and 2,018 in the second; 3% responded 'yes' when asked the question if they stammered. With the UK population currently (as of 2021) at 66 million, the original 1% incidence figure of stammering would give us 660,000 PWS living in the United Kingdom. However with the revised higher figure, this could be as high as almost 2 million people. Given this range, it is highly likely that most healthcare professionals will at some point during any typical year come into contact with a significant number of PWS.

The potential impact of living with a stammer on one's emotional well-being, self esteem, and willingness to participate in society is well documented. Smith and Weber (2017) discusses complex feelings of embarrassment, shame, frustration, fear, anger, and guilt associated with stammering, while Craig Blumgart and Tran (2009) demonstrate that stammering negative impacts quality of life measures in the domains of vitality, social functioning, emotional functioning, and mental health status. Sheehan (1970) popularised the iceberg analogy of stuttering, stating that 'stuttering is like an iceberg, with only a small part above the waterline and a much bigger part below'. The iceberg analogy is a useful tool in understanding a wide range of conditions that cause the patient to deal with and process a large number of thoughts and feelings (unseen, below the surface) caused by a proportionally smaller amount of physically visible symptoms and signs.

Sheehan goes on to explain that the tip of the iceberg is what most people think of as stuttering, but that the real bulk of the problem lies hidden and is only truly experienced by the PWS themselves. Its nature contributes to continued poor understanding among the general population of how big a problem stuttering can be.

Exploring and mapping out one's own 'stuttering iceberg' can be a very useful tool in therapy, helping the client understand the thoughts and feelings that go along with their stutter, in order for the clinician to help them tackle the condition as a whole. Blomgren (2013), with an adult population as opposed to paediatric, says that the theme of 'avoidance' will invariably come up as an issue to be placed below the surface. Blomgren (2013) states that 'for many who stutter, avoidance behaviours can be the most handicapping aspect of the disorder'.

Avoidance can be thought of as taking place at different levels, from sound level (e.g. avoiding any words that begin with D or G) and word level (avoiding proper nouns, names, words with a particular emotional load), up to role level (e.g. taking on a managerial role in the workplace, or offering to speak at a presentation), social level (avoiding certain social situations) or communication partner level (e.g. avoiding speaking with figures of authority). In the context of a medical appointment, one can see how different levels of avoidance behaviours have the potential to disrupt effective communication. Sound and word level avoidance may prevent the PWS from accurately describing their symptoms to the assessing clinician; they may avoid words completely or use circumlocutions to say 'easier' words but those which may not help pinpoint the problem. Role level avoidance may impede a PWS in the context of accompanying a relative, for whom they care, to a medical appointment, where they are required to take on the role of advocate or interpreter. Communication partner level avoidance may be the most problematic in the context of medical appointments; doctors typically have high status in society and therefore command and deserve a certain level of respect, which may be a trigger for some PWS. Situational level avoidance is commonly reported with reference to speaking on the telephone. As some healthcare booking systems still rely on this method, it may cause some PWS to avoid arranging appointments entirely.

Poor understanding of the complex levels of avoidance behaviours may have the effect of PWS being discharged for non-attendance, or being dismissed as unconcerned, unmotivated, or 'difficult', when really they need support or time to be able to engage.

In her book *Stutterer Interrupted; The Comedian Who Almost Didn't Happen* (2019), Nina Ghiselli discusses reframing the iceberg to suggest an alternative way of thinking about stuttering, highlighting the positives that have come from engaging with the stuttering community and embarking on a journey of self-discovery. In her version of the stuttering iceberg, emotions such as 'fear', anxiety', and 'shame' are replaced with more positive experiences such as 'acceptance', 'pride', 'courage', and 'community'.

Considering the significant incidence of stammering in the United Kingdom, and the impact it can have one one's self-esteem and confidence, it is easy to see how this may pose challenges in making healthcare fully accessible for this population. Perez, Doig-Acuña and Starrels (2015) carried out a qualitative study of PWS' experiences in navigating a healthcare system as service users.

Five broad themes characterised how their stammer affected their experiences

1. Discomfort speaking with office and medical staff.
2. Avoiding healthcare interactions due to stammering.
3. Reliance on a third party to navigate the healthcare system.
4. The need for trust and rapport with doctors to be built before discussing stammering.
5. Speaking assertively with doctors required self-acceptance of stuttering.

The last of these is achievable for a large number of PWS, but for many this will have required extensive speech and language therapy and/or immersion in self-help groups and community activities. Perez et al. (2015) conclude by highlighting the need for increased awareness and training for medical staff and physicians when caring for PWS. The risks involved in avoiding healthcare are self-evident; it is therefore imperative that clinicians and healthcare staff are able to adapt their discourse style in such a way as to be inclusive to a population with diverse communication abilities.

Clinical practice recommendations

- When a person is stammering, avoid finishing their sentence for them. Be patient and let the person finish. To complete an unfinished sentence for a speaker can be disempowering, and may lead to disengagement. It is also advisable to maintain eye contact with a person when they are stammering.
- Avoid giving advice for managing their stammer (e.g. 'take your time', 'take a deep breath'). Although well intentioned, this is likely to come across as patronising to somebody who has lived for many years with this condition and is already well versed in how to manage their own speech.
- Be aware that stammering is a neurological condition and is not caused by low intelligence, impaired language ability, or anxiety. Although the latter may exacerbate the condition, it is certainly not a root cause.
- Use person-first language. The preferred term for referring to somebody who speaks with a stammer is 'person who stammers' (PWS); this implies that you are seeing the person first and not the impairment.
- Consider the use of non-verbal practice management systems; e.g. appointment bookings, attendance confirmation. Systems that rely solely on speech and do not offer an alternative are more likely to disengage those who experience anxiety with their speech.

Clinical case examples

Names and locations have been changed to conceal identities.

Case study 14.1

A positive experience comes from a 46-year-old female who underwent surgery at a large teaching hospital in Scotland:

> At the pre-op talks I said I have a stammer as I'm usually fairly fluent, but didn't know how I'd be when I woke up. So I thought I'd better declare it in case I stammered a lot afterwards and they thought it was caused by the surgery. They were all fantastic. Once I got home I needed to speak to the consultant again on the phone and at some point got really stuck so I had to stop and take a breath. He just said 'it's ok, I'm here' and waited. Probably the most empathetic response I've ever had over the phone from someone who doesn't know me (but knew I stammer). I had to deal with doctors a lot on the phone afterwards and they were all great. One GP thought the line was breaking up and when I said 'no I have a

> stammer' she couldn't be more apologetic. It wasn't a problem for me she thought that, I might have done the same.

Her experience highlights an exemplary piece of communication from this doctor, who displayed patience, respect, was sensitive to the added pressures of speaking on the telephone, and did not offer any advice for her to produce speech fluently.

Case study 14.2

This case example comes from a client of mine, a 29-year-old gentleman who recounts a distressing interaction with a nurse at a health centre in London.

> I don't know if he was trying to put me at ease, but it certainly didn't come across that way. When I had to give my name, I blocked (as I tend to do on my name) and he laughed and made the usual clichéd joke of 'did you forget your name?'. When I explained that I have a stammer, he started saying how he stammers all the time so he knows what it's like. It's not like that. I was trying to explain that true stammering and tripping over your words are two completely different things. Then he kept finishing off my sentences when I was blocking, it was so frustrating. I get that it takes me a bit more time to get my words out, and it's the NHS and they have a busy caseload, but his whole attitude just put me in a bad mood the whole day, and it honestly put me off going to the doctors for like a year after that. I just don't need that kind of negativity in my life.

This example shows us how considerate and compassionate communication is key in engaging service users, and how poor understanding of communication disorders can turn people away, ultimately ending in poor outcome measures.

Case study 14.3

Another client, a 34-year-old civil servant, discusses his thoughts on current systems for engaging with their local GP Surgery.

> The GP surgery is literally the worst part of the entire system. Everything is rushed, staff are impatient, you get interrupted,

receptionists interrupt and humiliate you, and there is deep ignorance about how to treat people with communication differences and disabilities. The insistence on telephone 'fastest finger first' bookings is a major part of the problem. Sure, individual members of the system may not *intend* to be ignorant and hurtful ... When it comes to my stammer, interactions with the NHS tend to actively *worsen* my health. It means I actively avoid the GP unless the need is deeply urgent that it becomes worth putting myself through it.

A recent post on an online support group page for PWS on the topic brought up the almost unanimous view that touch-screen systems for checking in are a positive addition to GP surgeries. Reliance on phone systems for booking appointments also seem to represent an antiquated and outdated method that may exclude a wide range of communicatively impaired service users.

Communication guidelines

Do not finish a sentence for a PWS who is stammering on a word. While this action would almost universally be well intentioned, it is easy to see how this could be construed as rude or arrogant. The communication partner may guess wrongly, commit a faux pas, or undermine the intended message of the PWS. For some PWS, finishing off a sentence can be a helpful strategy, but express permission must be given by them before proceeding with this.

Maintain eye contact with a PWS when they are stammering. The key to good communication is showing engagement, and there's no more effective way of showing a person you are focused on them than by looking at them. Averting your eyes is likely to convey a sense of embarrassment or discomfort. Please note that this strategy is not internationally applicable, and is intended for a Western healthcare setting (the United Kingdom). Leith (1986) discusses how sustained eye contact is not typical or desired in some societies.

Avoid giving advice such as 'Slow down', 'relax', or 'take a breath'. PWS universally share stories of being told this and relay a sense of being patronised. It is likely that they are already fully aware of their strategies and techniques they need to employ in order to generate speech, and being told such things is likely to cause irritation.

Be patient, and understand that for PWS, delivering a message verbally may take a little more time. If you're able to show that you're relaxed, comfortable, and listening, the message is less likely to become compromised. PWS are not language disordered, nor do they have lower intelligence; they wish to be treated the same as any other service user.

If the PWS is your patient, always make them the primary person you are addressing. When a person with a communication difficulty presents in a medical setting accompanied by a family member, it can sometimes be tempting to speak instead to the family member, referring to the patient in the third person. Never let others speak for them, unless that is their express wish.

If you know that a person stammers, or if they are clearly struggling, it is OK to acknowledge it and ask the person what you can do that is helpful; e.g. 'I notice from your records that you stammer, is there anything that I should do that will make it easier for you while you're here?' or 'I can see you're struggling a bit today, what would you like me to do?' Often just acknowledging the communication is tough can help.

Try to use person-first language, so, e.g. 'Patient A is a gentleman who stammers' rather than 'Patient A is a stammerer'. This kind of language shows that you are seeing the person first rather than their difficulty. The stammering community is very vocal in supporting the notion that stammering does not define them as an individual; the language used to refer to the individual should reflect this.

Listen to *what* is being said rather than *how* it is being said. Stammering is a relatively rare but well-known condition that the vast majority of people will recognise, and may even be able to relate back to a past experience or a person that they know. It's natural to want to remark on a condition that the listener feels familiar with, but the content of the PWS's speech must always take precedence over its form.

Never assume it is ok to joke about a person's stammer; only when express permission is granted, and only then after a close rapport has been established between the clinician and the speaker. Most PWS have heard the jocular 'did you forget your name?' when they stammer on their own name; indeed, it causes eyes to roll in tired recognition among self-help and support groups when stories such as these are recounted.

If it is relevant to the PWS' situation or clinical presentation, do not be hesitant in asking them about their stammer. Ask them if there is anything you can do to make sure communication between you flows more effectively. Ask if the person's speech may be affected by the presenting condition which brought them into the medical setting.

Avoid assigning positive or negative values to fluent or dysfluent speech respectively. It should be assumed that a PWS will prefer to say 'my speech is dysfluent today' rather than 'my speech is bad today'. For example, if an interaction with a PWS is increasing their dysfluency, it would be advisable to say 'I can see your speech is becoming less fluent' rather than 'your speech is getting worse'.

Try to slow your own speech; not so slowly as to sound unnatural, but slow enough to convey that communication between you is unhurried and free flowing.

If you have not understood what the PWS says, ask for clarification. It is always preferable to be open and honest and state that you have not understood, and ask for the message to be repeated. To assume you have heard the PWS correctly and continue may save embarrassment, but it would undermine their capacity and the communication that occurs between you.

Do not praise a PWS for their speech if you think a particular utterance sounded good or was produced fluently. Instead, focus on the message of what was conveyed and respond to that.

Do not show pity or express that you 'feel sorry' for the PWS. For many people, especially those who have undergone successful therapy programmes, having a stammer can be reframed as a 'gift', a positive experience. To automatically assume it is a negative thing may be to undermine this.

If you have personal experience with stammering (e.g. you are a PWS yourself, you stammered as a child, or have a family member or close friend who stammers), be forthcoming in sharing this. Be conscious though that this does not necessarily mean that you understand what it is like to be in your patient's situation, just that you have been previously acquainted with stammering and that this is not your first time speaking with a PWS. Also be mindful that all people have certain *non-fluencies* present in their speech (tripping over your words, getting 'tongue-tied'), but this is a very different experience to living with stammering as a neurological condition.

Consider resources from or a referral to stammering self-help groups. There are many national and local organisations that hold support groups, conferences and get-togethers for PWS to share their experiences, yet many PWS are unaware of their existence. Signposting in the first instance to the British Stammering Association is advised; their website contains a comprehensive list of free-to-attend groups, both online and in person.

Remember that every stammer is different; for some, a stammer will be overt (visible), whereas others may be covert; that is to say the PWS has learnt how to conceal their stammer, which may come as a result of great effort.

Acknowledge discrimination and highlight the rights that a PWS has. The website Stammering Law www.stammeringlaw.org.uk is an excellent resource created and maintained by a PWS and former solicitor. Here can be found many interesting case examples and practical advice.

Summary

This chapter has proposed a set of practical guidelines for effective communication with PWS; an overriding theme of the clinical guidelines and practice recommendations has been, as supported by St Louis et al. (2017), to *treat stuttering as a non-issue*. Like all people with any form of impairment, be it physical or communicative, people who stammer seek parity and equal opportunities in relation to access to healthcare, which should extend to the interactions they have with healthcare staff. Another theme is to exercise sensitivity as to how you should react to a person's stammer; e.g. the guidance to never finish a person's stammer is universal, though it may be for some people that this is helpful; this should be pursued only if given express permission to do so. It is also important to consider interaction with a healthcare system in a wider context, beyond one-to-one spoken communication with staff; new technologies allow for non-verbal booking systems, check-ins etc., which should feature in any update to a healthcare setting's infrastructure. Finally, awareness raising continues to be an ongoing goal of the stammering community; healthcare workers should be encouraged to seek out extra information and receive in-house training from PWS where available. A recommended reading list is included below of further resources where more information on stammering can be sought.

Recommended reading/resources

1. British Stammering Association website: www.stamma.org.
2. Campbell, P., Constantino, C., Simpson S (eds) 2019, *Stammering Pride and Prejudice: Difference Not Defect*, J&R Press, London.
3. Ghiselli, N. 2019, *Stutterer Interrupted: The Comedian Who Almost Didn't Happen*, She Writes Press, Berkeley CA.
4. Action for Stammering Children website: https://actionforstammering-children.org.
5. Mitchell, D. 2016 *Thirteen Ways of Looking at a Stammer.* Germany: Stotteren & Selbsthilfe Landesverband Ost e.V.

References

Andrews, G., & Harris, M. (1964). *The syndrome of stuttering. Clinics in developmental medicine* (No. 17). London: Heinemann.

Blomgren, M. (2013). Behavioural treatments for children and adults who stutter: a review, *Psychology Research and Behaviour Management*, *6*, 9–19. Retrieved from: www.ncbi.nlm.nih.gov/pmc/articles/PMC3682852/

Canter, G. (2013). Observations on neurogenic stuttering: a contribution to differential diagnosis. *British Journal of Disorders of Communication*, *6*, 139–143.

Craig, A., Blumgart, E., & Tran, Y. (2009). The impact of stuttering on the quality of life in adults who stutter. *Journal of Fluency Disorders*, *34*, 61–71.

Ghiselli, N. (2019). *Stutterer interrupted: the comedian who almost didn't happen.* Berkeley, CA: She Writes Press.

Leith., W. (1986). Treating the stutterer with atypical cultural influences. In K. O. St Louis (Ed.), *The atypical stutterer: Principles and practises of rehabilitation* (pp. 9–34). New York: Academic Press.

Perez, H. R., Doig-Acuña, C., Starrels, J. L. (2015). 'Not unless it's a life or death thing': a qualitative study of the health care experiences of adults who stutter. *Journal of General Internal Medicine*, *30*(11), 1639–1644.

Sheehan, J. (1970). *Stuttering: research and therapy.* New York: Harper & Row.
Smith, A., & Weber, C. (2017). How stuttering develops: The multifactorial dynamic pathways theory. *Journal of Speech, Language, and Hearing Research, 60*(9), 2483–2505.
Starkweather, C. (2002). The epigenesis of stuttering. *Journal of Fluency Disorders, 27*(4), 269–288.
St Louis, K., Irani, F., Gabel, R., Hughes, S., Langevin, M., Rodriguez, M., Scaler , K., & Weidner, M. (2017). Evidence-based guidelines for being supportive of people who stutter in North America. *Journal of Fluency Disorders, 53*, 1–13.
Stamma (2020). *Stammering in the population.* Retrieved from: https://stamma.org/news-features/stammering-population
Yairi, E., & Ambrose, N. (2013). Epidemiology of stuttering: 21st century advance'. *Journal of Fluency Disorders, 38*, 66–87.

15

Communication, hearing loss, and deafness

Gareth Smith and Crystal Rolfe

Chapter contents:

- A global view of hearing loss
- A brief introduction to ear disease
- Clinical relevance
- Identifying hearing loss and deafness
- The challenging healthcare environment
- Communication tactics for health professions
- References

Blindness cuts us off from things, but deafness cuts us off from people.
(Attributed to Helen Keller, Deaf–Blind author and activist, 1880–1968)

Introduction

Hearing loss can be an isolating condition; cutting off individuals from family, friends and colleagues. It can lead to long-term psychosocial challenges such as depression and loneliness. It threatens independence and challenges the sense of self and social identity. It is a major barrier to accessing healthcare and leads to poorer outcomes for hard of hearing (HoH) and Deaf individuals. Conversely, whilst loss can be viewed negatively by those from a hearing world, deafness can also be celebrated as a unique cultural experience.

We will in this chapter explore hearing loss prevalence, impact and strategies for healthcare settings. We will discuss the demonstrable links between the adverse effects of hearing loss and the healthcare outcomes for people with the hearing loss. Further, we will discuss identification of people with hearing loss and how to support them in clinical interactions.

DOI: 10.4324/9781003142522-20

A global view of hearing loss

Over 5% of the world's population has disabling hearing loss, defined by the World Health Organization (WHO) as a moderate or greater loss (as described below). This is set to rise to over 900 million people by 2050 (World Health Organization, 2020). High income countries are greatly impacted and prevalence is even higher in low and middle income countries. In the UK for example, estimates suggest 1 in 6 people have a hearing loss of some degree. To give this some context against other long-term conditions; 1 in 16 people in the UK have diabetes and 1 in 79 people have dementia. Due to the ageing population, and following the global trend, prevalence of hearing loss is likely to rise in the UK to 16 million people (1 in 5) by 2035.

Hearing loss is the fourth leading cause of years lived with disability in males and seventh in females (GBD 2017 Disease and Injury Incidence and Prevalence Collaborators, 2019). Hearing loss can have consequences on interpersonal communication, psychosocial well-being, quality of life, and economic independence. In infants and children, hearing loss can impact speech and language acquisition and educational attainment. In adults, social isolation and stigma, abuse, psychiatric disturbance, depression, relationship difficulties, occupational stress, increased risk of dementia, and relative low earnings have been observed (Davis & Hoffman, 2019; Graydon, Waterworth, Miller, & Gunasekera, 2018; Livingstone, et al., 2020).

A brief introduction to ear disease

Hearing loss can be congenital or acquired at any point in life. There are varying descriptors that attempt to quantify hearing loss. The WHO defines hearing loss as mild (26–40dB HL), moderate (41–60dB HL), severe (61–80 dB HL), and profound (81 dB HL or greater). A normal conversation level, in a quiet environment, would be around 60 dB (A), therefore someone with a moderate hearing loss would hear that conversation at a whisper level, and someone with a severe hearing loss would be unlikely to access the conversation, based on sound alone, at all. We can further define hearing loss as a factor of frequency/intensity and link this to access to speech sounds. In simplified terms, a high frequency hearing loss will limit access to consonant sounds – i.e. the beginnings/ends of words, whilst low frequency hearing loss will remove access to vowel sounds, taking away the 'power' of speech.

Whilst these definitions can be helpful, even mild and unilateral hearing losses can cause significant difficulties for individuals and hearing loss levels are poor predictors of hearing disability (Graydon et al., 2018). Further to defining the 'level' of hearing, hearing loss can be described as transient or permanent and can be related to the anatomy of the ear; broken down into outer-ear, middle-ear, and inner-ear, as well as central or brain function.

In children, transient hearing impairments are common. Middle-ear conditions account for much of the temporary hearing losses in children and tend to be short-lived: 8 out of 10 children in the UK, for example will experience an episode of 'glue ear' by age 10 (NDCS, 2020). Permanent hearing loss in children is less common. In the UK, approximately 1 in 1000 children are born with permanent hearing loss of a moderate – profound nature as identified by new-born hearing screening. By school age, this has risen to 3.5 in 1000 (Bamford et al., 2007).

In adults, a range of factors can cause hearing loss: noise-exposure, ototoxicity, and late-onset genetics causes to name a few. The biggest factor associated with hearing loss in adults is age. Presbyacusis, or age-related hearing loss, is progressive and irreversible. The hearing loss is often bilateral, symmetrical, and starts to affect high-frequencies first and progresses across the frequency range, towards mid and lower frequencies as time progresses. The slow progression of presbyacusis often results in the affected individual being unaware of their hearing loss in the early stages.

As age increases, the prevalence of hearing loss correspondingly increases: 45.6% of 70–79 years olds will have a significant hearing loss, 67% of 75–79 year olds, with increases in prevalence thereafter (78% of 80–84 year olds and 80 >85 year olds) (Lin et al., 2011).

Hearing loss: an unmet need

The often slow and insidious nature of the condition can mean that the person with a hearing loss will not acknowledge or recognise it in the early stages. It may take up to 10 years for someone with a hearing loss to receive help (Davis et al., 2007). Early coping mechanisms often externalise the hearing loss; phrases such as 'everybody mumbles' or 'the sound on the TV isn't working properly' can be early indicators of an unrecognised hearing loss. There is a dearth of information on unrecognised hearing loss in adults, given that they will not present for intervention if they do not recognise a hearing problem, and once recognised there may be further delays in taking action. Further, unlike new-born hearing screening programmes, there are no national screening programmes for adult-onset hearing impairment. An example of prevalence is provided by De Iori, Rapport, Wong, & Stach (2019) who recruited a control group for a hearing loss study. The adults in the control group reported normal hearing, however on testing, 33% of the group in fact had hearing loss.

Even once a hearing loss is acknowledged, the uptake of interventions such as hearing aids is low. In the United States, only 40% of those with moderate hearing loss use hearing aids, with average time from candidacy to hearing aid adoption at 8.9 years (Simpson et al., 2019).

Unmet hearing loss does not only affect the HoH individual but has wider psychosocial consequences for their spouses, partners, close family members, and care-givers. Changes in the relationship caused by limiting social activities, denial of the hearing loss, and the need for communication partners to act as communication 'go-betweens' all added to the stress felt by both the person with the hearing loss and their significant communication partners (Barker, Leighton, & Ferguson, 2017).

Clinical relevance

Hearing loss

People who are HoH are more likely to require health interventions. Children with additional needs are 40% more likely to have a hearing loss. There is a well-established association between hearing loss and poorer physical, psychosocial and cognitive health (Wells, et al., 2020; Lin et al., 2011). To highlight two examples; falls in the elderly are three-fold more likely in patients with hearing loss, even if that hearing loss is mild (Lin & Ferrucci, 2012). Dementia also has a strong correlation with hearing loss (Lin, Metter, & O'Brien, 2011; Thomson et al., 2017) and treating hearing loss in mid-life is one of the modifiable risk factors that may reduce the incidence of dementia (Livingstone et al., 2020).

Deafness

Much of the information within this introductory section is set within a context of hearing loss in a hearing world; demonstrated as a problem to be addressed and fixed through technology and rehabilitation. There is however an important group that health practitioners must acknowledge and understand: Deaf People, Deaf Community and Deaf Culture. In this context the capitalised 'D' often signifies people who were born with severe to profound hearing loss at, or very near to, birth whose main form of communication is sign language.

British Sign Language (BSL) or Irish Sign Language (ISL) is the preferred language for over 87,000 Deaf people in the UK. Sign language is not homogenous and its basis is not rooted in the language of the country in which it is used – for example, ISL is heavily influenced by French Sign Language. The Deaf community enjoys a rich cultural experience rooted within language. Poetry, art, story-telling, and satire to name a few. There are Deaf sports teams, competing from local to international levels (British Deaf Association, 2020).

Identifying hearing loss and deafness

Having established that many people attempting to access healthcare services may have a hearing loss or identify as Deaf, recognising those that might need modified or enhanced communication strategies is the next step.

Firstly, and often over-looked, is to ask the service user if they have a hearing loss or are Deaf. There are critical points at which to gather this information to ensure ideal communication.

Visually, healthcare professionals (HCPs) can consider if the service user is wearing any hearing technology; hearing aids, cochlear implants, or bone-anchored hearing aids for example. It should however be recognised that Deaf service users, whose main mode of communication is sign, may not use hearing technology.

If HoH service users are not asked in advance, or if they do not recognise a hearing loss, there are signs to be alert for both in your conversations or from the service user's history. Presented here are some signs to be alert for:

- Difficulty hearing in background noise such as pubs and restaurants.
- Having to turn the TV up so that others complain about the volume.
- Asking people to repeat themselves.
- Unaware of conversation when the speaker is not facing the individual.
- Speech sounds muffled or people do not speak clearly.
- Avoiding social situations.
- Withdrawal from conversation.
- Mishearing, and inappropriate responding.
- Unable to hear environmental noises such as bird song.
- Reporting tinnitus – noises in the ear, ringing, buzzing, whooshing etc.
- Difficulty hearing on the telephone.
- Intently watching the face of the speaker.

(RNID, 2021; RCGP, 2021)

When HCPs recognise the signs of hearing loss they can discuss this with service users. Various models of onward referral are in operation internationally; in many countries access to audiology services is via a GP or direct access via the private sector.

The challenging healthcare environment

People with hearing loss and that are Deaf, report lower levels of communication between themselves and HCPs and poorer overall healthcare compared to those with normal hearing. It is difficult for them to engage in discussions, particularly in noisy environments with unfamiliar medical terminology. Doctors can also become frustrated with communication difficulties or are unaware of communication tactics (Mick, Foley, & Lin, 2017). Often, the experiences of Deaf and HoH people accessing healthcare are similar; they face barriers to access and once they have accessed healthcare, they are met with systems and HCPs who do not optimise the opportunities for communication. A report in 2013, looking at Deaf access to healthcare, demonstrated it was challenging to even access NHS services at a Primary Care level: 33% respondents reported not accessing services as they found making appointments very difficult, 36% felt it wasn't worth making appointments as the communication was poor. Whilst 86% of the respondents would prefer to communicate through an interpreter, only 51% reported they had access to this communication method. Just under half reported they communicated with HCPs by writing things down, although none preferred to communicate this way (SignHealth, 2013). Pharmacies comparatively seem to provide more accessible information to Deaf people and this may be because a third are offered a private room away from noise (Ringham, 2012).

Lip-reading

People who are Deaf or have hearing loss rely heavily on visual cues including facial expressions and lip-reading to understand what is being said. It can be difficult or impossible to follow what is being said when they do not have access to these visual clues. This creates challenges making an appointment or during a consultation, hospital stay, or follow up. Whilst these visual cues, including lip-reading, are essential for some to communicate, skills vary considerably so they have varying levels of success. Facial hair, accents, and lighting can have an impact on its accuracy (National Association of the Deaf, 2021).

Accessing an appointment

Deaf and HoH service users will often struggle with using the phone to arrange appointments. Bailey (2018) found that nearly half (44%) of survey respondents contact their GP surgery by phone to book an appointment but less than a quarter (23%) said the phone was their preferred method of communication. The other half (47%) visit their GP surgery in person to book appointments, but only 14% said they prefer to book appointments this way. One-quarter (26%) said that they ask a family member, friend, or support worker to call their GP surgery on their behalf, but only 7% said they wanted this. Lip-reading may be difficult when making an appointment in person if the receptionist is attending to the computer or behind a screen. It is challenging to hear in background noise, such as waiting rooms, for most people with hearing loss. Once at the surgery, a third of respondents reported no arrangements were made to improve communication despite most of them having indicated they had hearing loss in advance. No allowances were made for calling them from the waiting room and once in a consultation practitioners turned their backs when talking (Stevens et al., 2018). One in seven people have missed an appointment because they didn't hear their name called in the waiting room (Ringham, 2012). Knowing there is a risk of this, Deaf people can find waiting rooms very stressful.

During the consultation

Ringham (2012) found that, following a GP appointment, more than one-quarter of service users had been unclear about a diagnosis or the health advice they were provided and one-fifth (19%) about their medication. Over half reported that the main reasons for this were: the GP not facing the patient (64%), the GP not always speaking clearly (57%), and the GP not making sure the patient had understood what had been said (51%). Far fewer were unclear after an appointment with a practice nurse. The same study surveyed BSL users and found that almost two-thirds did not get a BSL interpreter, despite asking, that they had to remind the GP of their communication needs, and almost half felt confused about their condition. When there is a sign language interpreter, the right level of interpreter is often not provided (AoHL, 2014).

Lip-reading can be difficult throughout the consultation as HCPs often look at the computer, notes, or move around the room to get a piece of equipment. It can be particularly difficult when lying down (Middleton et al., 2010).

Use of masks can be extremely challenging for people with hearing loss and sign language users due to the barrier to lip-reading, reading facial expressions and the muffled speech . The WHO (2020) highlighted that the use of masks in healthcare settings created potential harms and risks that should be noted.

Video call consultations may be more challenging than face to face appointments. RNID (2020) found 70% didn't feel they would hear well during a remote appointment. It may be easier than a face to face appointment with an HCP wearing a mask. People with severe hearing loss may need captions on these platforms.

In multi-professional meetings, it can also be difficult to identify the direction of sound and who is talking when there is more than one other person.

Service users often struggle along with the conversation and don't have the confidence to speak up.

Hospital settings

Hospital in-patient settings pose considerable challenges for Deaf and HoH people. A systematic review looking specifically at patient-provider communication in a hospital setting found that patients identify a wide range of communication difficulties. Included within these challenges were difficulties understanding consultations, hearing in background noise, HCPs speaking too fast, not making eye contact and not facing the patient during consultations. They found hearing loss could lead to significant delays in treatment. There was also significant non adherence to treatment plans (Shukla et al., 2019), with an RNID report finding 43% of Deaf and HoH service-users not feeling fully involved in decisions about their care (AoHL, 2014).

Middleton et al. (2010) highlight the particular difficulty in following conversation in hospital theatres when dulled by sedation medication, without glasses and hearing aids. People with hearing loss and deafness can become more isolated in hospital than others if they can't communicate with other patients. Hospital media services may not have subtitles and phones may not have loop systems, amplifiers, or text (discussed in the recommendations section) adding to the feeling of isolation.

Ambient noise levels in hospital can make hearing very difficult even for people with normal hearing. There may be alarms, multiple discussions taking place, and poor sound insulation (Stevens et al., 2018).

A report in 2003 found that Deaf BSL users are at a severe disadvantage when attending Accident and Emergency services due to difficulties communicating. Difficulties are found whilst queuing to be seen, understanding or communicating with staff, and they may fail to understand vital information, risking their safety. Many staff did not understand their communication needs. The study found that when a sign language interpreter was present almost all obstacles to communication were removed. Often family members were asked to assist with communication. Sometimes service users were happy with this but others were not as they may be asked to translate serious illness or injury. This was especially difficult when children were used to interpret (Reeve, 2003).

Challenges experienced by people with hearing loss and who are Deaf in these settings will also be experienced with a range of other HCPs such as dentists and paramedics, especially those that wear masks or in noisy environments.

Mental health services

A meta-analysis (Gill & Fox, 2011) found the therapeutic relationship between service users who were Deaf and their therapist was challenged in psychotherapy services. There were problems with service issues (difficulty locating mental health services); communication with other workers (trying to contact the office); communication between therapist and client; lack of knowledge (unfamiliar terms difficult to translate into sign language, or belief the therapist lacked knowledge of Deaf culture); how the client perceives the therapist's feelings (feeling HCP was uncomfortable or had unethical views towards Deaf culture); the use of an interpreter (clients concerned about confidentiality due to the size of the deaf community); and the role of family and friends (when used as an interpreter due to confidentiality and therefore restricting what they disclosed).

Access to public health information

People who are HoH may not be able to hear public health messages on television and radio. Sign language users may not be able to access information widely available to others, if it has not been interpreted from written or spoken language into sign language. Consequently, they may not be able to make an informed choice about treatments and health behaviours.

Getting it right

Many countries have legislation in place to ensure that people with disabilities, including deaf people, can access health services. In the UK the Disability Discrimination Act 1995 and Equality Act 2010, required the NHS to make 'reasonable adjustments' for deaf people so that information is available in an accessible format. Additionally, the Accessible Information Standard requires NHS services, private providers funded by the NHS and adult social care services in England to identify a person's communication needs and put measures in place to meet them. In America, the Americans with Disabilities Act 1990 requires the healthcare provider to ensure that effective communication takes place between themselves and the patient.

Communication tactics for health professions

The RNID (2020) provide simple tips to communication. Where lip-reading is possible:

- Ensure there is adequate lighting.
- Face the person you are speaking to.
- Get the person's attention before speaking.
- Use normal lip movements, facial expression, and gestures.

For some people lip-reading can be exhausting, and particularly difficult for those with additional needs, such as visual impairments and cognitive impairments, so it is important not to rely on this (National Association of the Deaf, 2021). If the service user is unable to use visual cues to lip-read, for example on the telephone or if the HCP is wearing a mask, the following tactics can be used (RNID, 2020):

- Speak clearly – avoid shouting or speaking unnecessarily slowly.
- Say things differently if people ask you to repeat what you've said or do not understand.
- Check understanding by asking the person to repeat the information back.
- Use plain language and be straight to the point.
- Reduce background noise as much as possible.
- Where possible, also provide written information.
- If requested, speak to a relative or friend.

The HCP should establish rapport with the service user, ask open-ended questions, cover one thing at a time, and minimise medical terminology. If moving around the room they should ensure that they stay in the service user's line of sight. For physical examinations where the HCP will be moving around the room, they could agree in advance how they will indicate that they are starting a conversation, for example touching the service user's arm (Middleton et al., 2010).

Where masks are necessary, provision of clear masks or face shields should be made if approved versions are available for the type of setting and procedure. This enables lip-reading but light reflections can still create barriers.

It is important not to assume that writing things down or providing written information is effective. In many countries the average reading age is low. For example, in England 16.4% of adults are described as having very low literacy levels (Natonal Literacy Trust, 2017). For most people who use sign language, it is their first language and the syntax and grammatical structures are often very different and not equivalent to spoken languages (The Association of Sign-Language Interpreters, 2020).

Deaf awareness training should be available for all HCPs adapted to the needs, environment, and service users they support.

Utilising technology

There is a range of devices and technology that can enhance communication. It is useful to know whether the service user usually uses any devices, if they have brought them, and if they are working. Hearing aid(s), cochlear implants, or other implantable devices are most commonly used. These devices do not restore hearing and, besides, 20% of people who have hearing aids do not use them (Dillion et al., 2020). Hearing aids need regular maintenance and cleaning. If the service user is unable to hear well the hearing aid(s) may need maintenance or fine tuning or a new hearing test may be needed. These issues can all be rectified if the service user returns to their hearing aid provider. Sometimes the service user may simply need reminding to use their hearing aid (s) during the appointment.

If a service user without a known hearing loss is struggling to hear, a hearing check should be completed, with a handheld screener or online (RNID, 2021). Research shows that people are willing to take up a hearing screen/check if it is recommended by a GP (Rolfe & Gardner, 2016) or whilst in hospital (AoHL, 2014). If the screening tool or observations suggest a hearing loss, referrals to audiology or ENT must be made for a full diagnostic test. In the UK hearing tests and hearing aids are free on the NHS. Hearing aids can also be purchased via private aid companies.

If the service user doesn't have working hearing aid(s) or devices with them, a personal listening device may aid communication for that appointment. HCPs should ensure they have one available to them as standard equipment within the surgery, ward, and departments.

There is a wide range of rapidly evolving technology for people who are deaf which can be accessed from a range of commercial organisations.

Loop systems (Telecoil or T-coil) work in conjunction with a hearing aid. If a switch on the hearing aid is activated it changes the aid to pick up sounds through the loop systems microphone and reduce background noise. Loop systems should be available in the reception and consultation rooms or a portable loop system for the latter when needed. It is important that these are working, switched on, that staff know how to use them, and service users know they are available, indicated with a widely recognised symbol.

The following technology may also be useful:

- Live speech to test apps: these have variable levels of accuracy so understanding must be checked.
- Remote video appointments with live captioning: these may be easier than the telephone as it will enable the service user to lip-read. This software has variable accuracy so understanding must be checked.
- Telephone or app relay: this allows the service user to type what they want to say and read the response from the HCPs.
- Video Relay Services for British Sign Language users: this allows an interpreter to support remotely by video.
- Emergency SMS messaging: this allows Deaf people to text the emergency services in the UK.

It is vital to be prepared to make and receive calls in these non-standard ways and to accept text, email, and online messages.

Equipment should be used throughout the session, even for seemingly less important transactions. This will avoid stress and ensure the service user is confident they have picked up all the information needed.

The healthcare environment

Getting the environment right is simple but effective. Visual display boards or vibrating pager systems are very important so that it is clear to the service user in a waiting room when it is their turn and where to go. If this is not possible, ensuring the service user can see the receptionist can be useful. The amount of hard surfaces should be reduced or limited and soft furnishings used where possible. Rubber stops for chairs and acoustic panels also help. Where necessary the HCP should move the consultation to a quieter room or corner of the ward, shut windows and doors to reduce ambient noise. The amount of light in the room should be maximised and seating set up considered so that the HCP's face is in the light and visible to the service user throughout. Moving about should be limited. Where possible the appointment should be held with a small group and in a quiet area.

Types of communication support

There are various types of communication support for people who are Deaf. Many do not use sign language but some HCPs may think of this as the easy solution (Hearing Loss Association of America, 2021). Getting the wrong type of communication support or strategy will not help any more than getting an interpreter in the wrong language. HCPs need to be aware of the differences to ensure the right type of communication support is booked. For example, HCPs need to check whether a BSL, ISL, or ASL interpreter is required, or if the service user is Deaf–Blind, and their communication preference. If there is a lot of medical language communication professionals may need specific experience in a medical setting.

Sign language users will typically need a sign language interpreter. In the UK the National Registers of Communication Professionals working with Deaf and Deafblind People (NRCPD) ensure there is a safe standard of practice. Only registered sign language interpreters should be booked and caution should be taken if booking a trainee. Staff members that are not fully qualified in sign language should not be used as interpreters because of the high risk of error conveying vital information. It is not ethical to ask family members to act as interpreters for several reasons including risks to the quality of the information passed on, because it could breach confidentiality, they may need to communicate inappropriate information, and it could impact on their mental health and their relationship with the service user (The Association of Sign-Language Interpreters, 2020). Sign language is a 3D language and therefore remote interpretation is not always appropriate and could increase the risk of misunderstandings, which can be serious. However, remote interpreter services are available if an in-person interpreter is not available and this is preferable to not having one. Availability of interpreters varies widely. In the UK demand in many areas far outstrips supply (The Association of Sign-Language Interpreters, 2020). Healthcare providers have contracts with interpreting companies and charities that include sign language as well as spoken language. Cultural needs should also be considered when booking an interpreter; for example, gender and the nature of the appointment. The HCP should speak in the first person to the service user not to the communication support. If gloves need to be worn, clear or white gloves should be provided rather than blue gloves as they can cause a distraction (The Association of Sign-Language Interpreters, 2020). There are also deaf translators who can work between written language and sign language.

Lip speakers repeat what is being said. They usually do this silently but can be asked to use their own voice if the patient has residual hearing. They reproduce rhythm, flow and tone, and facial gestures. They may also finger-spell the first letter of the word if needed.

Speech to text reporters, also known as palantypists or stenographers, type what is being said verbatim. This appears on a screen in front of the service user. The speech to text reporter may be in the room or remote.

Having procedures in place to support communication bookings can make this simpler and more timely (Ringham, 2012).

Specific healthcare settings

These principles can be applied to various healthcare settings. Research in hospital wards (AoHL, 2014) recommends that in addition to good communication tactics and personal listeners, screening devices and hearing aid maintenance kits are useful. Pink plastic hearing aid storage boxes were particularly beneficial to ensure hearing aids were not lost. Lost aids were a particular barrier to communication because many people have custom-made earmoulds and were without their aids whilst new ones were made. In Accident and Emergency services things can be written down whilst waiting for communication support to arrive, if service users cannot or do not want to communicate through family or friends. Pictures may help if the service user cannot read written language. These tactics should only ever be used temporarily in an emergency, even if it appears that the service user is communicating well. An interpreter must be arranged urgently.

Dentists should improve communication by lowering their masks where possible, learning simple signs, and reducing background noise (Champion & Holt, 2000).

RNID (2020) recommend several ways to improve communication in care settings: screening should be carried out through portable screeners kept on site or by online checks; hearing aid(s) should be recorded in each individual's care plan along with any accessories and written instructions on how to use them, (provided when issued) and hearing aid(s) should be checked regularly for function and fitting. Care settings should also help to get the environment right.

Tele psychiatry is indicated not to compromise the quality of care for Deaf service users and therefore this can be used to overcome barriers that service users face in remote locations or through a lack of interpreters in their area (Crowe et al., 2016).

Public health messaging should be subtitled and translated into sign language. This should include key government announcements, television adverts, and important letters.

Knowing your service user's needs

It is essential to know what service user's communication needs are. Best practice is to proactively ask all service users what their communication needs and preferences are when they register. Examples of communication action plans and communication passports can be found online. A physical or digital note/symbol could also be created for patient records. This should link to a description of hearing; hearing devices used; equipment needed;

communication support. If cancelling an appointment, care needs to be taken to communicate via the service user's preferred method. Leaving an answerphone message can cause unnecessary distress. It could also lead the service user to ask for help from friends and family which could breach confidentiality and impact the autonomy of the patient.

Clinical practice recommendations

1. Understand Deaf and HoH service user's needs from the start of the journey and record those needs
2. Understand basic communication tactics
3. Have access to technology and use it
4. Set up the environment to maximise the view of faces and minimise noise
5. Know how to book appropriate communication support

Summary

For HoH service users, HCPs should start with the mantra, 'How can I help you hear me?', and for Deaf services users, 'How do you prefer to communicate?'. From there, communicate with people using the right communication tactics and communication support; utilising technology and getting the environment right is essential. This is vital for the service user to make an appointment, know when they are being called from the waiting room, communicate clearly during the appointment, and understand follow up information such as test results and management plans.

Case study 15.1

Stephanie, who has moderate deafness, received a letter asking her to call the surgery to arrange a medication review. Stephanie was unable to hear well on the phone which made her very anxious. Stephanie asked her friend to call the surgery to arrange the appointment for her, after a long wait her friend got through to the surgery but the reception team refused to talk to her because she wasn't the patient even though it was explained to them that Stephanie couldn't make the call. The receptionist suggested that she could call Stephanie instead. Stephanie's friend requested that Stephanie could email the surgery to arrange the appointment – the receptionist said that they were not able to do that. Stephanie made a written compliant to the Practice Manager. Following a face-to-face meeting with the Practice Manager in response to the compliant, it was agreed that Stephanie could e-mail to make appointments.

Adjustments that would have helped: The GP surgery needs a variety of options for arranging appointments. These could include phone, text, email, and face-to-face. The options for arranging appointments need to be publicised to all patients. The reception staff need to undertake basic Deaf awareness training.

Case study 15.2

David attended A&E; he is Deaf and uses BSL. Staff communicated by paper and pen that David needed an urgent operation and may die with or without it as it was a high-risk procedure. They asked him to sign a Do Not Resuscitate order (DNR). After waiting on a trolley due to a lack of beds, and unable to effectively communicate with those around him, David found an interpreter's number and gave it to the hospital. The booking was made but then the hospital called to cancel it saying they were coping fine with pen and paper. The interpreter called the hospital to explain why interpreters were vital for full consent and patient understanding. When the interpreter arrived at the hospital David was hoping to go home and had not understood the severity of the situation.

Adjustments that would have helped: an interpreter should have been booked when David arrived at A&E. It is appropriate to try pen and paper when waiting for the interpreter. The hospital should not wait for the service user to ask for an interpreter or for them to find the contact details themselves.

References

AoHL. (2014). *Caring for people with hearing loss: a framework for change.* London: AoHL.

Bailey, T. (2018). *Good practice?* London: AoHL.

Bamford, J., Fortnum, H., Bristow, K., Smith, J., & Vamvakas, G. (2007). Current practice, accuracy, effectiveness and cost-effectiveness of the school entry hearing screen. *Health Technologies Assessment*, *11*(32). https://doi.org/10.3310/hta11320

Barker, A., Leighton, P., & Ferguson, M. (2017). Coping together with hearing loss: a qualitative meta-aynthesis of the psychosocial experiences of people with hearing loss and their communication partners. *International Journal of Audiology*, *56*(5), 297–305.

British Deaf Association. (2020, December 1). *What is deaf culture.* Retrieved from BDA: https://bda.org.uk/what-is-deaf-culture/

Champion, J., & Holt, R. (2000). Dental care for children and young people who have a hearing impairment. *British Dental Jour*nal, *189*, 155–159.

Chodosh, J., Weinstein, B. E., & Blustein, J. (2020). Face masks can be devastating for people with hearing loss. *British Medical Journal, 370*. doi:https://doi.org/10.1136/bmj.m2683

Crowe, T., Jani, S., Jani, S., Jani, N., & Jani, R. (2016). A pilot program in rural telepsychiatry for deaf and hard of hearing populations. *Heliyon, 2*(3). www.cell.com/heliyon/pdf/S2405-8440(15)30432-1.pdf.

Davis, A. C., & Hoffman, H. J. (2019). Hearing loss: rising prevalence and impact. *Bulletin of the World Health Organization, 97*(10), 646–646A.

Davis, A., Smith, P., Ferguson, M., Stephens, D., & Gianopoulos, I. (2007). Acceptability, benefit and costs of early screening for hearing. *Health Technologies Assessment*. https://doi.org/10.3310/hta11420

De Iori, M., Rapport, L., Wong, C., & Stach, B. (2019). Characteristics of adults with unrecognized hearing loss. *The American Journal of Audiology, 28*(2), 384–390.

Deafness and Hearing Loss Toolkit. (2021, January 29). Retrieved from Royal College of General Practitioners: www.rcgp.org.uk/clinical-and-research/resources/toolkits/deafness-and-hearing-loss-toolkit.aspx

Dillion, H., Day, J., Bant, S., & Munro, K. (2020). Adoption, use and non-use of hearing aids: a robust estimate based on Welsh national survey statistics. *International Journal of Audiology, 59*(8), 567–573.

GBD 2017 Disease and Injury Incidence and Prevalence Collaborators. (2019). Global, regional, and national incidence, prevalence, and years lived with disability for 354 diseases for 195 countries and territories, 1990–2017: a systematic analysis for the Global Burden of Disease Study 2017. London: *The Lancet*, 1789–1858.

Gill, I. J., & Fox, J. R. (2011). A qualitative meta-synthesis on the experience of psychotherapy for deaf and heard of hearing people. *Mental Health, Religion & Culture*, 15(6), 637–651.

Goldin, A., Weinstein, B., & Shiman, N. (2020, April). Speech blocked by surgical masks becomes a more important issue in the era of COVID-19. Retrieved from The Hearing Review: www.hearingreview.com/hearing-loss/health-wellness/how-do-medical-masks-degrade-speech-reception

Graydon, K., Waterworth, C., Miller, H., & Gunasekera, H. (2018). Global burden of hearing impairment and ear disease. *The Journal of Laryngology & Otology, 133*, 18–25.

Hearing Loss Association of America. (2021, February 19). Patients/Providers. Retrieved from Hearing Loss Association of America: www.hearingloss.org/hearing-help/communities/patients/

Lin, F. R., Thorpe, R., Gordon-Salant, S., & Ferrucci, L. (2011). Hearing loss prevalence and risk factors among older adults in the United States. *Journal of Gerontology, 66*(5), 582–590.

Lin, F., & Ferrucci, L. (2012). Hearing loss and falls among older adults in the United States. *Journal of the American Association Internal Medicine, 172*(4), 369–371.

Lin, F., Metter, J., & O'Brien, R. (2011). Hearing loss and incident dementia. *Journal of the American Association Neurology, 68*(2), 214–220.

Livingstone, G., Huntley, J., Sommerlad, A., Ames, D., Ballard, C., & et al. (2020). Dementia prevention, intervention, and care: 2020 report of the Lancet Commission. London: *The Lancet*.

Mick, P., Foley, D., & Lin, F. (2017). Hearing loss is associated with poorer ratings of patient–physician communication and healthcare quality. *Journal of the American Geriatric Society, 62*(11), 2207–2209.

Middleton, A., Niruban, A., Girling, G., & Myint, P. K. (2010). Communicating in a healthcare setting with people who have hearing loss. *British Medical Journal, 341*, c4672.

National Association of the Deaf. (2021, February 19). *Position statement on health care access for deaf patients.* Retrieved from National Association of the Deaf: www.nad.org/about-us/position-statements/position-statement-on-health-care-access-for-deaf-patients/#_edn1

National Literacy Trust. (2017). National Literacy Trust. Retrieved from https://literacytrust.org.uk/information/what-is-literacy/

NDCS. (2020, December 1). Research and Data. Retrieved from www.NDCS.org.uk: www.ndcs.org.uk/information-and-support/being-deaf-friendly/information-for-professionals/recognising-the-signs-of-hearing-loss/

Orji, A., Kamenov, K., Dirac, M., Davis, A., Chadha, S., & Vos, T. (2020). Global and regional needs, unmet needs and access to hearing aids. *International Journal of Audiology, 59*(3), 166–172.

RCGP. (2021, January 29). *Deafness and hearing loss toolkit.* Retrieved from Royal College of General Practitioners: www.rcgp.org.uk/clinical-and-research/resources/toolkits/deafness-and-hearing-loss-toolkit.aspx

Reed, N., Betz, J., Kucharska-Newton, A., Lin, F., & Deal, J. (2019). Hearing loss and satisfaction with healthcare: an unexplored relationship. *Journal of the American Geriatric Society, 67*(3), 624–626.

Reeve, D. (2003). *Access to health services for deaf people: summary report for A&E un*its. Manchester: ResearchGate.

Ringham, L. (2012). *Access all areas.* London: AoHL.

RNID. (2020). *Communication tips for health and social care professionals.* Retrieved from RNID: https://rnid.org.uk/information-and-support/support-for-health-and-social-care-professionals/communication-tips-for-healthcare-professionals/

RNID. (2020, November 11). *GPs to help deaf patients navigate remote appointments.* Retrieved from RNID: https://rnid.org.uk/about-us/media-centre/press-releases/gps-to-help-deaf-patients-navigate-remote-appointments/

RNID. (2020). *Guidance for residential care homes.* Retrieved from RNID: https://rnid.org.uk/information-and-support/support-for-health-and-social-care-professionals/guidance-for-residential-care-homes/

RNID. (2021, January 31). *Signs of hearing loss.* Retrieved from RNID: https://rnid.org.uk/information-and-support/hearing-loss/signs-of-hearing-loss/

Rolfe, C., & Gardner, B. (2016). Experiences of hearing loss and views towards interventions to promote uptake of rehabilitation support among UK adults. *International Journal of Audiology, 55*(11), 666–673.

Shukla, A., Nieman, C., Price, C., Harper, M., Lin, F., & Reed, N. (2019). Impact of hearing loss on patient–provider communication among hospitalised patients: a systematic review. *American Journal of Medical Quality, 34*, 284–292.

SignHealth. (2013). *Research into the health of deaf people.* England: SignHealth.

Simpson, A., Matthews, L., Cassarly, C., & Dubno, J. (2019). Time from hearing aid candidacy to hearing aid adoption: a longitudinal cohort study. *Ear & Hearing, 40*(3), 468–467.

Stevens, M., Dubno, J., Wallhagen, M., & Tucci, D. (2018). Communication and healthcare: self-reports of people with hearing loss in primary care. *Clinical Gerontologist, 40*(5), 484–494.

The Association of Sign-Language Interpreters. (2020, June 1). *Guidelines for booking interpreters in healthcare settings during the COVID pandemic*. Retrieved from ASLI: https://asli.org.uk/wp-content/uploads/2020/06/Best-Practice-for-Booking-Interpreters-in-Healthcare-settings-during-Covid-19-FINAL.pdf

Thomson, R., Audoung, P., Miller, A., & Gurgel, R. (2017). Hearing loss as a risk factor for dementia: a systematic review. *Laryngoscope Investigative Otolaryngology, 2*(2), 69–79.

Wells, T., Nickels, L., Rush, S., Musich, S., Wu, L., Bhaattarai, G., & Yeh, C. (2020). Characteristics and health outcomes associated with hearing loss and hearing aid use among older adults. *Journal of Aging and Health, 56*, 724–734.

Wilson, B. S., Tucci, D. L., Merson, M. H., & O'Donoghue, G. M. (2017). Global hearing health care: new findings and perspectives. *The Lancet, 390*(10111), 2503–2514.

World Health Organization. (2020, March 1). Deafness and Hearing Loss. Retrieved from World Health Organization: www.who.int/news-room/fact-sheets/detail/deafness-and-hearing-loss

World Health Organization. (2020, December 1). Mask use in the context of COVID-19. Retrieved from World Health Organization: www.who.int/publications/i/item/advice-on-the-use-of-masks-in-the-community-during-home-care-and-in-healthcare-settings-in-the-context-of-the-novel-coronavirus-(2019-ncov)-outbreak

16

Conclusion and reflections

Michelle O'Reilly and Riya Elizabeth George

Chapter contents:

- Summarising core messages
- Summarising the book content
- Summarising the practitioner messages
- Final thoughts and reflections
- Conclusion

Summarising core messages

Communication is fundamental to the function of society and is a cornerstone of all healthcare practices. For practitioners working in a healthcare setting, effective communication with their client group is essential to the work, the process, and the outcomes. In an era of shared decision making, patient-centred care, patient rights, and quality improvement, there is a greater emphasis in contemporary health on engaging people in their healthcare. Good practices in communication can facilitate rapport building, promote medication adherence, encourage future appointment attendance, and impact longer-term outcomes.

Despite the vital and instrumental role of communication, it is arguably the case that many healthcare practitioners rely heavily on anecdotal evidence, their clinical experience, and any component of their training that focused on communication to inform their expertise in their everyday interactions with their client group. Many healthcare practitioners in modern contexts engage in evidence-based practice and seek to find some time to explore the research and scientific evidence to help contribute to their field but may find less work focused on communication or may not always consider this as a central interest. Furthermore, when engaged with communication-specific evidence, much of this relies on certain theoretical

DOI: 10.4324/9781003142522-21

approaches or models that do not always fully account for the diversity of patient or client populations, or diversity in communication need. This is especially pertinent in the context of atypical communication, where one party within the health interaction setting communicates differently in some way. Healthcare practitioners are likely to frequently encounter atypical communicators, and adjustments are important to promote a competency framework and to encourage engagement.

Engaging and practising atypical communication can be challenging, especially when the evidence base has not provided a full and agreed definition of the concept. Nonetheless, despite some critical tensions in this area, there is consensus to an extent that when one interlocutor or more has an impairment that has consequences for the process of social interaction it can be considered atypical (Wilkinson, 2019). In other words, when an individual has communication that has not developed in the normative way or is impeded by a disability or disorder.

Individuals with atypical communication are likely to have complex needs and thus will require significant support from the healthcare practitioner during the healthcare interaction (Goldbart & Caton, 2010). In offering such support it is important that the healthcare practitioner recognises the individuality, the uniqueness, the specific aspects of the person and does not roll out the same approaches and methods to communicate with all atypically communicating persons. This can be difficult for the busy healthcare practitioner, especially if their training in this area has been limited or if they have less experience in these kinds of social interactions. Nonetheless, it is helpful to recognise the asymmetry that exists in the healthcare setting, and to realise that in practice this is worsened for those with a communication disability (Law, this volume). Healthcare practitioners are facing increasing restrictions in time, resources, capacity, training, and so forth, and this can make the communication situations more challenging and risks overlooking the benefits of changing communication styles to help ease the interaction.

Notwithstanding the huge resource issues faced in modern healthcare practice, we have illustrated in this book the central importance and benefits for healthcare practitioners to engage with the communication literature and research. The value of knowledge, recognising and reducing stigma that is so often imbued with disability, and taking time to reflect on one's own practice can make a big difference to people's lives. Healthcare practitioners can benefit greatly from placing a stronger emphasis on the importance of communication skills and training, and from reflecting on their own communication styles and practice, especially in the context of atypical communication. Empirical research from a range of different disciplines and methodologies can provide a valuable foundation for that learning, and this book is a good starting point to think about the diversity of atypical communication.

Summarising the book content

This book has covered a wide spectrum of issues, conditions, healthcare settings, and challenges for atypical communication. The different authors have represented a range of different disciplinary backgrounds, clinical skills and expertise, methodological preferences, and theoreties. In the chapters, authors have worked to provide a clear, clinically relevant set of practices and recommendations that audiences can translate for the field they work in, which will be helpful in informing good practice going forward. While there has been a broad range of population groups and issues covered across chapters, they are anchored by a commitment to thinking about communication, and particularly thinking about the challenges that atypical communicators can bring to healthcare settings. Following our own introduction to these wider issues at stake, the book manages to identify areas of practice in healthcare that would benefit from reflection and further engagement with the need to focus on atypical communication. As editors, we value the combined clinical and academic expertise that distils these complex areas into straightforward practice-based messages for the audience.

In Part I of our book, we focused predominantly on the theoretical and social debates that are pertinent to the field of atypical communication. Here we saw a contextualisation of the social and cultural context of meaningful conversations, as it was recognised that communication is fundamentally social. During this part of the book, there were important critical considerations of language and its role in communication, as well as cultural, multimodal, and context-dependent aspects of the healthcare interaction. During this section of the book, there were necessary considerations of the wider framing of power and asymmetry imbued in healthcare interactions and how this translates within specific healthcare contexts. Noteworthy here was highlighting the potential risk that healthcare practitioners may make assumptions about the person in front of them and how consequently this can negatively impact process and outcomes.

During this section of the book, there was some focus on storytelling and how this is a communication tool of value when interacting with an atypical communicator. The promotion of a two-way process, engagement of the patient or client, and the importance of taking time to understand things from their perspective were all important take-away messages from this part of the book. Additional to storytelling, was some reflection on the value of new digital technologies; with the rise of machine learning, digital technology, and digital media, there have been new opportunities for healthcare providers to find new and innovative ways of engaging atypical communicators in their care. While such technologies do not ameliorate the communication challenges that exist within healthcare settings, they do potentially provide a mechanism for facilitating things in the future.

The second part of the book focused on a specific population and the associated benefits and challenges of practice with children and their families.

Multi-party interaction can be complex, and frequently children can become secondary in their care, with the risk that practitioners focus on communicating with their parents. However, child-centred practice is a modern healthcare endeavour and healthcare practitioners are increasingly aware of the importance of engaging children in the consultation and process. This is especially important as children and young people with atypical communication are frequently seen in healthcare settings and require strategies to be in place to support their engagement. In this way healthcare practitioners can start to think more carefully about how they might continue to develop their skills to support such diverse communication needs.

This part of the book focused on children, and authors pointed out how it may be the case because of developmental stages and chronological ages, the atypicality in communication may not necessarily be overt or obvious. Their communication competencies and abilities are developing at that age, and therefore some attending to style and strategies to engage is necessary anyway with this population. It may be the case that further care and attention is needed to identify any atypicality and to respond appropriately. Furthermore, the multi-party nature of the conversation will require some sensitivity in managing parental communication need and child or young person needs. This part of the book explored some of the communication barriers that families can face when accessing the healthcare system and how the quality of care was important to those families.

The third part of our book was more focused on specific conditions, examining atypical communication in progressive neurological disorders. There are a range of neurological conditions that can impact a person's communication ability, such as multiple sclerosis, motor neuron disease, Alzheimer's, and Parkinson's disease. These conditions can result in language impairments and pragmatic deficits and thus changes in communication caused by these conditions will need attention from healthcare practitioners, especially in helping reconfigure impairments in terms of competencies. The communication impact of these conditions extends beyond speech and includes challenges with cognition, language, and non-verbal expression. It is therefore arguably incumbent on healthcare practitioners to ensure that the voices of those impacted are heard and understood, and that they continue to play a role in their own healthcare practice. To do this effectively, healthcare practitioners need the resources and tools to be able to communicate effectively. Without such training and effort on the part of the healthcare practitioner, there could be a breakdown in the relationship, an eroding of rapport, and a significant impact on the efficacy of care and treatment.

In Part IV of the book the authors provided more specific practical guidance on specific conditions resulting in atypical communication. Although there is some diversity in this category, the chapters focused on conditions of a stroke, aphasia, learning disabilities, autism spectrum condition, stammering, and deafness. Thus, this section of the book focused on those chronic conditions in children and/or adults that result in a communication impairment. In this part of the book, authors provided clarity on definitions of the types of conditions they were introducing and placed those in a wider social context in terms of the role of society, stigma, systems, and consequences for impaired individuals, such as isolation and impact on mental health. In so doing they illustrated the necessity of the role of healthcare practitioners to recognise these, but also to not contribute to the negative impact and outcomes by reinforcing stereotypes, disability, deficit, and stigma. The authors promoted the importance of disability rights, person-centred care, and valuing their voices in practice and research, and illuminated the central role of the healthcare practitioner in achieving that.

Summarising the practitioner messages

A central facet of this book has been the important practical messages for practitioners, identified by the authors within each chapter. Here in this conclusion, we simply synthesise and cluster the core recommendations made by the authors of this book, and strongly recommend that you read the original chapters, rather than solely rely on our short summary of their key recommendations. What we provide here by summary, is merely intended as an overview of some of the key practical guidance messages that have been identified from the book. In so doing, we are providing some overarching and general guidance for attending to atypical communication as a category, and not pointing to specific conditions, individual needs, or age of the population.

- Things to find out

If there is information about the client or patient available to you before the appointment this can be helpful. It may be that in their records there are already suggestions for facilitating the healthcare interaction, or information that you can use to facilitate the current appointment. If there is nothing in the record, then it might be worth asking some simple questions about facilitating communication before you start the main appointment.

It is worth spending time with the client or patient to find out what they already know about the context and appointment, as that will provide a foundation for care, and give an opportunity to correct any misunderstanding. This is also an opportunity to find out what they expect, what their goals are, what they fear and so forth.

- Emotional aspects of the interaction

It is important to attend to the emotional context of the communication and be empathic with the person attending the appointment. Be open and honest with them about the condition, the situation, and any treatment. It will be helpful to be patient and kind, which can be more challenging than it seems with time constraints, targets, and limited resources. Sometimes the client or patient will need pauses between questions and information to process and understand what they are being told, so allowing those will be important.

- Communicative style

There are simple things that can be done with communication style and language that might facilitate the healthcare interaction. Slow down the pace of speech to give the person a chance to process, be aware of their bodily and facial reactions to give clues as to concern, confusion, and so forth, and be prepared for a reaction. It is important to check with the person that they understand what they are being told and, where there are doubts, ask them further questions and encourage them to repeat it back to you in their own words. When speaking, it is necessary to be clear and concise.

Speaking directly to the person whose appointment it is, is also important. This is especially true for certain vulnerable populations like children or those with learning disabilities, who can be marginalised in a healthcare interaction by being overlooked or not spoken to directly. Using next speaker selection techniques, such as the client's/patient's name directly as a tool for engagement and checking in to see if they agree with their parent or carer can also help to keep them engaged in the interaction. Remember that it may be necessary to rephrase the question or request for the person, rather than simply turning to the carer and dismissing the person as not being able to understand. This is not to underestimate the value of the caregiver or parent, as they will know the client or patient very well and can be instrumental in smoothing the communication process.

For those populations where it is more challenging to engage or build rapport, it may be useful to use specific participatory strategies, like subjective units of distress scales (Wolpe, 1969; Kiyimba & O'Reilly, 2020), where there is scale of one-to-ten, or social stories (Gray, 2015), or drawings and asking the person to represent visually what they think or feel, or using objects like toys, or digital tools.

Active listening will be crucial when working with those with atypical communication. Hearing and reflecting back in a way that is responsive and demonstratively showing engagement can be a useful communication tool (Hutchby, 2010). Try to avoid directly correcting them if they make linguistic or pragmatic errors and instead clarify or reframe what is being presented. Likewise, try to avoid finishing their sentences for them or presuming to know what they are trying to say.

- Clinical reflection

Most healthcare practitioners are reflective by training and expertise, and this can be a useful tool in communication too. Reflecting on one's personal and professional values can raise awareness of any assumptions being made and can encourage a critical reflection on one's own communication skills. Such reflections may help identify where adaptations are needed to improve on communication with atypical communicators to help the interaction become more meaningful and more equal.

- Culture and diversity

Being mindful that intercultural communication is not simply about language, but also reflects norms and expectations is important in the healthcare interaction. It might be useful to discuss this openly.

Additionally, no single group is homogenous just because they are anchored together by a specific condition or disorder. Be mindful of the uniqueness of the person in front of you and adapt to their specific needs.

- Communication modality and medium

It may be the case that the client or patient requires some technical adaptations to facilitate communication, such as an interpreter, signer, or machinery. Furthermore, it is useful to account for preferences and constraints on traditional face-to-face appointments. In-person meetings may not be practical or may not be possible and digital modalities can provide useful alternatives. However, it is necessary to be mindful of the digital literacy of the client or patient, as well as the challenges of digital inequalities that exist in all countries, even those with high income.

It may be the case that the digital literacy of the healthcare practitioner also requires some attention. Identifying gaps in one's own knowledge and recognising training needs is a positive endeavour for practice.

- Multi-modality

So much communication is non-verbal and so it will be helpful to be mindful of your own multi-modal communication strategies. Think about what your facial expressions are showing, your hand or arm gestures and their meaning, and the way you are holding your posture. These can signal to the person that you are in a rush, or have not got time, and your impatience may be on show.

It is also important to be observant of the multi-modal communication of the client or patient sat with you. They may be struggling to express themselves, may be uncomfortable, embarrassed, or attempting to mask their emotions. Try to take steps to ease any discomfort, reassure them, and smile.

Final thoughts and reflections

Any good practitioner, academic, and researcher benefits from engaging in an exercise of reflexivity. As editors of this volume, we have been engaged with a broad range of experts and have been communicating with those authors to bring this volume together. To edit this book and to illustrate the importance of writing about atypical communication, we have been immersing ourselves in the evidence base and the clinical expertise of our contributors. To bring this book to a close, we therefore present our own reflexivity, to illustrate our own personal positions, epistemological frameworks, motivations, and experiences that inevitably will have shaped the way this text came to be.

Michelle has professional expertise and experience in child mental health, working in the University of Leicester and Leicestershire NHS Partnership Trust. Here she takes a personal positionality to convey to the audience her position and motivation in producing this book. The switch is therefore made to the personal pronoun.

> For over 20 years I have been undertaking research with children and young people about their engagement with services, such as family therapy and child mental health assessments, and focusing on specific mental health areas, such as autism, self-harm, anxiety, and well-being. In so doing, I have worked with various children and young people who are constructed as vulnerable or marginalised, such as refugees, homeless, looked after, those in the majority world, orphaned, street, and so on. Yet, this professional expertise and experience all began with personal insights and personal motivations, because of being a sibling of a brother diagnosed with autism.
>
> My main personal experience of atypical communication lies with living with and supporting my autistic brother over the years. Inevitably, my interdisciplinary approach to mental health has created dilemmas and questions for me for my research in this field, as all that I do is inevitably coloured by my personal experiences. In terms of autism, my shifting sociological, psychological, and medical framing of the condition are not always congruent, and the experiential epistemic position occupied simply complicates this perspective further. On one hand, the sociologist and psychologist within me takes a more critical academic position on autism, as I promote a competence and rights-based framework for autism and lean toward a neurodiversity approach for constructing autism. My social constructionist epistemology informing my methodological choices and guiding the direction of my research critically questions the medicalisation of autism and of mental health more generally. However, my personal experiences, witnessing the distress a disability can create for individuals and families, and encountering the resource and service challenges for accessing support, tempers any hard-line academic position I might occupy. Furthermore, working with psychiatrists, psychologists, nurses, and allied health professionals in my occupation has clearly highlighted to me just how much practitioners genuinely care about their clients or patients. Yet, the systemic and organisational frameworks,

policies, rules and regulations, financial commitments, and managerial input can sometimes mean that important aspects of the patient or client get lost, and this does not sit well with me.

I was only young when my brother was diagnosed, and the memories of the 'battle' my family went through to secure the label remain ingrained for life. In the research literature there is no end of reference to parents who 'battle' with services and different practitioners before they finally get the appropriate diagnosis and the necessary support, and this seems to be a continuous message in the evidence for decade after decade. I find it challenging to understand why after all the years since my own parents battled for help, very little seems to have really changed, despite the much greater awareness and literature on autism now. It is this kind of engagement with the literature, juxtaposed with my own personal lived experience that motivate me to continue to write about autism, continue to highlight the autistic voice and their families, and to continue to use qualitative methods to contribute to the wider field of mental health. It is this founded desire to help families and those with communication challenges that led to my involvement in this very practical book.

Riya has professional expertise and experience in working in a range of healthcare settings, particularly mental health and palliative care. She is currently working at Queen Mary University of London, specialising in teaching clinical communication skills and diversity education to medical students and doctors. Here she takes a personal positionality to convey to the audience her position and motivation in producing this book. The switch is therefore made to the personal pronoun.

I was born in Kerela, South India and came to the United Kingdom at an early age. The sudden need to blend contrasting cultures in a way that made sense to me required time and reflection. Language, accent, dialect, articulation, and the expression of words were closely intertwined with my personal experiences as well as my developing professional interests. The binary position of classifying communication into typical and atypical for me continues to pose more questions than answers. Do the communication profiles of typically developing individuals reflect the natural variation in language and communication competence or do they signify a qualitatively different and abnormal developmental trajectory? I pose this question in Chapter 1 when I first discuss the influences of culture and diversity on our understandings of communication development.

My educational philosophy is located within a social constructionist perspective; this states that there is no one absolute truth as the context is relevant. These approaches do not attempt to look for signs and symptoms, which can lead to a classification of an ethnic group or other social category; they avoid reducing complex terms such as culture, diversity, and social issues to a list of characteristics. The philosophy behind these models or frames of thinking recognise that different people interpret the world differently, so that even two individuals in the same group, who experience the same event, may take very different meanings from it. The philosophy behind this is that there is no single objective reality to be discovered. It acknowledges that individuals construct their own version of these terms culture, diversity, and society, dependent on the various social discourses of which they are aware or in which they participate. These approaches are more interested in the relationship between different components of culture and their meanings to individuals.

My social constructionist epistemology informing my educational values, methodological choices, and guiding the direction of my research critically questions the medicalisation of disease. Despite the movement away from a reductionist biomedical perspective, the literature suggests its philosophy remains deeply entrenched, resulting in serious consequences for the teaching of communication skills and diversity issues in the field of medicine and healthcare. The biomedical model assumes disease and illness are fully accountable to measurable biological factors. Engel (1977, p. 2) describes its approach as 'a process that moves from the recognition and palliation of symptoms to the characterisation of a specific disease in which the aetiology and pathogenesis are known and the treatment is rational and specific'. By shifting the focus from care to cure, the topics of communication and diversity as perceived through a biomedical lens, is categorised in a similar way to disease. It becomes reduced to a set of observable traits and characteristics pertaining to assumed homogenous patient groups, which can be learnt as '*facts*' (Sharma, Pinto, & Kumagai, 2018) or lists of '*dos and don'ts*' for particular cultural groups (Chirico, 2002). These traits and characteristics become surrogates for the human experiences associated with different patient groups. From the first chapter through to the end of this book, we hope it begins to challenge the assumptions made by the endemic practice of categorisation (typical versus atypical) in communication development and encourage greater attention and reflection towards the diverse social context in which we converse with people.

Conclusion

We conclude this book in a similar way to how we started it, by saying that communication is at the heart of everything a healthcare practitioner does. We argue that there is a continued need to think about, write about, and research healthcare communication and to pay special attention to atypical communication. We argue that it is crucial that the voices of those persons with communication disabilities, impairments, challenges, are at the centre of our knowledge and understanding of healthcare interaction. We need to move away from deficit-focused ideas about atypical communication and promote equality and opportunity for those individuals to be actively involved in their own healthcare and related decisions, even if that requires substantial communicative support.

The COVID-19 pandemic has likely changed the landscape of healthcare and healthcare interactions forever, and health inequalities, digital inequalities, disadvantage, marginalisation, stigma, oppression, and economic resources are likely to dominate health in coming decades. Through this book, the contributing authors have highlighted the importance of taking a person-centred approach, of making reasonable communication adjustments, of recognising the individuality and uniqueness of the person, of compassion, care, and humanity in care. The authors have used a range of communication evidence, with some showcasing their own work to illuminate valuable insights for the field. We consider ourselves lucky to have such skilled and interesting contributions to this edited collection.

We now turn over to the reader to consider, reflect, and digest the broader issues at stake for atypical communicators in healthcare settings. We, as editors, and the authors have encouraged proactive engagement with the wider literature and other resources to help with practice. We have promoted critical thinking as we have navigated and presented different areas of concern for communication. We have been transparent about our own positionalities, and authors have identified their clinical and academic expertise. We hope that the audience has found benefit from reading this text and that the audience takes time to reflect on those practice-based messages.

References

Chirico, S. (2002). Towards cultural competency. Retrieved 7 October 2002 from www.fons.org/networks/tchna/chirico.htm

Engel, G. L. (1977). The need for a new medical model: a challenge for biomedicine. *Science*, *196*(4286): 129–136.

Goldbart, J., & Caton, S. (2010). *Communication and people with the most complex needs: what works and why this is essential*. Manchester, UK: MENCAP.

Gray, C. (2015). *The new social story book: 15th anniversary edition*. Arlington, TX: Future Horizons.

Hutchby, I. (2010). Active listening: formulations and the elicitation of feelings-talk in child counselling. *Research on Language and Social Interaction*, *38*, 303–329.

Kiyimba, N., & O'Reilly, M., (2020). The clinical use of subjective units of distress scales (SUDs) in child mental health assessments: a thematic evaluation. *Journal of Mental Health*, *29*(4), 418–423.

Sharma, M., Pinto, A. D., & Kumagai, A. K. (2018). Teaching the social determinants of health: a path to equity or a road to nowhere? *Academic Medicine*, *93*(1), 25–30.

Wilkinson, R. (2019). Atypical interaction: conversation analysis and communicative impairments. *Research on Language and Social Interaction*, *52*(3), 281–299.

Wolpe, J. (1969). *The practice of behavior therapy*. New York: Pergamon Press.

Tribute to Professor James Law, OBE

Professor James Law, OBE, sadly passed away as this book was being created. Below is a tribute to his tremendous work in the field of communication.

James was Professor of Speech and Language Sciences at Newcastle University, a role he held since 2010. In 2003 he published a seminal Cochrane Review on speech and language therapy interventions, and from 2008 to 2012 was also responsible for carrying out the biggest review of speech and language support for children in England, as one of four academics who led the Better Communication Research Programme – a project arising from the *Bercow Review of Services for Children with Speech, Language and Communication Needs*, and which led to the development of the *What Works for Children with Speech and Language Needs* database.

His work was also instrumental in the application of public health approaches to speech and language therapy in general, and child language in particular. This approach was motivated in part by his passionate belief in the need to tackle inequalities in society.

James was one of the world's leading researchers into child language development and disorders, and particularly in the application of large population cohorts to this field. His recent work includes leading the Cost Action European research network to enhance children's oral language skills across Europe, as well as supporting the profession to consider how to use telehealth to deliver paediatric speech and language therapy services in response to the COVID-19 pandemic.

James was tireless in his efforts to bring evidence-based practices to services for children with language difficulties across the UK, Europe, Australia, and beyond. He gave his time, knowledge, and energy to countless SLTs and researchers with the aim of increasing the capacity of the profession worldwide to conduct high quality research that could improve the lives of children and young people with language and communication needs.

James understood that research can only bring benefits if it is recognised in policy and used in practice. His ability and dedication to building partnerships across disciplines and sectors ensured that his influence extended across academia, into government and public policy research, at home

DOI: 10.4324/9781003142522-22

and abroad – in this way bringing real world benefits to children with language and communication needs.

In 2008 James was awarded a Fellowship of the RCSLT in recognition of his contribution to the field; in 2018 he was awarded an OBE for services to speech and language therapy. In 2021 James received an Academic Distinction Award from Newcastle University, recognising his outstanding impact within the university, nationally and internationally.

Index

Note: **Bold** page numbers refer to tables and *italic* page numbers refer to figures.

For Product Safety Concerns and Information please contact our EU
representative GPSR@taylorandfrancis.com
Taylor & Francis Verlag GmbH, Kaufingerstraße 24, 80331 München, Germany

www.ingramcontent.com/pod-product-compliance
Ingram Content Group UK Ltd.
Pitfield, Milton Keynes, MK11 3LW, UK
UKHW022318250926
475702UK00046B/921
* 9 7 8 0 3 6 7 6 9 6 1 2 2 *